Diabetes Desserts Cookbook

by Amy Riolo
Award-winning author and chef Co-author, *Diabetes For Dummies*

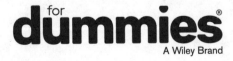

Diabetes Desserts Cookbook For Dummies®

Published by: **John Wiley & Sons, Inc.**, 111 River Street, Hoboken, NJ 07030-5774, www.wiley.com

Copyright © 2025 by John Wiley & Sons, Inc. All rights reserved, including rights for text and data mining and training of artificial technologies or similar technologies.

Media and software compilation copyright © 2025 by John Wiley & Sons, Inc. All rights reserved, including rights for text and data mining and training of artificial technologies or similar technologies.

Published simultaneously in Canada

For general information on our other products and services, please contact our Customer Care Department within the U.S. at 877-762-2974, outside the U.S. at 317-572-3993, or fax 317-572-4002. For technical support, please visit https://hub.wiley.com/community/support/dummies.

Wiley publishes in a variety of print and electronic formats and by print-on-demand. Some material included with standard print versions of this book may not be included in e-books or in print-on-demand. For more information about Wiley products, visit www.wiley.com.

Library of Congress Control Number: 2025934289

ISBN 978-1-394-30956-6 (pbk); ISBN 978-1-394-30958-0 (ebk); ISBN 978-1-394-30957-3 (ebk)

SKY10100492_031925

Recipes at a Glance

Base Recipes

- Basic Tart Crust 120
- Dark Chocolate Ganache 124
- Homemade Pie Crust 119
- Light Fruit "Ganache" 125
- Vanilla Cream Custard 122

Fruit-Based Desserts

- Avocado, Yogurt, and Mango Salad 144
- Baked Spice & Almond Stuffed Apples 132
- Broiled Figs & Balsamic Reduction 133
- Broiled Pineapple with Yogurt and Honey 140
- Cantaloupe in White Balsamic Vinegar 131
- Cherries with Goat Cheese and Pistachios 142
- Fresh Fruit Kabobs 130
- Grape, Goat Cheese, and Almond Skewers 146
- Kiwi and Raspberry Trees with Honey 135
- Mixed Berry Compote 134
- Poached Pears with Vanilla and Cardamom Cream 141
- Roasted Plums with Mascarpone Cheese 143
- Seasonal Italian Fruit Platter 145
- Summer Berry and Fresh Fig Salad 136
- Turkish-Stuffed Apricots 139
- Watermelon "Cake" 137
- Watermelon, Cantaloupe, Kiwi, Feta, and Mint Mosaic 129

Brownies & Bars

- Blackberry Lemon Bars 154
- Blueberry and Lemon Oatmeal Bars 156
- Dark Chocolate & Extra-Virgin Olive Oil Brownies 149
- Date, Dark Chocolate, and Cashew Bars 150
- Gingerbread Spice Squares 159
- Orange and Almond Bars 155
- Quinoa, Cranberry, and Pecan Bars 158
- Ricotta, Chocolate, and Orange Brownies 151
- Strawberry-Studded Blondies 153

Cookies

- Almond Orange Biscotti 173
- Carrot Cookie Bites 177
- Chocolate Chip Almond Butter Cookies. 165
- Chocolate Oatmeal No-Bake Cookies. 182
- Chocolate, Pistachio, and Cranberry Biscotti 166
- Hazelnut Cookies 170
- Honey Citrus Cookies 176
- Italian Pine Nut Cookies 179
- Lemon and Walnut Biscotti 168
- Meringues 178
- Moroccan Sesame Cookies 175
- Oatmeal Cookies 181
- Oatmeal Cranberry Cookies. 183
- Pistachio Macaroons 171
- Tuscan Cantucci 172

Spoon Desserts & Puddings

- Almond and Cherry Clafoutis. 208
- Apple Cinnamon Crisp 199
- Blueberry Cream Cobbler. 197
- Cherry Chocolate Bread Pudding 189
- Chocolate Almond Pudding 188
- Chocolate Orange Rice Pudding 190
- Citrus and Cinnamon Rice Pudding 194
- Mixed Berry and Mascarpone Parfaits. 205
- Passionfruit Tiramisu. 202
- Pumpkin Gingerbread Trifle. 204
- Ricotta and Berry Cheesecake Torte 206
- Strawberry Basil Crisp. 200
- Strawberry Shortcake 203
- Sweet Holiday Couscous. 192
- Sweet Peach Cobbler. 198
- Vanilla Cardamom Panna Cotta 187
- Vanilla Pudding with Berries 191
- Wheat Berry Pomegranate Pudding with Pistachios. 195
- Yogurt Custard with Apricots and Pistachios 193

Truffles and Sweet Bites

🍳 Chocolate Peanut Clusters 212
🍳 Chocolate Swirl Bark 218
🍳 Chocolate-Covered Stuffed Dates 220
🍳 Coconut Chocolate "Fudge" 216
🍳 Dark Chocolate–Covered Cherries 222
🍳 Date, Almond, and Cocoa Balls 211
🍳 Peanut Butter and Coconut Bombs 213
🍳 Quinoa and Macadamia Clusters 217
🍳 Stuffed Figs Dipped in Chocolate 221
🍳 Yogurt Kisses 214

Frozen Desserts

🍳 Banana and Peanut Butter "Ice Cream" 235
🍳 Blackberry Banana Soft Serve 242
🍳 Chocolate "Ice Cream" 233
🍳 Coffee Ice Cream 232
🍳 Espresso Granita 238
🍳 Frozen Peanut Butter and Vanilla Cups 241
🍳 Lemon Granita 237
🍳 Orange and Greek Yogurt Creamsicles 229
🍳 Pineapple Frozen Yogurt Pops 227
🍳 Pistachio Honey Ice Cream 234
🍳 Raspberry Sorbet 239
🍳 Red, White, and Blue Creamsicles 243
🍳 Strawberry Swirl Ice Cream 231
🍳 Strawberry, Yogurt, and White Balsamic Semifreddo 228
🍳 Vanilla Frozen Yogurt 225
🍳 Vanilla Gelato 226

Pies & Tarts

🍳 Almond and Apricot Tart 253
🍳 Apple, Raisin, and Nut Strudel 249
🍳 Blackberry Lemon Pie Pots 257
🍳 Cinnamon-Scented Apple Pie 254
🍳 Creamy Lemon Crostata 248
🍳 Key Lime Pie Jars 256
🍳 Mixed Berry Crostata 247
🍳 Strawberry, Citrus, and Ricotta Tart 252

Sweet Drinks

⊘ Almond and Banana Smoothie 267
⊘ Apricot and Ginger Cooler 265
⊘ Creamy Chai 270
⊘ Hot Spiced Chocolate 269
⊘ Moroccan Avocado Smoothie 261
⊘ Papaya, Banana, and Orange Smoothie 266
⊘ Pineapple Cardamom Crush 262
⊘ Spiced Hot Cider. 271
⊘ Zero-Proof Sgroppino 264

Cakes

⊘ Angel Food Cake. 276
⊘ Apple, Cinnamon, and Olive Oil Cake. 279
⊘ Banana Chocolate Chip Cake. 283
⊘ Carrot Pecan Spice Cake. 277
⊘ Chocolate and Pumpkin Snack Cake 282
⊘ Gluten-Free Chocolate Cupcakes 286
⊘ Italian Sponge Cake. 275
⊘ Mini Flourless Olive Oil and Chocolate Cakes. 285
⊘ Orange, Almond, and Olive Oil Cake 280
⊘ Upside-Down Kiwi Cake 281

Table of Contents

INTRODUCTION 1
About This Book. 1
Foolish Assumptions. 3
Icons Used in This Book 3
Beyond This Book 4
Where to Go from Here 4

**PART 1: DISCOVERING DELICIOUS
AND NUTRITIOUS DESSERTS** 5

CHAPTER 1: **Defining Diabetes-Friendly Desserts** 7
Exploring Blood Glucose Levels. 7
Looking at how sugar affects the mind and body 8
Regulating your blood sugar while enjoying desserts 9
Creating a Lifestyle That Supports Diabetes Desserts. 9
Eating right — Focusing on macronutrients 10
Fitting diabetes-friendly desserts into your diet. 10
Having the right ingredients on hand. .11
Choosing healthful desserts when not home 11
Preparing and Eating Delicious Dessert Recipes 13

CHAPTER 2: **Understanding Sugar's Role in the Body** 17
Noting How the Body and Brain Use Sugar. 17
Listing the types of diabetes 18
Understanding the basics of diabetes 18
Taking control of your behavioral health. 19
Examining the Causes of Sugar Cravings. 20
Understanding cravings often lead to impulsive eating 20
Curbing sugar cravings: The how-to. 21
Recognizing what to eat when you're craving sugar 22
Making easy substitutions 22
Preparing yourself to give up your sugar cravings. 23
Adding "Sweet" Lifestyle Strategies to Your Day. 24
Tapping into your happiness hormones .25
Utilizing the emotional guidance scale. .26
Selecting Healthy Ingredients Directly Impacts Your Diabetes. 27
Discussing glycemic index and load 27
Using better ingredients to make better choices 28
Making Desserts Healthful with These Ingredients 30
Fresh fruit. 30
Almonds, almond butter, and almond flour 32

Pure cinnamon. 32

Other sweet spices 33

Dark chocolate. 34

Extra-virgin olive oil (EVOO) 34

Unsweetened peanut butter 34

Tree nuts. 35

Greek yogurt. 35

Seeds. 35

Whole-grain flours. 36

Identifying Ideal Desserts for People with Diabetes 36

Desserts Redux — Making Desserts Diabetes-Friendly. 40

CHAPTER 3: **Keeping Blood Glucose Balanced
While Eating Desserts**. 43

Regulating Blood Glucose Levels 43

Shining a spotlight on blood glucose 44

Measuring blood glucose at home 46

Comparing testing for people with type 1 and
type 2 diabetes. 47

Perusing the Best Diabetes Care. 48

Relying on professional help 48

Making a plan to seek help 50

Focusing on Problematic Foods 51

Spotting problematic dessert food. 51

Getting rid of problematic food and subbing it with
more healthful options. 52

Noticing your emotional triggers to food. 53

Satisfying your sweet tooth in a wholesome way. 54

Keeping Track of Your Goals 55

Starting a food and exercise journal. 55

Noticing patterns. 56

PART 2: INCORPORATING DESSERTS
INTO YOUR DIET. 59

CHAPTER 4: **Making Macronutrients Work Together**. 61

Understanding How Protein, Carbs, and Fat Affect What You Eat. . . .62

Going deeper into macronutrients. 62

Recognizing how your body uses nutrients. 64

Identifying the Best Proteins, Carbohydrates, and Fats 64

Taking a closer look at protein 65

Considering carbohydrates 67

Exploring fat. 72

CHAPTER 5: **Enjoying Diabetes-Friendly Desserts: The How and When**.................................73

Focusing on Timing...73
    Knowing the right time to eat dessert.....................74
    Making smart lifestyle choices.............................75
Strategizing Your Meals When You Have Diabetes..............76
    Planning your meals with dessert..........................76
    Preparing ahead: Adjusting desserts to make them more diabetes-friendly................................77
    Putting together sample meal plans with desserts.........78
Calming Your Feelings of Shame and Guilt....................83
Comparing Desserts: Eating Out and Store-Bought versus Homemade...85
    Looking at store-bought and restaurant desserts..........86
    Making homemade desserts (and a plan)....................87

CHAPTER 6: **Building a Pantry and Choosing Healthful Sweeteners**.................................89

Decoding Nutrition Labels......................................90
Stocking Your Kitchen with Diabetes-Friendly Dessert Ingredients...91
    Supplying your pantry......................................92
    Keeping your fridge stocked...............................93
    Freezing some foods.......................................94
Sweetening the Pot — Sweeteners...............................94
    Deciphering the good from bad..............................94
    Identifying healthful sweeteners...........................96
Swapping Out Healthful Sweeteners in Recipes................100

CHAPTER 7: **Fitting Homemade Desserts into Your Schedule**...105

Analyzing Your Schedule to Include Baking...................105
    Getting started...106
    Fitting baking into your schedule.........................106
    Creating a plan to make desserts..........................109
Making Desserts in Advance....................................110
Whipping Together Last-Minute Desserts.......................111
Reinventing Baking Day: Recognizing the Benefits to Baking with Others...112

**PART 3: PREPARING DIABETES-FRIENDLY
DESSERTS: THE RECIPES** 115

CHAPTER 8: Introducing Base Recipes to Your Kitchen 117
Baking Crusts 117
Whipping Up Custard 121
Making Ganache 123

CHAPTER 9: Focusing on Fruit-Based Desserts 127
Transforming Fruit into Dessert 127
Preparing Creamy Fruit and Dairy Desserts 138

CHAPTER 10: Making Brownies and Bars 147
Indulging in Chocolate Brownies and Bars 148
Savoring Fruit-Studded Brownies and Bars. 152
Whipping Up Whole-Grain Goodness Bars and Squares. 157

CHAPTER 11: Enjoying Cookies 161
Making Cookies: The Basic How-To Techniques. 161
Baking Cookies with Chocolate 163
Enjoying Nutty Cookies. 167
Traveling the World: Classic Cookies from around the Globe 174
Adding Oatmeal Cookies to Your Repertoire 180

CHAPTER 12: Preparing Spoon Desserts and Puddings 185
Making Panna Cotta and Puddings. 186
Creating Comfort Desserts: Crisps and Cobblers. 196
Adding Fruit to Traditional Dessert Recipes 201

**CHAPTER 13: Creating Truffles and Fruit-Based
Sweet Treats**. 209
Satisfying Your Sweet Tooth with Bite-Sized Treats 209
Pleasing Your Palate with Fudge, Clusters, and Bark. 215
Dipping Fruit in Chocolate 219

CHAPTER 14: Whipping Up Frozen Desserts .223
Having Fun with Frozen Yogurt. 224
Transforming Ice Cream into a Healthful Finale. 230
Trying Granita and Sorbet Recipes 236
Freezing Delightful Frozen Classics. 240

CHAPTER 15: Mastering Pies and Tarts. 245
Creating Crostata and Strudel. 246
Making Tarts and Pies. 251
Serving Jars and Pots 255

CHAPTER 16: **Sipping on Sweet Drinks**................................259

Crafting Some Sweet Fruit Sips 260
Cooling Down with Drinks 263
Warming Up with Hot Drinks....................................268

CHAPTER 17: **Baking Cakes** 273

Experimenting with Classic Cake Recipes 273
Baking Fruit Cakes...278
Relishing Chocolate Cakes 284

PART 4: THE PART OF TENS..287

CHAPTER 18: **Ten Ways to Enjoy Desserts When You Have Diabetes** 289

Relishing Desserts..289
Consuming All Three Macronutrients during Each Meal...........290
Monitoring Your Blood Glucose Levels 290
Eating More Fruit-Based Desserts..............................290
Paying Attention to Portion Sizes 291
Substituting Butter with EVOO Whenever Possible 292
Making It a Team Effort 292
Exploring New Tastes and Dessert Styles 293
Planning Ahead 293
Exercising on a Regular Basis 294

CHAPTER 19: **Ten Myths Debunked about Diabetes and Desserts**.............................295

Knowing Your Current Blood Glucose Levels Doesn't Matter......296
Exercising to Control Your Glucose Doesn't Help...............296
Increasing Medications Enables You to Eat Anything 297
Using Alternative or Artificial Sweeteners Is Okay 298
Preparing Desserts in Advance or Thinking about Them Is Taboo...299
Making "Healthful Desserts" Taste Good Is Impossible..........300
Planning for the Unexpected Isn't Necessary 300
Thinking That Desserts Can't Be Good for You..................301
Prepping Tasty Diabetes-Friendly Desserts Is Hard.............301
Avoiding What Is Problematic Is Difficult.....................302

CHAPTER 20: **Ten Best Ingredients for Diabetes Desserts** 303

Cinnamon..304
Dark Chocolate 304
Almonds and Almond Flour......................................305
Other Nuts 305

Extra-Virgin Olive Oil...306
Seeds..306
Citrus: Oranges and Lemons....................................307
Plain, Full-Fat Greek Yogurt..................................307
Fruit..308

INDEX..309

Introduction

Welcome to the world of desserts that lets you experience tasty and nourishing sweet treats at the same time. In addition to actual recipes, this cookbook contains information on nutrition, lifestyle hacks, and diabetes care to ensure that you're setting yourself up for success and to enable you to enjoy desserts more often without suffering spikes in blood sugar.

When discussing the topic of desserts for people with diabetes, two philosophies are prevalent:

>> People with diabetes must completely cut out all sugar and simple carbs — even natural sweeteners like honey — from your diet.

>> People with diabetes can eat whatever type of dessert you want, even a triple chocolate fudge cake filled with artificial ingredients and unhealthful fats, if it uses a sugar substitute.

Although this first option is better than the second, I'm realistic about the fact that most people wouldn't be able to sustain a sugar-free diet forever. I don't believe in artificial sweeteners, or other artificial ingredients for that matter. I also know that before determining what types of desserts are safe for people to eat, you must first consider the other foods that they eat during that meal and day, their activity level, and other factors, which are difficult to consider when writing a book that thousands of people whom you know nothing about will read.

When writing *Diabetes Desserts Cookbook For Dummies,* I incorporate useful information about diabetes and blood sugar levels along with delicious and nutritious recipes that you can rely on to help regulate your glucose without giving up good flavor. I hope you can utilize these recipes and also use some of the healing tips to live both a pleasurable and healthy life.

About This Book

Diabetes Desserts Cookbook For Dummies busts a common myth about diabetes — that desserts aren't allowed if you have diabetes or prediabetes! If you plan ahead and use whole ingredients, delicious options like cakes, cookies, and brownies are still on the menu. This book features approximately 125 flavor-forward, healthful treats that are mouthwatering enough for a menu but simple enough to make at home.

The secret to making diabetes-friendly desserts is in balancing your macronutrients and portion sizes along with adding ingredients that are most beneficial to people with diabetes. If you've been diagnosed with diabetes or prediabetes, cook for someone who has, or are just looking for healthier desserts, this handy guide introduces you to delicious, wholesome recipes that will satisfy. These recipes aren't watered-down versions of the classics you crave. They're the real deal, and they'll be a hit with kids, too.

This book is for anyone looking for dessert ideas for a diabetes-friendly diet. You don't have to give up on dessert. *Diabetes Desserts Cookbook For Dummies* has the healthful recipes and lifestyle tips that you need to continue enjoying the sweet things in life.

Here are a few guidelines to keep in mind about the recipes:

- » All eggs are large.
- » All flour is all-purpose unless otherwise specified.
- » All extra-virgin olive oil is the best quality possible.
- » All Greek yogurt is plain and full fat unless otherwise specified.
- » All cinnamon is pure (Ceylon) cinnamon.
- » All vanilla is pure vanilla extract unless otherwise stated.
- » All honey is raw.
- » All maple syrup is pure.
- » All date sugar and coconut sugar is organic.
- » All monk fruit sweetener is organic.
- » All salt is unrefined sea salt, which contains some raw minerals that help the body digest salt minus any unwanted additives. If you're swapping out regular salt, use an even smaller quantity.
- » All dry ingredient measurements are level — use a dry ingredient measuring cup, fill it using a spoon instead of scooping to the top, and scrape it even with a straight object, such as the flat side of a knife.
- » At the end of many of the recipes I add helpful tips, notes, and ways you can vary the recipe.
- » 🍅 If you need or want vegetarian recipes, scan the list of "Recipes in This Chapter" on the first page of each chapter in Part 3. A little tomato in front of the name of a recipe marks that recipe as vegetarian. (See the tomato to the left of this paragraph.)

This isn't a complete book about diagnosing and treating diabetes and its complications. Check out the most recent editions of *Diabetes For Dummies*, if you need diagnosis and treatment information, or *Diabetes Meal Planning & Nutrition For Dummies* (both by John Wiley & Sons, Inc.) if you want a deeper dive into meal planning and nutrition.

Consuming raw or undercooked meats, poultry, seafood, shellfish, or eggs may increase your risk of foodborne illness.

Foolish Assumptions

When writing this book, I made the following assumptions about you, my dear reader:

>> You believe that blood glucose levels are impacted by the foods you eat.

>> You need a refresher course on diabetes basics or in meal planning.

>> You're new to diabetes or prediabetes and want to get valuable information that can help you live your best life in addition to recipes.

>> You're committed to your health and looking for as many ways as possible to improve it.

>> You're already an expert on diabetes-related nutrition and have consistently even glucose levels, but you're wanting some new desserts in your meal plan or just need a refresher.

No matter, you can find out with a little planning, you don't need to sacrifice on desserts, even if you're living with diabetes.

Icons Used in This Book

The icons alert you to information you must know, information you should know, and information you may find interesting but can live without.

This icons points out essential information.

REMEMBER

TIP

This icon marks information that can save you time and energy.

DOCTOR SAYS

This icon provides medical advice — from my culinary medicine partner and technical editor of this book, Dr. Simon Poole — about the choices you have to optimize your treatment.

TECHNICAL STUFF

This icon gives you technical, scientific, or medical information or terminology that may be helpful, but not necessary, to your understanding of the topic.

WARNING

This icon warns against potential problems (for example, things to avoid when balancing blood sugar).

Beyond This Book

In addition to the content of this book, you can access some related material online. It contains important information that you may want to refer to on a regular basis. To find the Cheat Sheet, visit www.dummies.com and search for "Diabetes Desserts Cookbook For Dummies Cheat Sheet."

Where to Go from Here

Where you go from here depends on your level of interest and passion. Personally speaking, I never tire of looking for new ways to feel and eat better. Like all *For Dummies* books, this book is modular, meaning you don't need to read it from front to back cover to grasp what I'm talking about.

If you want information about topics like glucose and macronutrients, go to Chapters 2, 3, and 4. If your blood sugar is stable and/or you already know how to manage your diabetes and you're ready to try the recipes, head to Part 3. Or you can scan the Table of Contents or the Index to find a topic that piques your interest, flip to that chapter, and start reading.

1

Discovering Delicious and Nutritious Desserts

Know what role blood sugar plays in your body.

Understand how blood sugar affects your physical and mental health.

Discover the best ways to keep your blood glucose balanced while eating desserts.

Chapter **1**

Defining Diabetes-Friendly Desserts

The term "diabetes-friendly desserts" may seem like an oxymoron to many people. After all, aren't individuals with diabetes supposed to avoid desserts altogether? In order to answer that question, you need to first understand how sugar affects your health and realize that not all desserts are created equal. By discovering how to prepare nutritious and delicious desserts, you can keep your blood sugar in check and satisfy your sweet cravings in a healthful way which prevents overindulgence in desserts that aren't good for you.

This chapter serves as your entry point into the world of diabetes desserts. I preview what you can discover in this book, including sugar's effect on glucose and how to harness the power of healthful ingredients in desserts.

Exploring Blood Glucose Levels

Consuming sugars and simple carbohydrates plays a direct role on a person's blood glucose levels. *Simple sugars* consist of glucose, fructose, and sucrose. Carbohydrates are found in *simple,* readily available small molecular forms called sugars or are linked together in more *complex* carbohydrates. When the body handles glucose improperly, symptoms of diabetes occur.

A hormone referred to as *insulin* controls the level of glucose in your blood. This hormone is a chemical substance made in one part of the body that travels to another part of the body to open cells so that glucose can enter. If it can't enter the cell, it can't provide energy to the body.

Insulin plays a major role in regulating blood sugar, is essential for growth, and enables fat and muscle to develop. When you don't have a sufficient amount of insulin, or when insulin isn't working effectively, glucose starts to rise. If it rises above a certain level (specifically 180mg/dl (10>0 mmol/L)), glucose begins to spill into the urine and make it sweet. The loss of glucose leads to short-term complications of diabetes.

REMEMBER

Your blood glucose level is the level of sugar in your blood, a key measure in diabetes. Glucose can change in just 30 minutes time, especially before and after meals. That's why monitoring your blood glucose continuously is so important in order to make sure that your glucose levels are not too high or too low. Dehydration, fatigue, kidney problems, and others are direct results of having imbalanced blood glucose.

The following sections touch on the role that sugar plays in your mental and physical health and how to regulate your blood sugar while enjoying desserts.

Looking at how sugar affects the mind and body

As I discuss in Chapter 2, consuming too much sugar, not balancing simple carbs in meals, or eating sweet foods or drinks by themselves will quickly affect your mind and body. Blood glucose levels that are too high will affect your ability to function normally because your brain needs correct levels of glucose to function properly. Glucose that's too high or too low can affect your ability to think clearly. Glucose that's too low can even cause loss of consciousness.

There's no magic number for the amount of sugar that you should eat in a day. However, many health professionals believe that you should eat as little as possible and balance it with good quality proteins and fats to lower the glycemic load of the foods that you do eat and prevent blood sugar spikes.

Regulating your blood sugar while enjoying desserts

You can regulate your blood sugar in many ways besides medicine and insulin. As Chapter 3 examines, a healthy attitude, approach to life, and lifestyle in general make a big difference. Even your thoughts and emotions help prevent blood sugar spikes. Taking charge of your mental health as well as your physical health is important in order to regulate your blood sugar.

REMEMBER

Keep the following in mind when selecting desserts to eat when you have diabetes to regulate your blood sugar:

>> **Ensure that the desserts you're eating are as healthful as possible.** The recipes in Part 3 are a great place to start.

>> **Make your own desserts.** When you make your own, you can ensure you're using nourishing ingredients and natural sweeteners that don't spike blood sugar.

Although certain foods such as simple sugars and carbohydrates can cause blood spikes when eaten in large amounts and not balanced with other macronutrients — protein, carbohydrate (in this case complex carbs), and fat — everyone's body responds differently to various foods.

>> **Regularly monitor your blood glucose to make sure that your levels stay balanced.** If you notice any patterns of sudden rises or sudden dips when eating or drinking certain things, or even thinking certain thoughts or after having not gotten enough sleep, take the necessary action to ensure that it doesn't continue.

Creating a Lifestyle That Supports Diabetes Desserts

A diabetes diagnosis doesn't have to be a bad thing. Think of it as your body's alert signal letting you know that something is off. You deserve to enjoy the sweetness of life and good health. A diagnosis is your permission slip to take good care of yourself.

Luckily, many of the lifestyle changes that support being able to eat diabetes-friendly desserts include activities that help your mental and physical health in general, and are free and readily available. Engaging in pleasurable activities such as hobbies and other things you enjoy doing, spending time outdoors, exercising, getting plentiful sleep including daily naps, and spending time in communal and even volunteer activities are all easy lifestyle additions that help the body to metabolize sugar better in the first place.

Thinking positively, practicing gratitude, and doing breath work and yoga are all easy additions that pay off in the long and short term. Cooking diabetes-friendly meals, including desserts, is also much easier than it seems. Dr. Simon Poole and I outline our best tips in our other books — the most recent editions of *Diabetes For Dummies*, *Diabetes Meal Planning & Nutrition*, and *Diabetes Cookbook For Dummies* (John Wiley & Sons, Inc.).

If you've recently been diagnosed with diabetes or prediabetes, you may feel overwhelmed — in particular about eating desserts and making better food choices.

These sections examine the essential information that you need to know about creating a lifestyle so you can enjoy eating the desserts in Part 3.

Eating right — Focusing on macronutrients

Balancing *macronutrients* — carbs, fats, and proteins — is important to everyone, but for people with diabetes, it's essential, especially if you want to enjoy desserts. Every time you eat, you should ensure that you choose the best quality complex carbs (whole grains and sweet potatoes are two examples) healthful fats (extra-virgin olive oil, avocado, and nuts are examples), and quality, low-fat protein (fish, seafood, chicken, edamame, beans, and legumes are examples). Chapter 4 provides more details.

Fitting diabetes-friendly desserts into your diet

If you want to have your cake and eat it too, literally, then you have to balance the rest of your meals during that same day in order to avoid blood sugar spikes. Say you know that you're going out to dinner and you'll splurge on a small portion of dessert, then eat well-balanced meals for breakfast and lunch that incorporate a single serving of complex carbs with lean protein and quality fats.

Be sure to get physical activity during the day. At dinner, prior to the dessert, eat a meal that consists of healthful fats, lean protein, and lots of green leafy vegetables. That way the extra simple sugars and carbs in the dessert won't affect you as much as if you ate a dinner heavy with simple carbs and unhealthful fats.

Refer to Chapter 5 for more information about ways to include diabetes-friendly desserts into your diet.

Having the right ingredients on hand

Starting out with the right ingredients in your kitchen makes preparing diabetes-friendly desserts a cinch. Chapter 6 describes building a pantry and how to choose healthful ingredients. For dessert making, a good selection of flours, nuts, EVOO, dark chocolate, cocoa powder, and natural sugars such as organic coconut and date sugar as well as raw honey are good options.

Choosing healthful desserts when not home

When eating out, selecting the best desserts is so important. This decision can be tricky because many menu descriptions make things sound better than they are. For instance, although a restaurant dessert may be made with dark chocolate, it may also include unhealthy fats and lots of sugar. However, no one expects that you completely give up restaurant and purchased desserts. That said, try to avoid them as much as possible and opt for the recipes in Part 3.

TIP

If you're going out to eat, plan in advance by ordering a meal that's high in lean protein, healthful fat like EVOO, and carbohydrates like leafy greens, and non-starchy vegetables. Including these macronutrients in your meal help you to prevent blood sugar spikes when enjoying dessert. When you do decide to order dessert in a restaurant, try to share it with others or only eat a small portion of it. Restaurant portions are consistently much larger than actual portion sizes. Eating an entire dessert can cause spikes in your blood sugar.

Chapter 5 explains in greater detail what you need to know about store-bought and restaurant desserts.

MY STORY: MY PASSION FOR HELPING PEOPLE WITH DIABETES

I was 15 years old when my mom came home from the doctor with a diabetes diagnosis. Her doctor scribbled down some off-limits foods on a single sheet of a prescription pad and told her not to eat sugar. That was pretty much it. During those days, I used to cook dinner for my parents and me after school because my mom worked and got home late. I felt so limited by that list of things that we couldn't eat that I forgot to think about what we could. A few days after the shock wore off, I started making a list of the foods we could eat and vowed to make my mom recipes using those ingredients.

My first cookbook consisted of recipes that I figured would be safe for my mom to eat and delicious for the rest of us. Keep in mind that this was the early 1990s — long before internet recipes, online cookbooks, and apps were available. I relied on information that I could find in books. In those days many of the diabetes cookbooks were labelled "diabetic recipes" and were full of some of the sweetest desserts around, focusing on substituting sugar alternatives for sucrose.

I intuitively knew that artificial sweeteners weren't the way to go, even though they were very popular at the time and even though some doctors were recommending them. I turned to some traditional Italian desserts that were naturally less sweet and incorporated some nutritious ingredients like fruit and spices as much as possible. Little did I know that this necessity to find good food that's also good for you for my mom would lead to my current career.

About 15 years ago my quest deepened. I went from searching for ingredients that wouldn't cause blood sugar to spike for people with diabetes to looking for superfoods (like EVOO, broccoli, plain Greek yogurt, and berries) that are particularly beneficial for people with diabetes and would positively impact their health. Each discovery was like finding a jewel that would help my mom and other family members live and eat better.

Then I went through my own health challenges. I was diagnosed with Stage 3 Lyme disease that had wreaked havoc on my central nervous system. I had more than 40 medical symptoms and was legally disabled for three years. My prognosis wasn't good. People in my therapy group had arrived at Stage 4 and died of heart attacks. My doctor told me that even if I got rid of my symptoms, I'd never get rid of the illness in my blood. My existence was constant pain and suffering.

I tried every conventional and complimentary therapy I could looking for relief. But getting better was taking longer than I could handle. My prayers turned from asking for healing to asking for the courage to take my own life because I no longer believed that healing was possible. At that time, my doctor recommended that I speak to a mind-body therapist, the late Kathleen Ammalee Rogers. She explained that the breadth of her work relied on the philosophy that we all have the capacity to heal ourselves and that each disease was simply the physical manifestation of an old belief that no longer served us and needed to be cleared out from our bodies.

For the next year I continued regular visits with Kathleen as well as taking my prescribed medicines, seeing a top-tier chiropractor, and attending neuro-biofeedback sessions. I prayed, meditated, used positive imagery and nutrition, and everything else I could to heal.

Within that time, I learned so much about how both the body and mind work together in order to achieve better health. Today, I incorporate this philosophy into new challenges that I've faced since as well. After I healed, I vowed that if I lived and healed, I'd dedicate my life to cooking, writing, and sharing the positive things that I've learned with people. I believe in incorporating as many things as possible to feel your best, and I bring that attitude to this book.

My career has focused on writing and educating people about the Mediterranean diet and lifestyle and often about diabetes-friendly foods. I must admit, I never thought I'd write a book on diabetes desserts. I've already written or cowritten 19 books, most of them based on the Mediterranean diet, the Mediterranean lifestyle, and diabetes-friendly cuisine. In those books, desserts weren't the focus. Even in the *Diabetes Cookbook For Dummies* that I released last year with Dr. Simon Poole, I created desserts mostly out of fresh fruit, nuts, and cheese, which is what you should be consuming anyway.

Preparing and Eating Delicious Dessert Recipes

This cookbook includes dishes that are naturally healthful and can be enjoyed as a part of a nutritious meal more frequently. You aren't limited to bland and tasteless desserts. Diabetes-friendly desserts come in all sizes and shapes. Here are the main types of dessert recipes that I include in this book:

>> **Fruit-based desserts:** Enjoying fresh fruit for dessert helps you to reach the fresh fruit and veggies requirements of a healthful diet while enabling you to enjoy natural sweetness and prevent you from indulging in more unhealthful desserts.

Make fresh fruit and veggies the base of your diet. Even though various diets and meal plans recommend different quantities of consuming fresh produce, the Mediterranean diet, ranked the best in the world for eight years in a row at the time of writing this book, recommends 9 to 12 servings of fresh fruit and vegetables per day. In the United States, the recommended dietary guidelines are 1.5 to 2 cups of fruit and 2 to 3 servings of vegetables, which is notably lower than Mediterranean standards. Putting fruit into dessert is another step toward getting your daily quotient. Refer to Chapter 9 for fruit-based dessert recipes.

» **Brownies and bars:** They're quintessential American desserts that have become popular around the globe. Normally these treats are laden with butter and table sugar, though.

Chapter 10 explains how to swap out healthier whole-grain and nut flours. Polyphenol-rich EVOO is also the protagonist, as it is throughout the recipes in this book, adding flavor and healthful fats. These recipes also freeze well and make great host gifts. Plus, they bake up in a short time. Last minute guests? No problem!

» **Cookies:** Cookies are a popular international pick-me-up. Chapter 11 explores how to make classics and new varieties while incorporating nutrient-dense ingredients. Keep these recipes in mind for holidays. They make great edible gifts.

» **Spoon desserts and puddings:** These recipes are among the easiest desserts to prepare because they don't require baking. Chapter 12 uses dark chocolate, chia seeds, and other healthful ingredients to allow you to indulge in creamy sweet flavors without any consequence. These are great make-ahead desserts to enjoy anytime.

» **Bite-sized treats:** Truffles, chocolates, and chocolate-covered fruit are fantastic ways to indulge your sweet tooth and enjoy the nutritional benefits of antioxidants.

» **Frozen treats:** Whipping up gelato, ice cream, and sorbets on your own lends a gourmet finale to your meals. When relying on ingredients like plain, full-fat Greek yogurt, fruit, and dark chocolate, you can make these favorites more nutritious (refer to Chapter 14). Have one or more of these treats on hand to avoid less healthy versions in the warmer months.

» **Tarts and pies:** Both veteran and new bakers can discover how to master diabetes-friendly tarts and pies. Making some of the nutritious nut-based crusts in advance gives you an advantage so that you can make a fruit-based version when you need it. Check out Chapter 15 and save these recipes for special occasions and for sharing because they're showstoppers!

>> **Sweet sips:** Sweet-tasting beverages are a great way to end a meal, especially when they're full of antioxidant-rich fruit, dark chocolate, and spices. Chapter 16 has some recipes that you can enjoy when you need a quick pick-me-up or when you're entertaining.

>> **Cakes:** If you've never made homemade cakes before, don't worry, these are classic, foolproof recipes that have stood the test of time. Best of all, you can make the recipes in Chapter 17 in advance, freeze them, and then serve them at a later date when you need them. Keep them in mind for potlucks, when you host guests, and when you need to bring a dish to a gathering. After all, if you bring a nutritious dessert, you can ensure that you enjoy one at a party without having to explain your meal plan.

MAKING SMARTER DIABETES-FRIENDLY DESSERT CHOICES

When evaluating and selecting diabetes-friendly desserts, factor in specific guidance from a nutrition professional as well as patterns in your glucose readings. If you consistently have high blood sugar after eating a certain type of food, avoid it. But if your readings are consistent, and you're eating healthful foods, you can afford to enjoy a nutritious dessert every now and then.

The chapters in Part 4 can help you pick the best diabetes-friendly desserts. These chapters cover the following:

- **Ways to enjoy desserts:** Chapter 18 explains in plain English easy ways to enjoy desserts with a diabetes diagnosis.

- **Debunked myths about desserts:** Chapter 19 dispels the myths that you might have heard about diabetes and desserts.

- **Diabetes-friendly ingredients:** Chapter 20 discusses the best diabetes-friendly ingredients to stock in your pantry, fridge, and freezer for dessert making.

Chapter **2**

Understanding Sugar's Role in the Body

The best way to get a step ahead of diabetes? Be knowledgeable about it. Yes, knowledge is power. Understanding how your brain and body respond to sugar and how to avoid excess sugar in your diet can help you to live your best life.

This chapter explores how sugar metabolizes in your body and how you can curb sugar cravings, add sweetness to your life to impact your overall health, read packaging and nutritious labels, and give your favorite recipes a makeover.

Noting How the Body and Brain Use Sugar

Your brain is responsible for determining a normal level of blood glucose in your body. Your brain is extremely important to your existence, doesn't require insulin to absorb glucose, and usually gets whatever it wants or needs. But your brain is more concerned about operating with low blood glucose levels than about higher levels. High blood glucose causes problems in other ways.

Plus, the brain, just like the gut, is a driving force in your overall health. Italian has the saying "*mente sana, corpo sano,*" which means "healthy mind, healthy body." Although physical symptoms can and do affect the way you think, your thoughts can also help you be both healthy and sick, which is why it's important to use them carefully. An excess of sugar in the diet and poorly controlled blood glucose can influence your mind and thought patterns as much as it can your body.

The following sections shine the spotlight on diabetes, including the different types of diabetes, what diabetes is, and how you can take better care of your psychological, emotional, and social self when you have diabetes.

Listing the types of diabetes

Deciding to take an active role in balancing sugar levels in your brain and body is the only way to prevent, treat, and hopefully reverse type 2 diabetes. To understand your role, you must first know about the different types of diabetes:

>> Type 1 diabetes results when you lose the capacity to produce insulin.

>> Type 2 diabetes happens when your natural insulin is unable to do its job effectively.

If you were a car and insulin was gasoline, type 1 diabetes is having an empty tank, and type 2 diabetes is more like lost efficiency from clogged fuel injectors. Managing type 1 diabetes requires constantly adding gasoline; type 2 diabetes requires that you get your fuel injectors to work better.

Understanding the basics of diabetes

In reality, your body needs to keep a certain concentration of glucose circulating in your blood — what's considered a normal blood glucose level. *Glucose* is the favorite fuel of your trillions of cells and some really important cells like your brain cells that can't get their energy from anything else. Glucose in your bloodstream is all about energy — it's delivered right to every cell that needs it.

TECHNICAL STUFF

Glucose enters your blood after you eat carbohydrate foods including table sugar, which causes your blood glucose levels to rise. Your body has a way to return those levels back to normal by storing the excess for later. The stored glucose can be released back into the blood when glucose levels drop between meals, keeping a constant supply available for your brain. This kind of balance in a biological system is called *homeostasis.*

The hormone responsible for escorting glucose into storage and regulating blood sugar is *insulin,* and insulin is automatically released from special cells on your pancreas when blood glucose levels increase after eating. If insulin isn't available or isn't working properly, blood glucose can't be stored and blood glucose levels remain high. High blood glucose levels not only upset glucose homeostasis, but also begin to damage cells and tissue.

REMEMBER

Chronic high blood glucose levels is diabetes — literally. Chapter 3 includes a more in-depth explanation on diabetes. In the simplest terms, having diabetes means your blood glucose levels go up after eating and don't come down to normal levels in a normal amount of time.

High glucose levels not only mean that excess glucose can't get into cells to be stored, but glucose also can't get into cells to properly fuel energy needs. It also results in damage to blood vessels that causes disruption to the supply of oxygen, glucose, and other nutrients and hormones to cells. That means your microscopic cells, like the muscle cells you need to move, don't have access to their favored fuel and must turn to plan B or plan C for generating energy. Plans B and C are ordinarily temporary plans for times of shortage — generating energy without glucose is inefficient and even produces toxic waste products. In short, diabetes upsets your entire energy balance.

In addition to being diagnosed, the actions of taking responsibility for your health, making good choices, discovering how to balance meals, especially desserts, and incorporating physical exercise into your daily life are important. If you have additional questions about your nutritional needs or glucose levels, discuss them with your primary care physician, endocrinologist, diabetes care specialist, and nutrition professional.

Taking control of your behavioral health

Taking control of your psychological, emotional and social health is also essential for enjoying good physical health, despite the fact that it's rarely mentioned in that way in western conventional medicine. In most modern countries mental health is seen as something separate from physical health and as something that's only sought when people are going through a mental crisis. Things shouldn't have to get that bad before patients are advised to take care of their own mental health.

For example, many schools have programs that teach young children breathwork, yoga, meditation, and the importance of their thoughts. The children in those programs are then studied and the findings are right in-line with common sense. The children who are taught to use coping mechanisms for their thoughts and mental health get better grades, perform better in school, and enjoy better health.

It's never too early or too late to form healthful thought. Mastering your thoughts leads to mastering yourself. This doesn't mean that you have to control your thoughts all the time or that you should aim to avoid negative thoughts altogether. Negative thoughts are a normal and natural part of the human brain's functioning because they're hardwired to protect you from harmful situations.

Choosing better thoughts and directing your attention toward them, however, positively impacts your health. The next time you find yourself feeling negative thoughts — worry, afraid, scared, sad — acknowledge those feelings and try to shift your focus to things that you're grateful for and appreciate. Little by little this shift will become more and more of a habit and your thoughts will help you to feel better. See Chapter 5 for more details.

Examining the Causes of Sugar Cravings

Low blood sugar can sometimes lead to intense cravings for sweets, creating a vicious cycle where eating sweet foods and not properly balancing meals further spikes blood sugar levels. The more sugar you consume, more than likely you'll experience cravings later. As I explain in the section "Noting How the Body and Brain Use Sugar" earlier in this chapter, the body has a need for quick energy and managing that need can be difficult without proper meal planning, dietary control, and blood sugar monitoring.

The following sections explore what's behind sugar cravings, discusses how to identify your sugar cravings, and what ingredients you can use when you're craving to your advantage to give yourself the nutrients and support that your body needs.

Understanding cravings often lead to impulsive eating

Sugar cravings often lead to *impulsive eating* (also known as *binge eating* — a disorder that causes eating large amounts of food, eating too quickly, and eating when no longer hungry). That means that in the contest between your impulse to eat and your thinking brain, impulse usually wins.

Impulsive eating has a negative connotation in the modern world, but it doesn't have to. Hunger is your body's way of encouraging you to nourish yourself.

With industrialization, advertising propaganda, and the invention of fast and junk food, however, many people are no longer in control of their cravings. A late night TV ad may stir desires for a double cheeseburger with bacon, and a billboard may make a candy bar look like something you can't live without. When coupled with subliminal messages that these items provide "a break," "a complete meal," or "a sinful delight," giving into temptation can be easy.

Many times people crave certain food styles when they're truly craving an emotional state. Consider these examples:

>> Craving salty foods most (if their cortisol levels aren't unbalanced) can be a result of a need for adventure.

>> Craving comforting pastas and carb-rich products can indicate a need for comfort.

>> Craving sugary snacks and sweet treats most often is because of a lack of perceived sweetness in life.

If you identify with any of these scenarios, explore whether you're truly craving the emotion associated with that type of food.

Because your life changes, so do your cravings. You may have a particular craving for sweets more than normal while in a particular stressful period of life. When things get hard, you may find yourself craving more comforting foods.

Curbing sugar cravings: The how-to

You have sugar cravings? Welcome to the club! So does everyone else. Here's my favorite technique that you can use to curb them and use them to your benefit.

TIP

Take a few minutes to pause each time you have strong cravings for certain foods and do these easy steps:

1. **Sit with your feet flat on the floor and put one hand on your heart and the other on your belly and breathe in and out very slowly three times.**

   Ask yourself:

   - Why am I craving this food?

   - What is it that I'm truly craving?

   - If I had a magic wand and could be doing anything now, what would I rather be doing?

2. **Take a deep breath and write down your answers.**

Reminding yourself that your health is your first priority, ask yourself if you can achieve the desired emotion (comfort, love, sweetness) another way.

You can do other activities like call a friend, go for a walk, and listen to music that you love to get your mind off the cravings and break the negative habits. Chapter 3 discusses these activities in greater detail.

Recognizing what to eat when you're craving sugar

Certain foods provide the nutrients that you need, help you feel full longer, and or lend a perception of sweet flavor to make you crave sugar less. Here are some foods that help to beat sugar cravings in general (consuming them can help to curb your sugar cravings):

- Avocados
- Beans
- Berries
- Chia seeds
- Cinnamon
- Coconut
- Coconut oil
- Dark chocolate
- Dates
- Eggs
- Fresh fruit
- Fresh vegetables
- Lean meat and fish
- Legumes
- Lentils
- Nuts
- Oats
- Plain, full-fat Greek yogurt
- Sesame seeds
- Smoothie
- Sweet potatoes
- Trail mix
- Whole grains

Refer to the section "Making Desserts Healthful with These Ingredients" later in this chapter where I discuss many of these ingredients in greater detail.

Making easy substitutions

If you're in the middle of an intense sugar craving, don't have any of the desserts in Part 3 already prepared and want to satisfy your sweet tooth in the healthiest way possible, turn to these ingredients:

- A cupful of fresh berries with either ½ cup plain, full-fat Greek yogurt and a teaspoon of raw honey or a handful of almonds

- A few small pieces of dark chocolate (80 percent or higher)

- A piece of fresh fruit balanced with a few nuts, nut butter, or cheese if in between a meal

- Cinnamon tea — steep 1 teaspoon pure cinnamon in a glass of hot water or milk for 10 minutes, covered, strain into a mug, and enjoy

- A few juicy dates with some nuts or seeds

- A serving of trail mix — be sure it's no-sugar-added variety or make it yourself

- A homemade smoothie — refer to Chapter 16 for some recipes that balance sugar, carbs, and fats with no added sugar

- A small banana with a few teaspoons nut butter

If you're new at switching your diet into a more healthful one and are used to consuming ultraprocessed foods, fast food, and junk food, you may suffer from chemical addictions to the ingredients in those foods as well as the foods themselves. Continuing to consume them will increase your blood glucose fluctuations, which will in turn cause you to continue to have more sugar cravings.

TECHNICAL STUFF

Although scientists are now able to identify the harmful effects of specific chemicals used in fast food and ultraprocessed junk food and understand the horrible effects that they have on the human mind and body when consumed frequently and over a long period of time, there's little talk about how to transform the addiction that they cause. If you've made a habit of turning to these foods on a regular basis, chances are giving them up won't be easy, just as it isn't easy to give up smoking or alcohol.

Preparing yourself to give up your sugar cravings

If you want to overcome this sugar craving battle, you have to rely on a lot of willpower. Know in advance that you'll go through withdrawal from not eating the foods you crave. Prepare yourself to give up these foods by doing the following:

- Set yourself up for success. Go into your decision to avoid unhealthful food with conviction, knowing that it will save your health and happiness.

- Know your weaknesses. For example, if you're turning to ice cream and shakes, turn to Chapters 14 and 16 to make your own.

>> Eat as many healthful foods as possible. The ingredients I discuss in the section "Making Desserts Healthful with These Ingredients" later in this chapter can help to keep you full and satiated.

>> Prepare healthy alternatives. The recipes in Part 3 are a great place to start. Make sure you have ingredients and recipes on hand for when the craving strikes.

>> Consider that you may be addicted to ultraprocessed foods and junk food. These types of foods are fast, readily available, and offer a quick hit of fat, sugar, and additives. Identify other things you can do when the craving strikes that you enjoy, such as walk outdoors, drink some water, exercise, call a loved one, and so on.

>> Take time to identify healthful foods that you enjoy eating and eat those instead.

>> Identify fast casual restaurants and take-out options that use more healthful ingredients to enjoy on occasion.

Go easy on yourself. Cutting an addiction cold turkey doesn't work for everyone. Remember that everything is relative. If you eat junk food and processed food every day and are able to cut down to once a week and then once every other week, and then once a month, your body and mind will thank you for it.

Adding "Sweet" Lifestyle Strategies to Your Day

The Italian "*la dolce vita*" — which literally means "the sweet life" but is transliterated as "the good life" — is often associated with luxury vacations and idyllic times by non-Italians. To Italians, however, who are often voted the healthiest people in Europe, *la dolce vita* is both a mindset and a lifestyle.

From a cultural perspective, Italians try to extract the most sweetness out of life. That means doing what you love, spending time with those you love, watching and listening to things you love, and enjoying the best food as often as possible. Of course, Italians have to work, raise families, and deal with problems like everyone else. But a unique feature to the culture is to accept them as what the Stoic philosophers called *amor fati*, destined things that you can't change about your life.

Without railing against what they can't change, Italians often focus their attention to the things that they can do to make themselves, and those around them, happy and healthy.

MUSIC ADDS SWEETNESS TO YOUR LIFE

I mention listening to music that you love as a means to add sweetness to your life often in this book. According to the National Institute of Health, the use of music intervention therapy has been found effective in treating a wide range of health issues, including diabetes. Music has the power to heal people at a cellular level. In fact, listening to music that you love can lower your blood pressure and blood sugar levels. Scientists have even found that exposing cancer cells to Beethoven's *Fifth Symphony* stopped their ability to spread quickly and even slowed their growth by 20 percent more than when no music was playing.

Many Italian winemakers play classical music on speakers in their orchards to help produce healthier vines and prevent disease. You can do the same things with your own body. Even when you sleep, you can listen to certain musical frequencies that have healing power. Whether you choose your favorite rock music, classical music, or healing frequencies, know that music can be a powerful ally in enjoying the sweet life — without added sugar!

Your goal is to find your good life. The following sections share widely available and easy ways to add enjoyment to your life without consuming additional sugar. Watching a beautiful sunset, beautifying your surroundings, going to an exhibit to see beautiful artwork, and setting a beautiful table are all ways that you can influence your own happiness.

Tapping into your happiness hormones

Happiness hormones make you feel happier and therefore inspire you to make healthier, sweeter choices in your lives without turning to consuming sugar. If you're not already harnessing their power, here's what you need to know about them:

>> **Serotonin:** Known as the "mood stabilizer" and also called the "feel-good hormone," serotonin helps prevent depression and anxiety. Most of the body's serotonin is produced in the gastrointestinal tract. A healthful diet, meditation, sun exposure, walking in nature, and exercise such as running, swimming, and cycling can help release serotonin.

>> **Endorphins:** These endorphins referred to as "the painkiller" help with pain relief, stress reduction, and mood improvement. Endorphins are often associated with exercise and the euphoric feelings that people get when exercising extensively. Activities like eating dark chocolate, laughing, and being physically active can help release endorphins as can using essential oils that promote mood stability.

>> **Dopamine:** Known as the "reward chemical," dopamine helps you focus and have feelings of satisfaction and pleasure. Dopamine can be released by sunshine, getting adequate sleep, listening to music, completing a task, doing self-care activities, celebrating little wins, and eating — especially protein.

>> **Oxytocin:** The "love hormone" is known for its role in bonding and attachment. Oxytocin levels increase with physical and sexual contact, such as holding hands, cuddling, kissing, playing with pets, and giving and receiving massages. Giving compliments, holding a baby, and hugging are also great ways to increase oxytocin.

Additional activities that can help promote the production of these hormones include exercising, visiting new places, getting a massage, playing with pets, and cooking and sharing a meal with someone you love.

Utilizing the emotional guidance scale

The Greek philosopher Aristotle said "Educating the mind without educating the heart is no education at all." The Emotional Guidance Scale, refer to www.the modernmanifestation.com/post/using-the-emotional-guidance-scale-to-raise-your-vibration, can help you identify where you are emotionally and how you can feel better. By tapping into your heart as well as your mind, you can improve the way you feel. Being able to transform your negative emotions is a priceless gift you can give yourself — one that you'll reap many benefits.

The scale can assist you in determining your current emotional state. The EGS is a list of 22 emotions ranging from joy at the top spot to depression at the bottom. Each emotion in between has a set frequency associated with it. By identifying where you are on the scale, recognize what emotion you're feeling, you can then use various techniques to slowly move yourself up the scale and to a better feeling place. Chapter 3 offers additional ways to improve your emotions.

Know that in the course of a single day you can go up and down the scale as you feel a wide range of emotions. The key is to stay in the upper part of the scale with the better feeling emotions most of the day.

TIP

When you aren't able to overcome your negative emotions, dealing with a disease diagnosis and living day-to-day can be a challenge. Using the scale can help. Write down the emotions that you experience predominately in a day in the same journal where you track your blood sugar level readings, what you eat, and your exercise (refer to Chapter 3 for more details about tracking these details). If you find that certain emotions persist and you need help transforming them, seek a mind-body therapist, mental health professional, and/or spiritual guide.

HARNESSING THE POWER OF YOUR EMOTIONS

Several years ago I emceed a fund-raiser at the Italian embassy in Washington, D.C., on International Women's Day. The profits were divided between an organization that helped battered women in D.C. and a Milan-based organization that taught emotional education in schools to at-risk children. The students were taught to identify their emotions, overcome negative ones, and become socially well adjusted. The organizations tracked their progress through school and found that despite their limited financial backgrounds and challenges that the students faced, they were able to get better grades, have a good academic career, and stay out of trouble (which wasn't the norm in their environment).

For years I volunteered for an organization that attempted to insert this type of curriculum in American schools. I was in my 30s when I finally learned to harness the power of my emotions, so I knew having this skill would have helped me a great deal when I was younger. It's never too late to start, and delving into this topic will be useful for the rest of your life.

Selecting Healthy Ingredients Directly Impacts Your Diabetes

This section explains the importance of the glycemic index and loads when you have diabetes and helps you to understand why the ingredients you choose are important to your health.

Discussing glycemic index and load

The degree to which a carbohydrate, or sugar, results in a rise in blood glucose is called its *glycemic index (GI)*, but a more realistic measure of the effects of eating a food considers how quickly it causes a rise in blood glucose against the amount in a serving — described as the *glycemic load (GL)*. That's why making a concerted decision about the food you eat is so important.

For example. Raw honey has a lower GI than sugar. The GI measures how quickly a carbohydrate raises blood sugar levels. Honey has a GI score of 58, and sugar has a GI value of 60. That means honey (like all carbohydrates) raises blood sugar quickly, but not quite as fast as sugar.

Considering that watermelon has a much lower GL than its higher GI suggests that it's because of its high water content. Focusing on the low GI rating of particular foods and the low GL when combining them together in a recipe can help you maintain stable and optimal control of blood glucose.

DOCTOR SAYS

Exercise lowers blood glucose and boosts insulin sensitivity. Higher *insulin sensitivity* (which allows the cells of the body to use blood glucose more effectively and reduce blood sugar) can persist for 24 to 72 hours after exercising. Exercising and eating healthful desserts on occasion is a key to keeping blood glucose balanced.

Researchers at the University of Toronto originally developed the GI of carbohydrate-containing foods in 1981. Recognizing that different foods affect blood glucose differently, they fed carbohydrate foods to fasting volunteers and monitored their fasting blood glucose response over the following two hours. The blood glucose response to eating pure glucose serves as a benchmark, affecting levels more quickly and more profoundly, and a little math produces a GI number that compares other foods to glucose. The GI number of glucose is set at 100, so Table 2-1 lists the values.

TABLE 2-1

Listing GI Values

GI Value	Labeled
70–100	High
56–69	Medium
55 and below	Low

REMEMBER

A cookbook about diabetes desserts can't give you your insulin-to-carb ratio or your correction factor because these numbers are unique to you. Your doctor will start you with dosages based upon your size and age, and together you can fine-tune based on trial and error. Eventually, your dosages for eating or correcting blood glucose may be different depending on the time of day. That's why meal planning and testing your glucose before meals is so key. You won't know where you're going if you don't know where you're starting.

Using better ingredients to make better choices

You can achieve a healthy carbohydrate intake by eating modest portion sizes, making good meal ingredient combination choices, and abiding by the following list:

>> **Choose whole grains.** Whole grains contain everything that makes up the grain, which is the bran, the germ, and the endosperm. Refined grains generally only contain the endosperm. Choosing whole grains simply means choosing whole-grain breads, crackers, and pastas, or whole grains such as oatmeal, barley, quinoa, and brown rice.

>> **Select whole fruit.** Whole fruit contains healthy dietary fiber and no added sugar. You don't have to choose fresh fruit though. Canned or frozen fruit is excellent as long as it doesn't contain any added sugars (packed in syrup). The no-added-sugar warning goes for fruit drinks, too, of course, but you may be surprised to know that eating fruit by itself is a better choice than 100-percent fruit juice.

>> **Eat lots of vegetables.** Vegetables are especially important to people with diabetes because of their low carbohydrate content and rich nutrient content. Frozen or canned vegetables are excellent if you avoid added sugar, fat, or sodium. Always choose the no-salt-added option for canned vegetables. Pick a wide variety of textures and colors, and avoid adding sugar, fat, or sodium at home with salt, butter, margarine, or salad dressings.

>> **Limit sweets.** Added sugar pours concentrated carbohydrates into your diet and at the same time delivers no nutrients. Many processed foods contain ingredients such as high fructose corn syrup.

The following sections discuss two other important aspects of your diet.

Incorporating fiber into your diet

Fiber is the most complex of carbohydrates, often forming the structural elements of plants. Fiber is relatively indigestible by humans but is still an extremely important part of your diet. The two types of fiber are as follows:

>> **Insoluble fiber:** It provides bulk, which helps to move food residues through your digestive system.

>> **Soluble fiber:** It's able to dissolve in water. It also has beneficial physiological effects. The most accepted benefit of soluble fiber is in lowering bad LDL cholesterol levels — oat bran is well recognized for this benefit, and beans are a tasty source of soluble fiber, too.

Specific benefits to health from the fiber component of your diet are challenging to isolate because foods that offer fiber are also rich in biologically active phyto-chemicals and antioxidants. Having adequate fiber in your diet may lower blood pressure, reduce the risk for some colorectal and breast cancers, strengthen your immune system, and improve blood glucose control.

Americans typically consume only about 15 grams of fiber per day, but the recommended daily consumption is

>> **Women between 19 and 50:** 25 grams

>> **Men between 19 and 50:** 38 grams

The recommended amount decreases for both men and women over 50, but the more the merrier. Although a huge volume of fiber can lead to digestive irritation, if you can tolerate more fiber, get more fiber.

Including healthful fats

Fats are an essential part of your diet, and with diabetes, more than likely your meal plan recommends that you get 25 to 35 percent of your calories from fat. Don't concern yourself with eliminating fat from your diet. Doing so causes skin problems, weakened bones, vision issues, and maybe even trouble thinking. Too much of the wrong kind of fat, however, has clearly negative health implications. The trick is to consume more healthful fats that balance with complex carbohydrates and lean proteins to prevent blood sugar spikes. Chapter 4 discusses this topic in more detail.

Making Desserts Healthful with These Ingredients

In terms of desserts, rely on the following ingredients to make them healthful.

REMEMBER

The dessert recipes in Part 3 take advantage of many of these ingredients. Meat, fish, lentils, and such aren't ideal for a dessert book, but you can incorporate them into your daily diet with plenty of dark leafy greens and vibrant vegetables to make sure that you crave sugar as little as possible.

Fresh fruit

Many people with diabetes and prediabetes think that they can no longer eat fruit. Fortunately, this isn't true.

Fruit contains antioxidants and bioactive compounds that are beneficial to your health. Per Mediterranean diet and lifestyle guidelines, most of your diet should consist of fruits (and vegetables) — 9 to 12 servings of fresh produce is recommended.

People with diabetes or prediabetes should enjoy mostly green leafy vegetables and colorful nonstarchy vegetables with balanced amounts of starchy vegetables and fruit. Fruit is perhaps the purest carbohydrate, often without any protein or fat; virtually every fruit has at least ten times more carbohydrate than protein. If you discount a few outliers like avocado (which has so much fat and so little carbohydrate it's placed in the dietary fat group), fruit is mostly fat-free. A carb choice for fruit varies depending upon the fruit itself, and whether it's dried.

Spend some time learning which fruits have the highest GL and avoid them. Opt for fruits, such as the ones I use in this book, that are better choices for people seeking to balance their blood sugar. Most of the desserts in this book are based on or incorporate fresh fruit or unsweetened dried fruit.

TIP

Try to make a single serving of fruit your daily dessert and enjoy the recipes in this book less often. When eating fruit as a snack, balance it with a healthful fat and protein source, such as nuts, good quality cheese, or full-fat plain Greek yogurt in order to prevent your blood sugar from spiking.

Here are a few specific fruits to include.

Banana

Ripe, mashed bananas can add natural sweetness to smoothies, breads, cakes, cookies, muffins, and more. Even though bananas are a natural sweetener, enjoy them in small amounts and balanced with other high protein and healthful fat ingredients. Keep ripe bananas on hand to mash and use as a sweetener instead of table sugar when needed.

Citrus

Sometimes it's great to have something really sweet, and it's hard to top an orange when it comes to sweet. Citrus is a secret ingredient that my maternal great grandmother, Michela, used in her desserts, and one that I can't go without. Whenever you want to add more flavor to a dessert without additional sugar, think about incorporating citrus zest and a bit of juice. Lemons and oranges are the best:

>> **Oranges:** A medium-sized orange is one 15-gram carbohydrate choice, making one orange or ½ cup of orange juice an effective treatment for moderate *hypoglycemia* (also called *low blood sugar,* which is when your blood sugar falls below normal levels, usually 70mg/dl).

In desserts, oranges can add a sweet-holiday flavor. If you want the full bang for your nutrition buck, go for the orange instead of the juice. You get more fiber and a better dose of antioxidants. Try eating them as a snack between meals with a handful of unsalted, unroasted almonds or tossing orange segments into a salad of spinach and avocado in lieu of tomatoes for a change.

» **Lemons:** They're a great source of vitamin C, and like vinegars, their acidity decreases the GL when combined with carbohydrates in a meal. Adding a squeeze of lemon juice to water is a wonderful way of staying hydrated while balancing the body's PH levels. It's also a wonderful detoxifier and has antimicrobial properties.

Almonds, almond butter, and almond flour

Almond flour increases the flavor, texture, and nutritional value of many baked goods. Let me share a little secret: It's been a go-to of mine for years to make recipes gluten-free and delicious. Furthermore, in diabetes-friendly desserts, this addition has a special appeal because almonds contain both healthful fats and protein that serve to balance out the natural sweeteners in the recipes.

Some studies suggest that eating almonds can help lower and stabilize blood sugar levels in people with prediabetes and type 2 diabetes. One study found that eating 20 grams of almonds 30 minutes before meals for three months led to lower body weight and improved glucose variability. In addition, consuming almonds before a meal helps you eat less and absorb more nutrients from the food that you eat.

Pure cinnamon

Pure cinnamon, often labelled Ceylon cinnamon in the United States, has been shown to help regulate blood sugar levels. It's also an anti-inflammatory ingredient that's important for anyone dealing with any type of illness.

From a dessert and pastry standpoint, this research is exciting because cinnamon is a common baking ingredient. In addition, the taste of cinnamon has been shown to trick your taste buds into thinking that they're eating something sweet because many sweets contain cinnamon.

ADDITIONAL BENEFITS TO ALMONDS

Almonds also contain significant amounts of magnesium, potassium, and vitamin E. A Chinese study found that people with the highest dietary intake of magnesium and potassium had the lowest risk of type 2 diabetes.

Here are some other things to know about magnesium, potassium, and vitamin E for people with diabetes:

- People with type 2 diabetes are more likely to have magnesium deficiencies, especially if they have poorly managed blood sugar or a chronic illness. Ask your healthcare practitioner to check your magnesium and potassium levels on a regular basis to avoid complications.

- Your healthcare practitioner may suggest supplements for magnesium and potassium, but make sure that you enjoy as much as possible in your daily diets as well. The recommended daily amount of magnesium for adults is 320 to 360 mg for women and 410 to 420 mg for men.

- Randomized controlled trials have found that vitamin E significantly reduces levels of HbA1c, fasting insulin, and HOMA-IR in patients with diabetes, particularly type 2 diabetes. Also, in studies that were conducted in less than ten weeks, intake of vitamin E was found to significantly reduce fasting blood glucose. Patients with type 2 diabetes may take 400 to 700 mg/day of vitamin E in addition to medication. Check with your healthcare practitioner to make sure that it's safe for you to take vitamin E supplementation. Vitamin E can also be found in sunflower seeds, broccoli, kiwi, asparagus, spinach, avocados, red peppers, beet root, butternut squash, tomatoes, peanuts, and Brazil nuts.

TIP

Add cinnamon to a recipe to cut back on sweeteners. Make sure it's pure and use a teaspoon more than normal.

Other sweet spices

These spices include ginger, cardamom, and cloves. They have powerful antioxidant properties and lend sweet flavors to desserts without harmful effects and extra calories. You can combine them together to make a delicious anti-inflammatory spice mix and flavor enhancer.

Dark chocolate

Dark chocolate cacao's flavanols and theobromine may reduce the risk of cardiovascular disease, improve cognitive function, and protect against age-related decline. Cacao also contains potassium and zinc, which help maintain strong blood vessels.

Chocolates contain the following cocoa solids and cocoa butter:

>> Dark chocolate: 65 to 90 percent

>> Semisweet chocolate: 40 to 64 percent

>> Milk chocolate: 10 to 39 percent

Dark chocolate with at least 70 percent cocoa is considered high quality. Nowadays, you can purchase 80, 85, and 90 percent dark chocolate.

TIP

For people with diabetes or those looking to prevent diabetes, opt for the highest percentage possible. It gives you the most benefits of the pure cocoa, which ancient Aztecs and Mayans used as a superfood and was an important commodity.

DOCTOR SAYS

Dr. Simon Poole recently shared a 2024 study published in the *British Medical Journal* that found that dark chocolate is associated with a decreased risk of type 2 diabetes, which gives people with diabetes more reason to enjoy it.

Extra-virgin olive oil (EVOO)

In this book I refer to EVOO as the fat of choice, and for good reason. Good quality EVOO is indispensable for good nutrition, good flavor, and tradition in my kitchen. Lecturing about olive oil and diabetes is what led me to meet the co-author of many of my books in the *For Dummies* series. Dr. Simon Poole and I even wrote an entire book dedicated to it called *Olive Oil For Dummies* (John Wiley & Sons), which dedicates 326 pages to our favorite ingredient.

Unsweetened peanut butter

Unsweetened peanut butter has been shown to improve blood glucose control, prevent blood glucose spikes, and lower cholesterol levels in people with type 2 diabetes. Freshly ground peanut butter (without added sugar or salt) can be an excellent snack for people with diabetes.

WARNING

Stay away from peanut butters or any other nut butters or ingredients that have added sugar and salt in them. Many supermarkets have freshly ground versions that contain nothing but the nuts themselves. This is the best choice. Furthermore, avoid peanut butter (or any other ingredient) that contains the artificial sweetener xylitol, which is lethal to dogs.

Tree nuts

Some tree nuts contain enough protein, fiber, and fat to help you feel full. Nuts contain mono-and polyunsaturated fats — an ounce of nuts contains 13 to 22 grams of these heart-healthy fats. Walnuts, Brazil nuts, cashews, pecans, hazelnuts, and peanuts (okay, I know that peanuts are legumes) contain more mono-unsaturated fats. Although the fat in nuts is predominantly these healthy fats, any fat is calorie dense. A 1-ounce serving of unsalted nuts contains 150 to 200 calories. Be sure to purchase nuts that contain no salt or sugar.

Greek yogurt

Plain, full-fat, Greek yogurt, produced around the world now, is high in protein and vitamin B12, which is mostly found in animal products, making it a great protein choice for individuals who don't eat meat. The original Greek variety is made from a combination of goat and sheep milk, and those types of milks offer additional nutrient profiles. Even cow-based milk contains a healthful dose of calcium, vitamin B2 and B12, potassium, and magnesium.

I use Greek yogurt in many recipes in this book; in addition to enjoying it for breakfast and snacks, swap it out for sour cream and heavy cream in baking and in desserts. Greek yogurt provides body in recipes while giving them protein and a healthful source of fat that helps to balance the sugars in desserts.

Seeds

Seeds contain protein, fiber, and fat that like nuts, are filling and can help prevent the body from absorbing sugar and keep glucose levels in check. Seeds are a desirable element of diabetes management because research found that their consumption can be a favorable replacement for carbohydrate snacks because they improve A1C numbers and lower bad LDL cholesterol after 3 months.

Here are the seeds I suggest:

>> **Sesame seeds:** In addition to adding texture and flavor to your recipes, sesame seeds can play a role in assisting you to reach your target blood sugar levels. The antioxidants in sesame oil can reduce the amount of sugar in your blood. Tahini (ground sesame seeds) are a good option in addition to the seeds themselves.

>> **Flaxseeds:** Flaxseeds may help people with diabetes improve blood sugar control, decrease insulin resistance, and reduce cholesterol and triglyceride levels. Flaxseeds are rich in fiber, omega-3 fatty acids, and bioactive compounds.

>> **Sunflower seeds:** These seeds may also help with type 2 diabetes due to their nutrients and bioactive components including magnesium, chlorogenic acid and selenium content.

>> **Chia seeds:** They expand in liquid as they sit, which makes them a great choice for healthful puddings and compotes.

Sesame seeds, sunflower seeds, chia seeds, and flaxseeds are used quite extensively in this book. Be sure to purchase salt-free seeds when using.

Whole-grain flours

Flours — whole-wheat pastry flour, barley flour, oat flour, and whole-wheat flour — are healthful whole grains that offer complex carbs with lower GI that are more beneficial than all-purpose flour.

WARNING

Limit your use of unbleached, all-purpose flour because it's a simple carbohydrate that is low in fiber and cause spikes in blood sugar. This book relies heavily on almond and other types of flours with a low GI. When I do use all-purpose flour, I combine it with EVOO, which can reduce its GL, as well as ingredients that contain protein and healthful fats that help the spike in blood sugar.

Identifying Ideal Desserts for People with Diabetes

Determining which types of desserts are best for you depends upon your overall eating plan. If you're following a diet appropriate for diabetes (refer to Chapter 5 for sample meal plans), then you can afford to splurge on healthful desserts. Seek the help of a nutrition professional and your primary care physician and endocrinologist if you can't get your blood sugar levels to be balanced before enjoying desserts.

The importance of a well-balanced diet based on whole foods, exercise, and a positive outlook can make a huge difference in diabetes care. When those are in place, enjoying delicious and nutritious desserts can bring additional pleasure to your day.

The best desserts for people with diabetes:

>> Contain healthful ingredients such as whole grains, fresh fruit, lean protein, and healthful fats

>> Are free of artificial ingredients

>> Rely on raw honey and limited amounts of natural sweeteners (see Chapter 6)

>> Are made with nut-based or whole-grain flours

>> Incorporate low GI fruits, such as cherries, apricots, grapefruit, apples, pears, oranges, plums, and grapes that are specifically beneficial to those with diabetes

>> Rely on EVOO as a source of fat

>> Use eggs, full-fat plain Greek yogurt, and ricotta cheese, tofu, and nuts for added protein

>> Include seeds for additional protein and omega-3 fatty acids

>> Incorporate foods that contain bioactive compounds (refer to Table 2-2). This comprehensive chart created by Dr. Simon Poole, shares a list of *bioactive compounds* (polyphenols) that cause actions in the body that may promote good health. You can look through the different ingredients and learn what benefits they have to offer.

REMEMBER

After you get accustomed to the pleasures of healthful desserts, you won't be as enticed by the more artificially sweet, unhealthful fat-ladened ones. You'll also be more satisfied because you're meeting your sugar cravings in a more nutritious way.

TABLE 2-2   **Polyphenols in Foods and Possible Bioactivity**

Polyphenol Type	Example	Food Sources	Potential Health Benefits
Flavonols	Quercetin	Onions, apples, berries, broccoli, green tea, capers, citrus fruits	Antioxidant, anti-inflammatory, cardiovascular health, allergy relief
Flavonols	Kaempferol	Kale, spinach, broccoli, green tea, strawberries, fennel	Antioxidant, anti-inflammatory, cardiovascular health, anticancer properties
Flavonols	Myricetin	Berries, grapes, red wine, pomegranate, walnuts, red onions	Antioxidant, anti-inflammatory, brain health, anticancer properties
Flavanols (Catechins)	Epicatechin	Green tea, cocoa, red wine, apples, berries, cherries, pears	Antioxidant, cardiovascular health, blood sugar regulation
Flavanols (Catechins)	Epigallocatechin gallate (EGCG)	Green tea, matcha, apples, berries, cocoa, dark chocolate	Antioxidant, metabolic health, brain health, weight management
Flavanones	Hesperetin	Citrus fruits (oranges, lemons, grapefruits), tomatoes, parsley	Antioxidant, cardiovascular health, anti-inflammatory
Flavanones	Naringenin	Grapefruit, tomatoes, oranges, lemons, grapefruit juice, hops	Antioxidant, cardiovascular health, metabolic health
Flavones	Luteolin	Parsley, celery, chamomile tea, thyme, sage, peppermint	Antioxidant, anti-inflammatory, brain health, anticancer properties
Flavones	Apigenin	Parsley, celery, chamomile tea, artichokes, basil, celery seed	Antioxidant, anti-inflammatory, brain health, anticancer properties
Anthocyanins	Cyanidin	Blueberries, blackberries, cherries, grapes, cranberries, eggplant	Antioxidant, cardiovascular health, brain health, anti-aging
Anthocyanins	Delphinidin	Blueberries, cranberries, raspberries, blackcurrants, red radishes	Antioxidant, cardiovascular health, brain health, anti-inflammatory
Hydroxybenzoic acids	Gallic acid	Coffee, tea, blueberries, blackberries, strawberries, red wine	Antioxidant, anti-inflammatory, cardiovascular health, anticancer properties
Hydroxybenzoic acids	Protocatechuic acid	Green tea, apples, pears, cinnamon, cocoa, cherry, vanilla	Antioxidant, anti-inflammatory, metabolic health, brain health
Hydroxycinnamic acids	Caffeic acid	Coffee, whole grains, apples, pears, artichokes, lettuce, parsnips	Antioxidant, anti-inflammatory, cardiovascular health, anticancer properties

Polyphenol Type	Example	Food Sources	Potential Health Benefits
Resveratrol	Resveratrol	Red grapes, red wine, peanuts, mulberries, dark chocolate, pistachios	Antioxidant, anti-inflammatory, cardiovascular health, brain health
Secoiridoides	Oleuropein, oleocanthal, Tyrosols	Extra-virgin olive oil	Anti-inflammatory, cardiovascular health including oxidation of LDL cholesterol, antioxidant properties
Lignans	Secoisolarici-resinol	Flaxseeds, sesame seeds, whole grains, berries, cruciferous vegetables	Antioxidant, hormonal balance, cardiovascular health, anticancer properties
Lignans	Enterolactone	Flaxseeds, sesame seeds, whole grains, berries, cruciferous vegetables	Hormonal balance, anticancer properties, cardiovascular health

REMEMBER

LOWER YOUR A1C NUMBERS BY EATING WHOLE FOOD

Recent research suggests that eating a whole food diet for one month can significantly lower A1C numbers in diabetes patients as well as improve many other important health markers. At a recent panel discussion on the Mediterranean diet and the gut microbiome that I presented at Georgetown University, a researcher presented results from her study of Gulf War veterans. Prior to the study, the vets' brains were imaged, showing that they had diabetes and suffered from many other mental and physical diseases, often associated with war.

During the month-long study, participants followed a whole food diet, which meant that everything they ate had to be natural — organic fruits and vegetables, grass-fed meat, seafood, beans, nuts, legumes, herbs, spices, and so on. Ultraprocessed, junk, and fast foods were off-limits. Without making any other changes to their life, the results were overwhelming. After only a month the veterans had significantly reduced all the markers that they were suffering from, including diabetes, anxiety, post-traumatic stress disorder, depression, heart disease, and cholesterol.

I was both overwhelmed and overjoyed when the scientist shared her results. As someone who specializes in writing books about diabetes and the Mediterranean diet, I'm well aware of the power of eating well. But the startling results of these veterans who were suffering so much to have such a dramatic and unanimous response to whole foods in just a month was reason to celebrate — and it still is. Let them be a motivation for you as they are an inspiration to me.

Desserts Redux — Making Desserts Diabetes-Friendly

Everyone has a favorite dessert — or two — or three! Some of them are passed down in families, others are restaurant classics, or other are reminders of happy times. For me, making sweet treats with Nonna reminded me that you could turn any day into a celebration by serving a dessert. But things are different nowadays than they were when Nonna was a child. Born in the Great Depression and living through World War II, she and many of the people around her experienced scarcity. Sweets were a luxury.

She and her siblings were consistently underweight as young girls, and the doctor ordered them to gain weight by indulging in milkshakes, which were unaffordable. You can see how this type of childhood and living nearly a century ago would give sweets a special and almost sacred place in the heart. Even people who were financially well off enjoyed meals made of wholesome, natural ingredients because ultraprocessed wasn't introduced yet.

Even nowadays, when most of your diet is healthful, you can splurge on occasion, which is also in-line with the tenants of the Mediterranean lifestyle. If there's a sweet recipe or two that you enjoy only once or twice a year on an important holiday, I wouldn't dream of trying to change it. Just eat a little bit of it once or twice a year along with a balanced meal and enjoy the memories that they conjure up.

On a more frequent basis, however, give the desserts that you most enjoy a makeover so that you can enjoy them more often. Here are a few tips, by dessert category:

>> Make simple desserts based on fresh fruit the majority of your sweet treats (see Chapter 9 for fruit-based desserts).

>> Make brownies and bars with EVOO, nuts, and nut butters (refer to Chapter 10 for recipes).

>> Swap out almond flour, whole-wheat flour, or oat flour, or a mix for all-purpose flour.

>> Enjoy cookies (see Chapter 11) by using whole-grain flowers, oats, dark chocolate chips, and nut butters.

>> Prepare spoon desserts and puddings (refer to Chapter 12) using plain, full-fat Greek yogurt, chia seeds, and avocado for depth and texture instead of heavy cream and butter. Use dark chocolate instead of milk chocolate.

» Create truffles and fruit-based chocolate treats (see Chapter 13 for recipes) using antioxidant-rich dark chocolate and dried fruit with nuts and seeds instead of higher fat ingredients.

» Make gelato and ice cream (refer to Chapter 14) using whole milk, almond milk, and pure, full-fat Greek yogurt instead of heavy cream and raw honey or other natural sweeteners.

» Master pies and tarts (see Chapter 15) by using shells made out of almonds and whole grains and filling them with fresh fruits and nourishing ingredients.

» Sip on sweet drinks (see Chapter 16) made with health-boosting ingredients like Greek yogurt, fruit, seeds, and dark chocolate instead of ice cream, heavy cream, sodium, and added sugars.

» Swap out almond flour and oat flour in cakes (refer to Chapter 17) and use natural sweeteners and fresh fruit for sweetness.

Chapters 5 and 6 provide an in-depth look into ingredients, building pantries, and baking nutrient-dense desserts as well. Chapter 7 discusses how to fit them into your schedules.

Know that every step you take toward understanding the role of sugar in the brain and body and utilizing that knowledge to create and enjoy more nutritious desserts will pay off in the long run. Often times, people find out that they like the "remake recipes" better than the original ones. Yes, baking with these ingredients costs more than baking with artificial ingredients and packaged convenience foods, which is actually a good thing. When sweets were more costly in the olden days, people indulged in them less, and they had better health as a result. In addition, the healthful ingredients play a part in your overall well-being, which is priceless.

Chapter **3**

Keeping Blood Glucose Balanced While Eating Desserts

The best way to be able to enjoy desserts and good health is to balance your blood sugar levels. I like to think of it as a sweet reward for prioritizing my health. Imagine the freedom of taking control of what you eat — letting your food work to help your body perform at optimal levels while still being able to enjoy delicious food!

This chapter examines ways to regulate blood glucose levels, explains how you can take readings, examines the best diabetes care, identifies foods that can mess with your blood glucose, and discusses how you can track your goals.

Regulating Blood Glucose Levels

Writing a book about diabetes-friendly desserts and not sharing the latest information on measuring blood glucose would be a disservice to readers. Without balancing blood sugar, even the healthiest dessert recipe can cause harm, so it's important that I go over these basics before you decide what to eat. By knowing some basics on blood glucose and ways you can track your own blood glucose readings, you'll set yourself up for a lifetime of success — and the ability to enjoy sweet treats without consequences.

Shining a spotlight on blood glucose

Diabetes is a state of blood glucose imbalance related to insulin. In type 1 diabetes, insulin production capacity is completely lost, and in type 2 diabetes, cells become resistant to insulin. In both cases, blood glucose levels after eating carbohydrate foods don't come down to normal levels in a natural way.

The topic of diabetes includes so many complex terms and intricate, yet important details, that you can easily get confused, especially when you're dealing with a new diagnosis, have *prediabetes* (impaired glucose tolerance that precedes a diabetes diagnosis), or were never properly educated about diabetes, which is often the case. Making regular readings a part of your daily routine will make a big difference in taking charge of your health. The following sections give a brief rundown of important terminology and briefly explain the tests used to monitor blood glucose.

Exploring some science about glucose

The word *glucose* gets used often in diabetes care, but it's rarely explained. Glucose is a simple sugar that's extremely important to you as a source of energy. It's the key ingredient in a biochemical recipe that produces a powerhouse molecule *adenosine triphosphate,* best known by its initials ATP. ATP is your fuel, the source of the energy you use to move or to think or, for that matter, to generate the heat needed to remain a steady 98.6° Fahrenheit.

You get glucose from food, and you eat a lot more glucose than you might think, even if you don't have an overactive sweet tooth. Glucose actually isn't that sweet anyway. Virtually all the glucose you eat is locked in chains with other sugars or more glucose — referred to as *polysaccharides.*

Table sugar (known as *sucrose*) is one molecule of glucose and one fructose — a *disaccharide.* If the chains are longer, even to hundreds or thousands of glucose molecules, the molecules are starch or fiber. Taken together, sugars, starches, and fiber are carbohydrates, a word you're surely familiar with if you have diabetes (refer to Chapter 4 for more information).

As blood glucose levels begin to drop, the beta cells sense this favorable change and suppress their release of *insulin* (a hormone that lowers the level of glucose in the blood). In healthy individuals this process is incredibly precise, and blood glucose *homeostasis* (balance among the body systems needed to function properly) is achieved in a few hours. But getting glucose into cells and out of the blood is only part of the blood glucose homeostasis story.

Glucose is stored as *glycogen* in liver cells — your liver is a warehouse for extra glucose. Glycogen in liver cells isn't obliged to remain in liver cells as it is with muscle cells. Liver cells can release glucose back into your bloodstream. *Insulin resistance* happens when your muscles, fat, and liver don't respond to insulin properly.

Recognizing blood glucose levels

Testing your blood glucose levels tells you whether or not the levels are in normal range, have impaired glucose tolerance, or are diabetes. This test is always administered after fasting. Fasting blood glucose results accurately reveal your blood glucose level after having no food or drink for eight hours.

Table 3-1 lists the international diagnostic standards — what the different fasting blood glucose levels mean.

TABLE 3-1

Fasting Blood Glucose Levels

Fasting Blood Glucose Range	Diagnosis
60 to 99 mg/dl	Normal range
100 to 125 mg/dl	Impaired glucose tolerance, also referred to as prediabetes
126 mg/dl or higher	Diabetes if that result occurs on more than one fasting blood glucose test

TECHNICAL STUFF

In *common measure,* about 1 teaspoon of glucose dissolved in your 1½ gallons of blood is perfect. In *laboratory measure,* that's 4,000 milligrams (4 grams) of glucose in your 50 deciliters (5 liters) of blood equaling 80 milligrams per deciliter, or 80 mg/dl. Milligrams per deciliter, mg/dl, is the *standard measure* used in the United States and some other countries. An alternative unit, millimoles per liter (mmol/l), is the *international standard measure* for blood glucose levels and is used commonly in many countries, too. The difference in units isn't relevant, but mg/dl can be easily converted to mmol/l by dividing by 18. Therefore, 80 mg/dl and 4.44 mmol/l represent the same concentration when measuring blood glucose.

Another test more representative of a realistic response to food is available. Called an *oral glucose tolerance test (OGTT)*, this test measures blood glucose response after ingesting glucose (usually 75 grams) over a two- or three-hour period by testing fasting blood glucose levels before the test and testing at hourly intervals after the oral dose of glucose.

Table 3-2 lists the different blood glucose levels for the OGTT.

TABLE 3-2

OGTT Blood Glucose Levels

OGTT Blood Glucose Level	Diagnosis
Below 200 mg/dl after one hour and below 140 mg/dl after two hours	Normal range
Higher than 140 mg/dl but lower than 200 mg/dl after two hours	Prediabetes
Higher than 200 mg/dl after two hours	Diabetes

REMEMBER

A blood glucose level higher than 200 mg/dl on any random test is diagnostic for diabetes. Doctors recommend a variation of the OGTT for all pregnant women to test for gestational diabetes. Ask your healthcare provider which test is best for you.

Measuring blood glucose at home

Testing your blood glucose on your own has never been easier with the advances in medicine. Here are the ways you can test your blood sugar at home:

» **Test strip method:** This method, which has been around for decades, requires you to draw a very small amount of blood from your finger or other location (with some meters) and get a relatively accurate measure of blood glucose in ten seconds.

» **Continuous monitors:** Many technologically advanced devices offer real-time glucose numbers to your smart phone or watch continuously.

» **Closed loop technology:** More and more people with type 1 diabetes are wearing continuous glucose monitors, which sense glucose levels through a small wire inserted into the fluid just beneath the skin. Linking continuous monitoring to an insulin pump that responds and adjusts through an algorithm either in the device or an associated app to give real-time dosing according to need is a recent development that promises to revolutionize the lives of people who have type 1 diabetes.

Check with your healthcare provider to find out which options are covered by your insurance and make sure that you set up an appointment to learn how to use them properly. Don't be embarrassed to ask questions or to take time. Not getting them right would be detrimental. One of the biggest benefits of the new systems is that they offer the most accurate results and store your history so that you don't have to write down your own results as was necessary in the past.

The recorded reading history can be downloaded to a computer or transmitted to a physician's office.

Comparing testing for people with type 1 and type 2 diabetes

People with type 2 diabetes typically follow a different testing regimen than people with type 1 diabetes. Consider the following:

>> **Type 2 diabetes:** Testing usually follows a less stringent schedule, maybe only once or twice a day; however if you're new and want to take charge of your health and are trying to figure out when it's a good time to eat desserts, I recommend testing more. Doctors recommend more testing if low blood glucose levels are a potential side effect of medication (insulin or a few different kinds of pills). I (along with my coauthor Dr. Simon Poole) provide guidelines in *Diabetes For Dummies* (John Wiley & Sons, Inc.).

>> **Type 1 diabetes:** Testing blood glucose levels is extremely important for people with type 1 diabetes because they must make real-time self-treatment decisions about food and insulin dosing based upon the result.

If you have type 1 diabetes and don't have closed-loop technology, you should test before every meal and approximately two hours after meals with some frequency, a time frame referred to as *postprandial*. You should test before exercising, before bedtime, and anytime you may sense high or low blood glucose levels. Test anytime when someone who knows you suggests your blood sugar may be low — people with type 1 often lack self-awareness of hypoglycemia clues (such as sweating, dizziness, slurred speech) that are obvious to others. You should also test if you're consuming alcohol and simple sugars in excess because alcohol can trigger hypoglycemia and hypoglycemia can resemble alcohol intoxication.

No matter whether you have type 1 or type 2 diabetes, your healthcare provider may order an important blood test to give you a big picture view of your blood glucose control. This test, called hemoglobin A1C, sometimes called HbA1C or simply A1C, is used at least once a year to evaluate your average blood glucose levels over a two- or three-month period.

TECHNICAL STUFF

A1C is a measure of glycated (or interchangeably, glycosylated) hemoglobin — what percentage of your blood hemoglobin has reacted with glucose. A1C is an excellent predictor of your overall blood glucose control and consequently of your risk for diabetes-related complications.

Perusing the Best Diabetes Care

Practicing self-care and prioritizing your health are particularly important skills to know when you have a diabetes or prediabetes diagnosis. Often times, by choosing to care for and prioritizing yourself you can enjoy an unexpected outcome. The concentrated and focused care that you give yourself after the diabetes diagnosis can help you feel and live better than you did before. If that's your goal, you can make it happen. The first step is putting together a team of diabetes care experts.

DOCTOR SAYS

According to Dr. Simon Poole, an estimated 25 percent of people with diabetes remain undiagnosed — that's a significant number of people with diabetes not getting regular medical care. Even for those people who do get medical care, studies of patients, such as the Diabetes Attitudes, Wishes, and Needs (DAWN) study, have shown a troubling low level of adherence to taking medication, self-monitoring blood glucose, diet, and exercise, and keeping medical appointments. Make sure you know how to respond to emergencies in potentially life-threatening situations.

The following sections explore what professionals you can turn to for medical care and a timeline to help you seek help.

Relying on professional help

Avoiding the serious complications of diabetes requires a multidimensional approach directed at both prevention and intervention. The newest edition of *Diabetes For Dummies* by Simon and me (John Wiley & Sons, Inc.) gives a detailed overview of medical care. Here's a quick overview of healthcare providers of which you can take advantage:

>> **Primary physician:** Most people with type 2 diabetes work with a primary care physician who prescribes medication and routinely monitors for signs of diabetes-related complications in physical exams and laboratory work. A primary physician may or may not have access to in-house diabetes-related support resources like a registered dietitian, certified diabetes educator, or an organized patient support group. Your primary physician should, however, be willing to recommend or formally refer you elsewhere for these very important support services.

>> **Endocrinologist or diabetologist:** These specialized physicians are most likely working with people with type 1 diabetes or people with type 2 diabetes who have poorly controlled blood glucose or diabetes-related complications. They're the experts in diabetes treatment and likely have in-house health professionals to help with diet, exercise, blood glucose monitoring, and emotional support.

>> **Registered dietitian or certified nutrition specialist:** Because food and eating habits are so closely connected with weight, blood glucose, and the risk for heart disease, seeing an expert in medical nutrition therapy is important.

>> **Pharmacist:** Your pharmacist is perhaps your best resource for education about medications, not only those prescribed for diabetes, but also those prescribed for other conditions. Most important, your pharmacist knows how your variety of medications could interact. Diabetes is so prevalent now that many pharmacists are diabetes educators. If you're taking any supplements, be sure to ask your pharmacist about possible drug interactions with them.

>> **Certified diabetes educator:** A wide range of healthcare providers — physicians, physicians assistants, registered nurses, nurse practitioners, registered dietitians, pharmacists, clinical psychologists, podiatrists, and others — have studied and taken a comprehensive certification examination to provide a broad range of education and support to people with diabetes. Spending time with a certified diabetes educator, individually or in a group, for diabetes self-management education (DSME) can be helpful in tying together the many medical and lifestyle responsibilities you may struggle to balance.

>> **Podiatrist:** Getting regular foot exams and early treatment of potential problems by a podiatrist can literally be a limb saver. The loss of sensation and circulation problems makes your feet an easy target for minor infections that can become difficult to control. Anyone with *neuropathy* (nerve damage) should see a podiatrist regularly.

>> **Dentist:** Diabetes can increase the risk of gum disease, so regular visits to your dentist for examination and cleaning are imperative.

>> **Mental health professional:** Diabetes can feel overwhelming, and people with diabetes are significantly more likely to experience depression than the general population. Depression and stress deserve attention because depressed patients can diminish self-care behaviors.

Chapter 2 offers additional types of complimentary therapies that can assist you on your journey to better health.

TIP

Make sure each of these professionals sends a report to your primary physician and endocrinologist so that they know what care you're receiving.

After reading this list you may feel overwhelmed. After all, making appointments and seeking out so many professionals, while attending the visits and taking care of yourself can seem like a full-time job. Feeling that way is completely normal. When you're first diagnosed with diabetes or prediabetes and trying to figure out what you need to do, you can feel stressed out. You're probably working full time with a world of responsibility and demands.

Making a plan to seek help

If you have the ability to take a month off to jumpstart this process — to begin treatment with professionals — and organize everything, I suggest doing so. However, I realize that most of the people reading this book don't have that luxury. In order to avoid being overburdened, remember that change takes time, and each step that you make in the right direction will have big payoffs.

You may have done nothing or very little to take charge of your blood glucose and diabetes care, so by making small efforts when possible now, you can still cause positive changes. Declare to yourself that your health is important and you're going to take the steps necessary to feel your best. Table 3-3 lists a sample timeline that may help you.

TABLE 3-3 **Planning Your Care after Your Diagnosis**

Week	What You Can Do
Week 1	Seek out a primary care physician (if you don't already have one), make an appointment, and read the first five chapters of this book.
Week 2	Make sure that you have an endocrinologist and diabetes educator. You can call your insurance company and ask people you know for referrals or try looking online.
Week 3	Tell your dentist about your diagnosis and set up an appointment with a podiatrist if you don't have one.
Week 4	If you need help determining your best meal plan (which most people do), use your primary care physician or certified diabetes educator, insurance company, or the internet to find a registered dietician or certified nutritionist to help.
Week 5	Introduce yourself to the pharmacist at your local pharmacy if they don't know you, tell them about your diagnosis, and ask any questions you may have.
Week 6	If you need help staying on track with all this information in this section and the previous section, seek out a health coach that accepts your insurance plan. This professional can help you coordinate everything. Many insurance plans offer free periodic calls with diabetes experts that can help to remind you about important things to monitor.
Week 7	Seek out a mental health professional to help you cope with the diagnosis and any other issues that may be getting in the way of your health or be preventing you from achieving your goals.

Following this schedule gives you a complete team of professionals to accompany you on your health journey. Like anything else in life, you get out what you put in.

Focusing on Problematic Foods

One of the best ways to keep your blood glucose balanced is to avoid problematic foods. After all, an old-fashioned dieting technique was to keep problematic foods out of the kitchen and the home. If they're not there, you can't be tempted, right?

Unfortunately today junk food and fat-, sugar-, and sodium-laden restaurant foods are just a click away and can be delivered directly to your door. Yes, having less of the bad stuff will keep you on track, but you also don't want to create such a nutritionally pristine kitchen that you're forced to order out in order to satisfy cravings that you could have met in a more nutritious way at home.

A key to optimal health is that realizing that food is your friend. It's your necessity as a human being, and when eaten properly it can be both a source of healing and joy. Adopting the mentality to fill your cupboards, refrigerator, and freezer with items that promote both health and pleasure will serve you well in the long run. (Chapter 6 explains what healthful ingredients to include in your kitchen.)

The following sections help you identify the trouble foods, explain how you can get rid of them, recognize your emotional triggers to trouble foods, and discuss healthful substitutions for them.

Spotting problematic dessert food

Problematic desserts are those that contain table sugar or artificial sweeteners, refined flour, unhealthful fats such as vegetable oils and margarine, and those which don't contain protein. You also want to avoid foods with artificial colors and flavors. Chapter 2 discusses how to identify those problematic ingredients and replace them with wholesome ones in order to be able to consume desserts healthfully.

REMEMBER

In most cases, processed foods (meaning ones that come in packages that aren't a single ingredient like beans, rice, legumes, and so forth) are problematic. Read nutritional labels and look for high levels of sodium, sugars, cholesterol, and saturated fat. If the ingredient list contains items that you can't read or pronounce, you shouldn't be ingesting it on a regular basis.

Getting rid of problematic food and subbing it with more healthful options

Adopting a healthy relationship with food and the Mediterranean attitude toward sweets and off-limits foods will help you to live better, longer, while enjoying yourselves in the process.

REMEMBER

Strict diets aren't sustainable in the long run. You can't completely cut out things you love forever. These types of plans often leave people feeling discouraged. I can't tell you how many readers and followers of mine do what I refer to as clean sweeps in their kitchens, stock up on healthful items, and then fall back into their old comfort zone of junk food and unhealthy take-out dishes within days.

The key is to get rid of the old but also to introduce new items that you enjoy eating. Find out how to coax the most flavor out of them and set aside time to work with them so that you don't need to fall back into old habits.

TIP

To rid your home of problematic foods, try this process:

>> **Start slow, if needed.** These foods may have been a part of your life for a long time. If you're used to eating a lot of junk food and processed food, chances are you've developed a chemical addiction to the ingredients in them. Some people report feeling better when eating junk food — that's because they're addicted to it. Chapter 2 offers tips to overcome this addiction which is key to long-term health.

>> **Think about replacing the unhealthful items with better choices.** Chapter 6 identifies healthful ingredients you can add to your pantry, fridge, and freezer.

>> **Know thyself.** If you need to finish off a less-than-good-for-you item in your cupboard or refrigerator, by all means, rid your home of it. Then think about what it is in those desserts that you enjoyed and find a healthier alternative to enjoy. For example, Greek yogurt makes a better sour cream alternative and almond and oat flour are better than all-purpose flour.

>> **Throw away any packaged white (shelf-stable) bread, packaged sweets, box mixes for desserts, sugary drinks, and any other processed items.** If you feel as if you can't go without any of these items, make a list of them and detail why you love them (refer to the next section where I discuss this point further).

You can eliminate popular baking ingredients that are problematic and substitute them with more healthful ones. Table 3-4 identifies some.

TABLE 3-4

Swapping Out Problematic Baking Ingredients

Commonly Used Baking Ingredients	Diabetes Friendly Swap-out
Sour cream	Greek yogurt
Milk chocolate	Dark chocolate
Artificial sweeteners and table sugar	Raw honey, maple syrup, allulose, coconut sugar, date sugar
Canned or sweetened fruit	Fresh fruit

Chapter 6 gives you a shopping list of healthful ingredients to use when making desserts. That chapter also provides specific information when you want to substitute sweeteners to make more diabetes-friendly desserts.

Noticing your emotional triggers to food

After you figure out which unhealthful foods you tend to enjoy the most, think about when you tend to consume them and why. Doing so may seem counterintuitive, but identifying the reason why you have an affinity toward an unhealthful food can help you find better replacements and let go of harmful ingredients.

Take a few minutes to truly understand the emotional triggers to food. Emotional eating has come to represent a psychological state where food becomes a means for coping with feelings of anger, sadness, loneliness, and even happiness. Eating in excess as a response to feelings can be emotionally and physically unhealthy, but responding emotionally to eating is something altogether different. It's truly part of your chemistry. Take for example that cookie your mother gave you when you scraped your knee. Or the ice cream cone you got when you brought home good grades in the second grade? Your good behavior was often rewarded with sweets, candy, and frozen desserts. Don't blame your parents or caregivers; they got the same reinforcement when they were children. (On the other hand, eating an ice cream cone occasionally won't have negative effects on your overall health. It's what you do most of the time that matters.)

REMEMBER

Even though people often associate emotional eating with a negative connotation, it doesn't have to be that way. You can use your innate cravings and triggers to both soothe yourself and eat nutritious foods — that's the basis of the discipline of *culinary medicine*.

TIP

To help identify your emotional triggers to food, do the following:

1. **Make a list of the recipes or foods that you crave often.**

2. **Figure out why.**

3. **Identify whether the foods are good for you, and if they have a healthier alternative.**

   If so, then you can continue to make enjoy them. On the other hand, if they're not healthful, you can identify what it is about them that you enjoy and look for a better-fitting replacement.

4. **Note whether you're drawn to particular foods when you feel a certain way; if you do, look for healthier options.**

   For example, researchers believe that creamy foods are most comforting when you're stressed or scared. In this case, Greek yogurt, avocados, and sugar-free frozen yogurt can be a great dessert swap for unhealthful foods and could help keep your glucose in check.

   You may find that at times you crave sweet foods. As humans, milk is our first taste in infancy. The sweetness of the milk triggers the sweet receptors in our brain, which in turn makes us associate sweet flavors with reward, empowerment, and good feelings throughout life. Recognize that human beings are all conditioned this way, and how, as an adult, you can incorporate healthful, natural sweet flavors, such as the ones in Part 3 without the harmful effects of too much sugar or chemical sweeteners.

Satisfying your sweet tooth in a wholesome way

A common misconception is that people with diabetes crave sugar continuously or eat copious amounts of sweets. In my 35 years of research and first-hand experience cooking and crating recipes for people with diabetes, I don't find that to be true. In general, many people with diabetes eat less sugar than individuals who don't have the diagnosis. Don't overlook that other illnesses, stress, hormones, sleeping patterns, and other factors all influence a diabetes diagnosis, not just eating sugar alone.

That said, after you're diagnosed with diabetes, you want to make sure you eat the right kinds of sweeteners and simple carbs. Not just foods bring sweetness into your life (see Chapter 2). Here is a quick overview of some activities when incorporated daily, believe it or not, will help you turn to sugar and sweet foods for satisfaction even less:

» Listen to music that you love.

» Choose sweet and kind words, use positive affirmations, speak gently to others, and read poetry.

» Engage in activities you enjoy.

» Spend time thinking about the things that you love and feeling as if they were part of your life.

» Replace fear with love in as many aspects of your life as much as possible.

» Indulge in the sweet things in life; remind yourself of sweet memories, linger in the sweetness of small successes.

» Keep a daily gratitude journal. Write down all things big and small that you're grateful for every morning, no matter how simplistic they may seem. Chapter 5 discusses the importance of practicing gratitude.

For example, something as simple as plumbing and electricity are always on my gratitude list, and I give thanks for how they positively impact my life. Sure, most people have them nowadays, but I'm thankful for their invention and the convenience that they bring into my life. Even kings and queens didn't have these luxuries a few hundred years ago. Remember the old adage "the more that you're grateful for, the more you have to be grateful."

Keeping Track of Your Goals

Tracking your daily progress and goals is the best way to encourage yourself to seek success. In the section "Measuring blood glucose at home" earlier in this chapter I discuss the use of continuous glucose monitoring systems to track your glucose levels and the capability that allow your doctor and healthcare team to download the data. But they are only numbers. In order to truly understand what helps and hurts you on a daily basis, you need to keep a food, exercise, and even a gratitude journal, to go along with the meter readings.

Starting a food and exercise journal

Starting a food and exercise journal can assist you and your wellness team in having the full picture of what influences your health.

The following steps can help you keep your own food and exercise journal:

1. **Decide whether you prefer to record things electronically or with a pen and paper.**

2. **Open a file on your phone or computer or get a notebook and dedicate to your health journal.**

3. **Each day, record the food that you eat at each meal, your glucose levels, and which type of exercise or activity that you did that day.**

   You may even want to write the type of day that it was as you experienced. Was it especially happy, stressful, sad? Did anything out of the ordinary happen?

   I even like to write down any encompassing thoughts. If they were good ones, I can continue thinking them. If something was troubling or worrisome, I seek help — you can ask your therapist, pray for guidance, or turn to a close confidante — on how to look at them in a different way that positively impacts my health.

4. **Do this daily and you can start to spot patterns that can be beneficial in choosing which items are best to continue doing and which need to be transformed.**

You can keep a gratitude journal in the same place you track your goals. Each day jot down three to five things in your life — something as simple as feeling the warm sunshine or cuddling under a blanket with your dog — for which you're thankful. Refer to the previous section for more information.

Noticing patterns

After a few months' time of keeping a food and exercise journal, you'll begin noticing patterns. You can see how what you do — what you eat, how you exercise, and how you think — can affect your blood sugar and give you the clues to continue what you're doing or make some changes.

All your actions are your choice — even if they're habitual.

When you suffer from physical symptoms, which many people with diabetes do, you may feel like everything is happening to you and at times you've lost control of your thoughts, bodies, and actions. Feeling that way is completely normal. Your old thought patterns, behaviors, and likes and dislikes took a lifetime to form, and at some point even the ones that lead to disease and illness probably served you in some way, or you may have believed that they served you. Receiving a disease diagnosis or beginning to have physical symptoms is your body and/or your mind's way of telling you that something needs to change.

REMEMBER

After years of mind-body therapy for an "incurable" (one that had no known medical cure) illness that I was fortunate enough to transform through years of dedication and commitment, I now see illness and disease as dis-ease, a state in which the body and mind aren't at ease. As a result, the first thing I do when I feel discomfort now is to say and affirm to myself: "I am willing to change." You'd be amazed at the way in which new treatments, good habits, and the ability to make healthy changes flood into your life by affirming this simple statement.

Tracking your results demystifies the negative patterns and illuminates the good ones to inspire the change that will lead to the good health that you deserve.

2

Incorporating Desserts into Your Diet

Explore macronutrients — carbohydrates, fat, and proteins — and how they can work together when you're eating desserts.

Understand how and when you can enjoy desserts when you have diabetes.

Put together a diabetes-friendly pantry and select healthful sweeteners.

Discover how you can schedule homemade diabetes-friendly desserts.

Chapter **4**

Making Macronutrients Work Together

Many people don't realize the crucial role of consuming balanced amounts of macronutrients — carbohydrates, fat, and protein — plays in the diet of someone with diabetes. The term *macro* means big, and macronutrients are certainly of big importance. But the term macro is used when referring to carbohydrates, fat, and protein primarily because you need them in big amounts. The macronutrients are what build you, protect you, and fuel your many activities. And the macronutrients store energy you know as calories.

The quality and quantity of macronutrients is also important to diabetes and to your overall health. In this chapter, you discover why carbohydrates, fat, and protein are so important to what you eat, especially in choosing desserts, and how your body utilizes macronutrients.

Understanding How Protein, Carbs, and Fat Affect What You Eat

When you have diabetes or prediabetes, knowing as much as you can about the three macronutrients — protein, carbohydrates, and fat — is imperative. By including the best possible versions of these macronutrients in your meals, you can better balance your blood sugar.

You're probably confused as to what constitutes a complete meal with the examples that television commercials and billboards blast and believe that specific marketing tactics are what constitute a meal. Although a burger, fries, and soft drink contain some degree of fat, carbohydrates, and protein, they aren't a complete and balanced meal.

REMEMBER

A complete and balanced meal (including a snack or dessert) uses a combination of foods from the three macronutrient groups to provide that balance. The key? Always consume the best types and amounts of foods that help you, the person with diabetes or prediabetes, stay properly nourished while keeping your blood sugar levels regulated. Refer to the section "Identifying the Best Proteins, Carbohydrates, and Fats" later in this chapter where I define protein, carbohydrates, and fat in greater detail. The more you can get familiar with what food you eat and how much of that food you consume, the better you can enjoy food and keep yourself healthy and satisfied.

Going deeper into macronutrients

Your need for varying amounts of carbohydrates, fats, and protein may vary depending on your physical activity, which you easily build into meal planning and food choices. Believe it or not, consuming the wholesome desserts in Part 3 on occasion (and others that follow these same principles) can help you to achieve your health goals.

The interactions between the macronutrients also have interesting effects. For example, adding a healthful source of fat such as extra-virgin olive oil (EVOO) to a carbohydrate in dessert recipes slows the rise in blood glucose due to delayed gastric emptying, beneficially influencing the speed and extent of the curve of blood glucose rise with a meal. In other words, the high quality fat source (EVOO) helps to balance out the carbohydrates in dessert recipes and can prevent a rapid rise in blood glucose.

Fats are also satiating, so in combination with other carbohydrates and proteins in a meal, snack, or dessert, they help you feel fuller more quickly. For this reason, the majority of the recipes in Part 3 contain all three macronutrients, so that you can enjoy them alone or without worrying that they aren't balanced. In the event that a dessert isn't balanced in this way because it would deviate too much from the classic version of the recipe, I provide instructions at the bottom of the recipe as to how you can enjoy the specific dish in relation to the rest of your meal.

Remember these other important points:

>> **Not all foods fall into a simple, one macronutrient category.** Beans, for example, offer proteins and carbohydrates. Full-fat Greek yogurt offers all three macronutrients in one serving.

>> **Not all macronutrients are the same.** You can choose high quality versions of each: lean proteins versus fatty ones, healthful fats versus trans fats, and complex carbohydrates versus simple ones.

>> **Just because something is a carbohydrate, remember that it still offers other valuable components.** Potatoes, for example, are also rich in important micronutrients such as vitamin C, potassium, and magnesium, and bioactive compounds with antioxidant and anti-inflammatory effects.

BEING AWARE OF FAD DIETS

Fad diets have been around for decades. One is the low-fat diet that encouraged people to reduce the risk of heart disease and eat foods low in fat. With the rise in obesity and type 2 diabetes, many health professionals began recommending a low-carb diet. There are variations on these themes, with keto diets advocating replacing carbohydrates with proteins, and others suggesting dieters increase fat consumption.

Instead of adhering to one of these fads, the recipes and nutritional information in this book rely on whole ingredients that have stood the test of time nutritionally and are in-line with the philosophies of the Mediterranean diet and lifestyle. One benefit is that this book doesn't contain recipes with *empty calories* (calories found in foods and beverages that provide little to no nutritional value). The majority of these recipes offer vitamins, minerals, and antioxidant properties, some of which help to regulate blood sugar and provide nutrients that are specifically needed by individuals who have diabetes and prediabetes.

Recognizing how your body uses nutrients

Knowing the health benefits that whole foods offer are more than just the sum of their parts. The way in which ingredients are paired together can also help to increase their health benefits.

In addition, prior to your metabolism kicking in to convert the macronutrients you absorb into useful components, your food undergoes significant processing by your trillions of gut microbes, which need to be healthily and happily balanced. Fermented foods, such as yogurts and quality cheeses, may be high in fat, but the beneficial effects they have on your microbiome are excellent for your health. For this reason I include Greek yogurt and cheese in many of the recipes in this book. Refer to the latest edition of my book with Dr. Simon Poole *Diabetes Meal Planning and Nutrition For Dummies* (John Wiley & Sons, Inc.) for more information.

Research has shown many of the traditional, heritage diets (such as the Mediterranean diet) around the world to be healthy. They share some important characteristics, which you can implement into what you eat daily for a more healthful diet:

>> They're low in processed foods and refined carbohydrates.

>> They comprise healthy (high quality) micronutrients.

>> They vary in actual amounts of carbohydrates, fats, and proteins

REMEMBER

Fresh produce is also a common denominator among heritage diets and even desserts. The majority of the desserts in this book are based on fresh fruit for this reason.

Identifying the Best Proteins, Carbohydrates, and Fats

To be able to enjoy delicious diabetes-friendly desserts with ease, you want to choose recipes that offer complex carbs, healthful sources of protein, and healthful fats. Because the sweeteners in diabetes-friendly desserts are considered simple carbs, make sure you balance them in meals and at dessert time. If you're planning to enjoy dessert, it's better to consume just good quality protein, a healthful source of fat, leafy greens, and nonstarchy vegetables prior. The following sections delve deeper into the three macronutrients and explain what you need to know when eating diabetes-friendly desserts.

Taking a closer look at protein

Just because a food has protein doesn't mean it's good for you. In fact, many so-called health experts are telling people to eat as much protein as possible, regardless of the source. That isn't wise advice, especially for people with diabetes or prediabetes. What's important, however, is identifying the best types of protein to use and incorporating them in all meals, snacks, and especially in desserts, to balance out the *simple carbs* like white bread, pasta, rice, potatoes (refer to the section "Picking your carbs wisely" for more details) that you consumed.

By adding protein to your meals and desserts you can help to keep your blood sugar from spiking. The following section explains how to do that.

Including protein in your meals and desserts

If you're someone with diabetes or prediabetes, make sure you consume the proper amounts of proteins and avoid the wrong types. During meals, choose eggs, lean poultry, fish, tofu, beans, legumes, and nuts. In desserts, you can add full-fat Greek yogurt, ricotta cheese, tofu, and nuts to add quality protein.

Proteins are extraordinarily complex, and the blueprint for assembling all the proteins you require is coded into your DNA. Protein molecules are primarily chains of *amino acids* (molecules that combine to form protein), and the chains can include many thousands of amino acid molecules, making some proteins very large.

The highest quality protein has amino acids that are readily available and easily absorbed during digestion. Some foods, called complete protein foods, such as quinoa, buckwheat, soybeans, and dairy, contain all the essential amino acids in sufficient amounts. Foods that don't contain all nine essential amino acids are called *incomplete,* and the missing essential amino acids are called the *limiting amino acid.* Lysine, threonine, and tryptophan are the most common limiting amino acids.

Nutrition researchers can give protein sources a score, based upon the abundance of essential amino acids, relative abundance of nonessential amino acids, the digestibility of the protein food, and the presence of allergens or compounds that inhibit amino acid accessibility. In the scoring contest, animal sources of protein often score highly.

Infusing powerful proteins in dessert recipes is easy. The recipes in this book rely on ingredients for protein such as eggs, soy and tofu, almonds and nuts, quinoa, Greek yogurt, and ricotta cheese to balance out the simple sugars.

Recognizing the importance of eating protein

Proteins have several healthful and essential functions in the human body. Consuming high-quality protein does the following, which are important in particular in people with diabetes or prediabetes:

>> **Regulates blood sugar:** Protein slows down the digestion of carbs and delays their absorption into the blood.

>> **Serves as transporters and messengers:** Antibody proteins, part of your immune system, capture and hold foreign bodies, including bacteria and viruses, and hemoglobin transports oxygen to cells around the body. Important protein hormones, like insulin, send signals to cells — to allow glucose molecules to pass through the cell membrane.

>> **Maintain key muscle mass:** Eating protein after resistance training stimulates muscle protein synthesis for up to three hours.

>> **Keep key metabolic functions humming along:** Consuming protein helps you to burn more calories around the clock, boost metabolism, and maintain lean muscle.

Meeting vegetarian/vegan protein needs

Even though animal sources of protein are ideal for people wanting to consume protein in their diet, I know that some people are vegetarian and vegan and choose not to eat animal protein for a number of reasons.

If that's the case with you, the soybean, often served green as edamame or prepared as tofu, is a high-quality and complete protein. Four ounces of edamame or tofu will give you 14 grams of high-quality protein, twice the protein of a large egg or an 8-ounce glass of milk. Incorporating soy into a vegetarian or vegan diet can assure that all essential amino acids are consumed in sufficient amount. If you live in the United States, I recommend seeking out organic soy.

Many other plant sources of protein are available as well, and a healthy diet — whether a person is a carnivore or not — should always include plant sources of protein. Beans and other legumes, nuts, and grains all can contribute to daily protein requirements. Quinoa offers 6 grams of protein in a ¼ cup (45g) (dry) serving, along with the essential amino acids to make it a complete protein.

Vegetarians who don't consume eggs or milk and vegans do need to get protein from a variety of complementary sources to assure they get a complete range of essential amino acids or learn to love soy.

With increasing vegetarian and vegan substitutes on the market, manufacturers tend to add artificial preservatives and flavor enhancers that may be detrimental to your health. Some of these products can be classified as processed or ultraprocessed foods. If you see a long list of additives in the ingredients list, I advise caution. Choose whole foods such as beans, legumes, soy, and others rather than artificial items just because they have protein added to them.

Considering carbohydrates

Contrary to popular belief, carbohydrates — carbs for short — when they come from good sources are good for you and essential. Nonetheless, the media has demonized them. *Cutting carbs* (significantly removing all sources of carbohydrates from your diet; refer to the section "Counting carbs" later in this chapter) while still consuming saturated fat, artificial food, and sweeteners seems to be a lifestyle choice of many. Before labeling carbs as off-limits or labeling specific foods as carbohydrates and others as not, it is important to know what carbs truly are. Carbohydrates aren't only in junk food, bread, pasta, and pastries; they're also present in vegetables, fruits, and whole grains that our bodies need to function properly.

Carbohydrates account for approximately half of your daily calories, and carbohydrate foods are the foods that have a direct impact on your blood glucose. For that reason, understanding how they work, choosing them wisely, and counting carbs can help you to make the most out of your meals. The next sections discuss these important points.

Getting the lowdown on carbs — How they work

Carbohydrates, specifically molecules of the carbohydrate glucose, are your body's favored fuel, and even though your cells can, and do, extract energy from protein and fat, glucose is the best choice. Glucose enters your bloodstream after you eat carbohydrates through absorption sites in your small intestine, and the rising glucose level in your blood signals special beta cells in the pancreas to release the hormone, insulin. Insulin stimulates cells, especially muscle, fat, and liver cells, to allow glucose molecules to pass through cell membranes where it can be stored inside of these cells for fuel when needed.

Cells store glucose in a molecule called *glycogen*, and glycogen is ready at a moment's notice to jump into a metabolic cycle that spits out the power pack molecule *adenosine triphosphate (ATP)*, the real fuel for everything requiring energy. Glycogen is your most accessible source of energy, and carbohydrates in your diet keep the supplies ready when needed.

The role of carbohydrates in your body isn't limited to energy although diabetes tends to focus attention on that role. These are also important:

>> *Glycolipids* (glucose plus lipids) are a component of cell membranes.

>> *Glycoproteins* (glucose plus proteins) help protect your sensitive tissues with mucus.

>> *Sugar lactose,* a component of DNA, is produced in the milk of nursing mothers and helps humans and animals get the energy needed for growth, temperature regulation, and strenuous activity like crying.

Believe it or not, plants are actually carbohydrate factories, and you can thank plant carbohydrates for providing the fuel that you need every day to run your body. Many plant foods including fruits and many vegetables, beans, and legumes that contain carbohydrates also happen to come along with essential vitamins, minerals, antioxidants, and other compounds that work to keep you healthy.

UNDERSTANDING COMPLEX CARBS

When choosing carbohydrates as a person with a diabetes diagnosis, it's important to consider the different types of carbs as well as think about the glycemic index and glycemic load. As the number of chained-together molecules of simple sugars gets longer, the carbohydrate foods are called *complex.* (On the other hand, simple carbs are white pasta, rice, breads, and so forth.) Here are the two main types of complex carbs:

- **Starches:** They're where plants store their excess glucose, and the chemical bonds connecting the simple sugars in starch are easily broken by your digestive system.

  Whereas starches can be refined and isolated from their source for dietary purposes like sugar, its use is usually limited to thickening agents like cornstarch. You're much more likely to get your dietary starch from the whole food, because starch itself is relatively tasteless. Starches are prevalent in potatoes, corn, peas, beans, lentils, hard-shell squashes, quinoa, rice, wheat, barley, oats, and the flours and refined products from grains.

- **Nonstarchy vegetables:** These veggies contain much less carbohydrate than the starchy ones, and in that regard are essential parts of diabetes management by contributing volume without fat, and by having a reduced impact on blood glucose. Greens of all varieties, including peppers, cucumber, summer squashes, green beans, carrots, broccoli, cauliflower, artichoke, turnips, fennel, and asparagus, are a few of the nonstarchy vegetables that can color your plate and deliver vitamins and healthy antioxidants to your body.

Carbohydrate stores 4 calories of potential energy per gram, and excess carbohydrate in your diet is stored as fat. Excess consumption of carbohydrate, especially fructose, can also act to raise levels of low-density lipoproteins, the so-called bad *LDL cholesterol*, and blood triglycerides. For this reason, limiting the total amounts of desserts that you consume and opting for desserts that use complex carbohydrates like whole grains rather than simple ones (for example, all-purpose flour) on a regular basis is important. (Check out the nearby sidebar for more discussion on complex carbs.)

Picking your carbs wisely

If you have a diabetes or prediabetes diagnosis, your task to enjoy optimal health is to manage your intake of carbohydrates that keeps those variations in blood glucose levels close to normal. Your meal plan recommends that you get as much as 50 percent of your daily calories from carbohydrate foods, but not all carbs are created equal.

REMEMBER

Carbohydrates include simple sugars like glucose and also sugar molecules joined in chains that form starches and fiber. Depending on how quickly the carbohydrates you eat are broken down during digestion and on the mix of carbs with other macronutrients when you eat, blood glucose can rise very rapidly or very slowly. Managing your diabetes means managing carbohydrates.

TECHNICAL STUFF

The word "sugar" doesn't just refer to table sugar. To biologists and chemists, the word sugar describes a particular kind of organic molecule belonging to a category of similar molecules called carbohydrates. Carbohydrates — the word actually means carbon with water — often follow the formula $C-H_2O$, and the numbers of carbons and hydrogens and oxygens can go into many thousands when joined together.

Sugars are the simplest carbohydrates. Here's a brief overview of the main types of sugar molecules:

>> **Monosaccharides:** In the world of food, they're the simplest of the simple sugar molecules. Glucose and fructose are two monosaccharides that are among the most known molecules.

>> **Disaccharides:** They're two monosaccharides joined together and include sucrose, common table sugar, the milk sugar lactose, and maltose, a sugar familiar to beer drinkers. Table sugar is one molecule of glucose, and one molecule of fructose.

>> **Oligosaccharides:** They contain up to ten monosaccharides in a chain and are common in legumes like beans.

Carbohydrate digestion works to break chains of sugar molecules into their monosaccharide-building blocks. In your diet, simple sugars and disaccharides can be absorbed rapidly, and the glucose component can have an immediate effect on blood glucose levels. When sugars aren't naturally packaged in their original state like an apple or a beet — added sugars like sucrose — sole nutritional benefit is in the calories.

In an affluent society, added sugars usually add up to excess calories, and with diabetes in the equation the rapid rise in blood glucose levels makes control more difficult. Even among individuals without diabetes, this spiking of blood glucose and insulin levels seems to have long-term consequences. And diets high in excess, added sugar clearly contribute to obesity and increase the risk for diabetes and heart disease.

In plain English, it's best to eat sugar in its natural form, for example from fruit, instead of as a refined, added sweetener.

Counting carbs

Understanding the glycemic index and glycemic load (*glycemic index* is a specific value used to measure how foods increase blood sugar levels whereas *glycemic* load is a number which estimates how much eating a certain food will raise a person's blood glucose — refer to Chapter 2 for more discussion about these two) and counting carbs are ways to ensure that you're consuming the proper amounts. When counting carbs, carbohydrates are packaged into 15-gram carb choices; one carb choice for a particular food always includes approximately 15 grams carbohydrate.

The measure of carbohydrate-containing foods — dairy or plant — that includes your 15 grams of carbohydrate isn't the same from food to food. Refer to Table 4-1, which shows the weight, volume, or size of one carb choice for some different foods.

Keep in mind that desserts in general — other than a serving of fresh fruit — shouldn't be indulged in daily. You can enjoy balanced, wholesome versions such as the ones in Part 3 a few times per week as a part of a nutritious balanced diet and exercise plan.

TABLE 4-1

Measuring a 15-Gram Carb Choice

Food	One Carb Choice
Maple syrup	1 tablespoon
Oatmeal	¼ cup, dry
Beans	⅓ cup, cooked
Rice or pasta	⅓ cup, cooked
Unsweetened cereal	½ cup
Milk	1 cup *
Yogurt	1 cup
Baked potato	3 ounces
French fries	10 fries
Bread	1 slice
Bagel	½ small bagel
Popcorn	3 cups popped
Apple	1 medium sized
Banana	½ medium banana
Raspberries	1 cup
Honeydew melon	1 cup
Nonstarchy vegetables **	1½ cups cooked
Nonstarchy vegetables **	3 cups raw

* 1 cup milk is actually 12 grams carbohydrate but is considered 1 carb choice.
** Nonstarchy vegetables include asparagus, artichoke, beets, green beans, broccoli, cabbage, carrots, cauliflower, cucumber, greens, jicama, mushrooms, okra, pea pods, peppers, radishes, rutabaga, spinach, tomato, turnips, yellow and zucchini squash, and many more.

REMEMBER

Tracking the carbs that you eat and choosing complex carbs when possible is important. Here are a few tricks to make that easy:

» Determine with your nutrition specialist how many servings of carbs you specifically can enjoy in a day (this amount depends upon your weight, age, lifestyle, and glucose levels).

If your meal plan calls for four carb choices at your evening meals, for example, you include a total of four carbohydrate foods, each in a serving size that equals approximately 15 grams of carbohydrate. You can eat four different carb choices, you can have two 15 carbohydrate gram servings of the same food (along with two more carb choices of different foods), or you could have four carb choice servings of the same food too, although variety is best.

>> Your meal plan recommends a specific number of carb choices at every meal and probably a carb choice snack or two as well. Think of the carb choices as 12 or 13 tokens, each one good for a 15-gram carbohydrate serving during the day — 4 grams for breakfast, 4 grams for lunch, 4 grams for dinner, and 4 grams for a snack.

Exploring fat

Fat also has a bad rap, but you need fat in your diet for several reasons:

>> Healthful fats can help your body with many functions, including the following:

- *Adipose* (fatty) cells release some hormones, including leptin, a hormone that signals the brain when you've had enough to eat.

- Key vitamins, including vitamins A, D, E, and K, are fat soluble and transported to cells by fat molecules.

- Your brain is about 60 percent fat, and fat in the material that insulates nerves, called *myelin,* helps protect the electrical signals from interference.

- Fats constitute a part of every cell membrane, and fat can segregate toxins.

>> Fat also stores energy, and the role of fat for producing energy is relevant to diabetes. When glucose isn't available, your cells can convert fat into energy. That's yet another reason why you want to choose healthful fats, such as those found in extra-virgin olive oil (EVOO), avocados, Greek yogurt, eggs, milk, seeds, and nuts in dessert recipes.

Fats can be divided into two types:

>> **Unsaturated:** These fats have a neutral or beneficial effect on blood cholesterol balance. Think EVOO.

>> **Saturated:** They tend to raise levels of harmful types of cholesterol. Think margarine.

The health benefits related to unsaturated fat are both in the reduction of the risk for cardiovascular disease and for diabetes management. Unsaturated fats improve the ratios between bad LDL cholesterol and good HDL cholesterol, and polyunsaturated fat is associated with improved insulin sensitivity. For this reason, use good quality unsaturated fats such as EVOO when baking and creating diabetes-friendly desserts.

Chapter **5**

Enjoying Diabetes-Friendly Desserts: The How and When

In addition to what you consume, when and how you consume it plays a big role in how your body and glucose levels respond. Knowing the best time to eat desserts and incorporating a few tricks as to how you should eat desserts can enable you to enjoy them more often.

This chapter explains how you can use timing to your favor, plan meals and daily activities to allow for indulgences in healthful desserts, and recognize the health advantages of homemade desserts versus commercial varieties.

Focusing on Timing

Nowadays most people are aware that simply increasing a dosage of blood sugar–regulating medication or taking an extra dose of insulin isn't the appropriate way to enjoy desserts with diabetes. Figuring out what, when, and how to enjoy desserts is crucial to maintaining balanced blood sugar. Timing plays an important role in eating patterns and blood sugar levels for several factors. You need to know your blood sugar level at the time before you consume desserts to ensure that you aren't doing your body harm. Eating dessert during a time in the day when you're still likely to exercise is also helpful. By harnessing the power of time, you can enjoy healthful desserts with ease. The following help you to determine how to enjoy desserts and the best time to do so.

Knowing the right time to eat dessert

Contrary to popular belief, enjoying dessert with diabetes doesn't have to be difficult or tasteless. With a little effort and consideration, you may be surprised to find yourself eating better-tasting and more nutritious desserts than before. In addition, your body will respond favorably as soon as you give it the proper fuel it needs.

TIP

Enjoy small portions of nutritious desserts after a balanced meal if your blood sugar wasn't elevated when you tested prior to eating. Always test your blood sugar prior to meals because fluctuations can occur the most between meals. Here are a few tips to keeping blood sugar even when eating:

>> Eat a balanced meal or snack (see Chapter 4) every five hours or so, including before bedtime.

>> Test your blood glucose before meals and talk with your healthcare provider, nutritionist, and or endocrinologist if your levels aren't balanced.

Many how-to books suggest people with type 2 diabetes to test twice daily. The good news: Advances in medicine have made monitoring easier than ever. Talk with your healthcare provider about which devices are appropriate for you and your insurance plan. When you're beginning to regulate your blood sugar after a diabetes diagnosis, be sure to check your glucose levels before all meals, especially before eating dessert.

>> Keep a journal of your meter readings and what you eat at each meal. This way, you can spot patterns that cause your blood sugar to spike. Everyone is different, so knowing your own body's response is important.

>> Discover tips to keep your blood glucose regulated. Chapter 3 provides some helpful things you can do.

REMEMBER

Don't be afraid to ask for help! Putting these concepts together takes time, dedication, patience, practice, and a deep sense of worthiness and belief in yourself. Refer to the section "Strategizing Your Meals When You Have Diabetes" later in this chapter for specific suggestions.

Making smart lifestyle choices

What you do on a daily basis plays a huge role in determining your blood sugar levels. The following affects your glucose levels so you can enjoy delicious food and good health:

>> **Getting a good night's sleep:** A lack of quality sleep has a significant effect on your *endocrine system* (the part of your body that produces hormones), which in turn makes keeping glucose levels balanced more difficult. A lack of sleep also causes inflammation and lowers the metabolism, among other things. If you're not sleeping properly, seek relaxation techniques before bed and speak with your healthcare provider and/or therapist about strategies and techniques that can help to improve your sleep.

>> **Avoiding stress of all kinds:** Stress can cause many problems in the body, especially if the stress is chronic. Talking to a mental health professional, health coach, and close confidants while incorporating stress-reducing activities and thought patterns can help (refer to Chapter 2 for some tips).

>> **Focusing on what food you eat:** Eating food that's unbalanced in macronutrients — protein, carbohydrate, and fat (check out Chapter 4 for more on macronutrients) — and high in sweeteners and simple carbs can cause blood sugar to spike.

>> **Considering how often you eat:** Going long periods of waking hours without eating can cause your blood sugar to become imbalanced. Make sure you eat something balanced every few hours.

>> **Not properly monitoring blood glucose:** Be sure to have your endocrinologist or diabetes educator help you to learn how to test and when it's appropriate in relationship to your specific meal plan.

>> **Exercising:** Being physically active helps you to keep your blood sugar balanced when you eat desserts. Exercise lowers blood glucose and boosts *insulin sensitivity* (your body's ability to effectively respond to insulin). Higher insulin sensitivity can persist for 24 to 72 hours after exercising.

Walking, swimming, gardening, dancing, going for an evening stroll, cooking, baking, and participating in activities like yoga, Pilates, aerobics, and weight training are some ways to keep moving. Some other examples of aerobic exercise include playing pickleball, biking, shadow boxing or martial arts, and playing team sports such as volleyball, softball, and basketball. Pushups, resistance training, and even housework can count toward your daily activity goals and help you metabolize your food better.

Strategizing Your Meals When You Have Diabetes

Unless you're a nutritionist, athlete, or dietitian, the concept of meal planning may seem as antiquated as speaking about dinosaurs. Despite the numerous meal planning and tracking tools at your fingertips and the vast amount of information available, most people don't know the first thing about planning meals, especially from a nutritional standpoint.

REMEMBER

Considering the timing when you consume desserts in advance enables you to eat with both pleasure and health in mind. Planning ahead puts your thinking brain in charge and enables you to make better decisions for the future.

TIP

If you have trouble planning meals for yourself, seek out the help of a nutrition professional. If you already have a meal plan, but have difficulty sticking to it, a health coach could help. If you need help preparing the meals, personal chef services or the tips in this book can be handy.

The following section reveals how to plan meals properly in order to enjoy desserts without complications. I also include a section focused on sample meal plans.

Planning your meals with dessert

If you want to enjoy dessert and keep your blood sugar balanced, you need to make concerted choices. Here are a few things to keep in mind about planning meals (Chapter 3 gives specific information about how to keep blood sugar balanced while eating desserts):

>> **Eat a meal chockful of macronutrients.** Desserts, even the more healthful ones, contain carbs and fat. For this reason, when planning on enjoying dessert, consume a meal prior that consists mostly of nonstarchy vegetables, leafy greens, and lean protein with a bit of healthy fat, such as extra-virgin olive oil (EVOO), nuts, or avocado.

>> **Avoid consuming sweetened foods or foods heavy in simple carbs.** This is especially true the same day if you're planning on indulging in dessert.

   If you're consuming dessert alone — in between meals, be sure to choose from the ones that are noted to be balanced in Part 3. Otherwise, plan to consume a handful of almonds or another kind of lean protein along with them to prevent a blood sugar spike.

>> **Steer clear of drinking sweet drinks (that should be a standard anyway).** If you indulge in a sweet drink with a meal every now and then, consider it to be dessert.

>> **Use EVOO as your main fat of choice during meals.** Use it to flavor lean proteins such as fish, chicken, tofu, eggs, and vegetables.

>> **Vow to only consume desserts that you enjoy.** This might seem like a silly tip, but social pressure and the desire to partake in what everyone else is doing or not offending a host can often derail your eating plans. Eating something to make someone else happy isn't a good idea for anyone, but especially people with diabetes.

>> **Avoid impulse eating.** Planning meals in advance before you go out, keeping a refrigerator and pantry full of food for you in advance, and becoming organized can prevent you from making poor choices later on.

>> **Set aside a few minutes to plan your meals for each day.** Do it either the night before (if not earlier) or at breakfast for the full day. Doing so enables you to make sure that you're eating enough, getting the right ingredients, and aren't forced to decide when blood sugar spikes and you're crashing.

In a perfect world, you'd plan out what you were going to eat a week in advance, make a grocery list, and do the shopping to set you up for success. In reality though, doing so can be challenging for many people. Read Chapter 6 for what to add to your pantry so you're able to cook and bake healthful foods in minutes.

Preparing ahead: Adjusting desserts to make them more diabetes-friendly

You can prepare and add basic ingredients to your pantry, fridge, and freezer. You can then use those ingredients and make several adjustments to the recipes in Part 3 so they're more healthful than traditional desserts. You can use these methods as a general rule when creating your own recipes:

>> Incorporate powerful antioxidants in your recipes — EVOO, seeds, nuts, and fresh produce — all contain these fantastic bioactive compounds.

>> Swap out sour cream and other fatty ingredients for plain full-fat Greek yogurt.

>> Include almonds and other nuts for added protein and healthful fats and nutrients that balance out the carbs in the recipes.

>> Use ricotta cheese instead of other more fattening cheeses.

>> Add sweet-scented spices like pure cinnamon to recipes for flavor and blood sugar–balancing properties.

>> Use dark cocoa and cocoa powder instead of sweetened varieties and milk chocolate.

>> Use EVOO instead of butter and other oils that helps to lower the glycemic load among all its other amazing qualities.

Refer to Chapter 20 for additional recipe suggestions.

Putting together sample meal plans with desserts

The following daily menu items are by no means meant to limit the types of foods that you can eat in a day. Many of my readers have told me that they find it helpful having guidelines when embarking on a new eating plan. For this reason, I demonstrate a wide variety of foods that you can eat in the course of different days to ensure variety of flavors, textures, and nutrients in the diet. I always include a bedtime snack to help keep blood sugar levels even through the night. Here are my samples:

Day 1

Breakfast

Berry, almond, and flaxseed Greek yogurt bowls with raw honey and cinnamon

Green or herbal tea, coffee, or espresso

Lunch

Mixed salad greens with broccoli and citrus-marinated chicken or salmon

Apple, Raisin, and Nut Strudel (see Chapter 15)

Snack

Homemade hummus with crudites

Dinner

Asparagus, red pepper, and tofu stir-fry with soba noodles and sesame seeds

Snack

1 medium apple

5 almonds

Day 2
Breakfast

Egg white, red pepper, and broccoli omelet with 1 piece 100 percent whole-grain toast drizzled with EVOO

Green or herbal tea, coffee, or espresso

Lunch

Homemade bean, lentil, and legume soup

1 hardboiled egg with 2 cups salad or your favorite greens

Dinner

Grilled or roasted fish drizzled with EVOO and lemon juice, 2 servings nonstarchy vegetables like spinach, carrots, and/or broccoli

Vanilla Cardamom Panna Cotta (see Chapter 12)

Snack

½ cup plain, full-fat Greek yogurt with 1 teaspoon raw honey and ¼ cup fresh berries

Day 3
Breakfast

Poached egg and avocado toast with a Persian cucumber, cherry tomatoes, and EVOO

Green or herbal tea, coffee, or espresso

Lunch

Sizzling herb–infused shrimp and mixed peppers over cannellini bean puree

Dinner

Herbed chicken stew made with 2 nonstarchy vegetables

Fresh Fruit Kabobs (see Chapter 9)

Snack

1 cup raw or blanched broccoli and/or cauliflower with 2 tablespoons plain, full-fat Greek yogurt, hummus, or tzatziki

Day 4

Breakfast

Plain, full-fat Greek yogurt bowl with 1 teaspoon raw honey, 1 teaspoon cinnamon, ½ cup fresh or frozen blueberries, 1 teaspoon ground flaxseeds

Green or herbal tea, coffee, or espresso

Lunch

Cucumber and smoked salmon pinwheels or sandwiches with mixed green salad dressed with EVOO and lemon juice or vinegar

Handful of plain almonds

1 Dark Chocolate & Extra-Virgin Olive Oil Brownie (see Chapter 10)

Dinner

Seafood stew served over quinoa

Snack

¼ cup olives (rinsed if in brine) with added EVOO and spices of your choice

Day 5

Breakfast

1 Moroccan Avocado Smoothie (see Chapter 16)

Handful of almonds

Lunch

Roasted sweet potato, black bean, spinach, and quinoa bowls with EVOO and lemon juice or vinegar

Dinner

Homemade chicken and vegetable soup

1 serving Chocolate "Ice Cream" (see Chapter 14)

Snack

Celery sticks with 2 tablespoons fresh, no-sugar-added peanut or almond butter

Day 6

Breakfast

Oatmeal with walnuts, flaxseeds, almond milk, and ½ cup berries

Green or herbal tea, coffee, or espresso

Lunch

Baba ghanouj with crudites and roasted chickpeas

1 serving Date, Almond, and Cocoa Balls or Chocolate Swirl Bark (see Chapter 13)

Dinner

Citrus marinated salmon with 2 nonstarchy vegetables

Fresh greens salad with EVOO and lemon juice or good quality vinegar

Snack

½ cup tablespoons plain, full-fat Greek yogurt drizzled with 1 teaspoon EVOO and homemade, whole-wheat pita chips or crudites

Day 7

Breakfast

1 hardboiled egg, 1 Persian cucumber, 1 Roma tomato, 1 piece whole-wheat pita, 1 teaspoon EVOO

Green or herbal tea, coffee, or espresso

Lunch

Eggplant and chickpea stew over brown basmati rice

Dinner

Lentil soup

Green salad with EVOO and lemon juice or good quality vinegar

1 serving Chocolate Chip Almond Butter Cookies (see Chapter 11)

Snack

½ cup plain, full fat Greek yogurt

GUILT AND SHAME COMMON WITH DIABETES

Modern society wasn't built on pillars of health and happiness, which makes staying healthy difficult. Furthermore, modern societies were built on the notions of expanding economies and industrialization. Hence, people naturally need to find new normal ways of functioning in society in order to maintain their mental and physical health.

A study at the University of New Zealand found that people who felt guilty after eating a piece of chocolate cake felt more out of control emotionally, but these negative feelings didn't motivate them to have stronger intentions to eat healthy. Additional research finds that people who feel guilty feel fatter and that guilt actually causes people's metabolic rate to slow down, making them gain more weight from eating the same number of calories.

People with type 2 diabetes may also feel guilty or shameful about having diabetes in the first place. Type 2 diabetes is often considered a lifestyle disease — the innate interpretation that people who have diabetes are doing something wrong — which can be shameful to many people. Diabetes definitely has a stigma associated with it, but that stigma should be turned on its head when you consider the number of people in the world who are diagnosed with diabetes or prediabetes and who are undiagnosed; if you have it, you're not alone.

According to metaphysical beliefs, all types of illness and disease are caused by a misunderstanding — an old belief that no longer serves you — which has been stored in your body. Illnesses and physical limitations are simply a chance to clear out these old beliefs, learn to love yourself, and claim your birthright to live the healthiest life possible. One year, after learning about the harmful effects of feeling guilt, during Lent, I vowed to give it up. I just said to myself that I realized how harmful it is to me and that no good can come of it. Adopting this belief has helped me to get rid of my own shame and guilt about the serious illnesses I have, transforming my life. Oddly, it was one of the easiest things I ever did, and I'm grateful to have learned that doing so was an option.

Calming Your Feelings of Shame and Guilt

The 2003 Italian movie *Ginger and Cinnamon* portrayed the complications of life as seen through the eyes of a 30-year-old woman and her 15-year-old niece who she tried to teach life's most important lessons. One of her lessons was it wasn't the dessert itself but the "sense of guilt" that one felt eating it that caused people to gain weight.

Although you know that desserts can lead to weight gain, the sense of guilt that you may feel when eating or in general is rarely discussed in terms of overall health and well-being. According to *Psychology Today*, you may want to let go of and/or reframe these feelings because research suggests those who associate guilt with indulgence (versus seeing it as a celebration) "have a significantly harder time maintaining their weight."

Physical signs of guilt may manifest as difficulty sleeping, gut issues, muscle tension, and digestion issues. Obsessive-compulsive disorder (OCD), depression, and anxiety have a particular symbiotic relationship with guilt. If you're a person who is overwhelmed when you need to make a decision, suffer from low self-esteem, or put others' needs before your own, you probably experience guilt.

Although everyone's feelings are different, you can take some steps to free yourself from guilt or shame:

TIP

>> **Practice positive thinking and visualization.** Positive thinking requires you to believe that good can come out of any situation and look for the good things in life. Visualization involves closing your eyes for a certain amount of time each day to imagine things exactly as you would like them while feeling the sensations that you would feel if you were in those situations. These ways can neutralize the sense of guilt and free yourself from it. You're more than your body and mind, you're a system of energy and consciousness, and the more you can influence your energy and consciousness to feel good, the better off your overall health will be.

Chapter 2 discusses concepts, such as happiness hormones, which can help you feel better. Any little thing that you can do to increase happiness and release negative emotions will offer health paybacks. (Refer to the nearby sidebar for more information.)

Here are some suggestions to help:

- Get quiet and investigate the roots of your guilt. Are they really limited to chocolate cake, or are there deeper things that bother you?

- Inhale and exhale three deep breaths and ask yourself if those beliefs about shame and guilt are necessary. Do they make sense to you now? Are they based on an old belief that no longer serves you? If you find that it's not logical or needed to feel this way, vow to give it up. Whenever shame or guilt comes up in your life, let them go.

- Acknowledge that even though these feelings no longer serve you, they may have been helpful in the past. For example, feeling guilty or shamed about something can help a person be motivated to be especially "good" or "worthy" in other areas of life. Those negative feelings may have helped you to excel in other areas. Acknowledge that you don't need the negative thoughts to motivate yourself or to do well. In fact, after you start thinking more positively everything becomes easier.

>> **Communicate or write a letter to someone who is the source of your guilt.** Sometimes you can no longer communicate with that person. In this instance, writing a letter to that person in an uninhibited way allows you to release all your emotions. After you write the letter, don't send it, but instead burn it or rip it up as a symbolic way of letting go of the guilt.

SHOW YOUR THANKS WHEN EATING

Studies have shown that if people smell food being cooked prior to eating it, or hear it being described pleasantly in detail, they digest the food more slowly and feel fuller quicker. During the rule of the Abbasid caliphate in medieval Baghdad, court poets recited poems to diners prior to eating their food. Although this practice may have seemed pretentious to many, it was actually an intelligent decision at the time. In addition to providing entertainment for the people at the table, the poems made for a more healthful dining experience.

Even if you're not a poet and you're not a part of a royal court, you can still say and think positive affirmations, give sincere gratitude that you feel for your food, and listen to beautiful music while eating. Dining with others and talking about pleasurable things will also enhance the experience from a physical and psychological standpoint.

>> **Pivot your guilty feelings into something positive by being grateful for the lessons that the particular situation taught you.** Expressing gratitude is also an easy way to elevate your mood quickly. Mindfulness is a wonderful practice as well. Check out *Mindfulness For Dummies* by Shamash Alidina (John Wiley & Sons, Inc.) for more details.

>> **Consider the process of *conscious eating*, a term used to describe the act of slowing down and enjoying the food you eat.** Set aside time to appreciate the aroma of what you're eating, be cognizant of the way it looks, take time to make a meal look special, and savor it slowly. Taking part in these types of activities can improve your overall health.

Comparing Desserts: Eating Out and Store-Bought versus Homemade

Like all foods, not all desserts are created equal. As you can see by flipping through the recipes in Part 3, the recipes and ingredients offered in this book are different from what you find in most supermarkets, restaurants, and commercial bakeries. Although they all taste good, making homemade desserts allows you to not only ensure that you're consuming predominately what is safe, but that you're also enjoying ingredients that contain specific nutrients that are beneficial to those with diabetes.

Looking at store-bought and restaurant desserts

Neither supermarket chains nor most restaurants or bakeries normally offer healthful desserts. Scan the nutritional info on labels of store-bought purchased desserts and websites of chain restaurants, and you can see exactly how harmful many of their items can be. Because sugar and unhealthful fats are the easiest way to add flavor to food, many restaurants rely on them for inexpensive additions.

REMEMBER

Eating out more frequently is associated with obesity, higher body fatness, and higher body mass index. According to the USDA, eating lunch away from home adds 158 calories to the daily intake, while dinner increases it by 144 calories. Eating out also increases the amount of fat and sugar that people consume.

The job and function of these establishments isn't to heal people or to help them balance their glucose levels. Rather it's to offer sweet desserts that taste good and meet their customers' guilty pleasure needs.

Even though organic supermarkets and artisan bakers tend to use more natural ingredients than large chains, rarely do they offer desserts that are appropriate for someone with diabetes. Even if a dessert is labeled as sugar-free, it may still contain saturated fats and be high in artificial sweeteners that may be more harmful than table sugar and high in sodium, all of which are problematic for everyone but especially for individuals with diabetes.

REMEMBER

The portion sizes of desserts in supermarkets, at bakeries, and in restaurants are usually large enough to split in half, and in some cases quarters. Restaurateurs know the game: They increase the portion sizes, which allows them to also increase prices and make a significant profit. In addition, with so many restaurants now offering large portions of desserts, those restaurants that don't do the same seem less generous in their offerings. Allowing yourself to indulge on occasion will help to prevent feelings of deprivation, as will enjoying your one homemade dessert.

TIP

When eating out and considering a restaurant dessert, I suggest you do the following:

>> Go online and check out a restaurant's menu so that you can find items that are suitable to you and would make a nutritious meal prior to dessert.

>> If you're with a group of people who insists on getting dessert, offer to taste someone else's dessert instead of ordering your own.

>> Consider ordering a sorbet or fresh fruit. These are better options than the heavier desserts.

>> Share your dessert with others or eat a portion of it, if you decide to indulge in a heavier dessert. Eat it slowly, enjoy it, and resist the urge to feel guilty. Then follow up by eating some protein such as unsalted walnuts or almonds, edamame, ricotta cheese, plain Greek yogurt, and such to avoid a blood sugar spike and walk around or exercise a bit afterward.

Making homemade desserts (and a plan)

Homemade (from scratch) desserts are the best choice for you because of the following:

>> You can control the ingredients. You can use complex carbs, EVOO, Greek yogurt, fresh fruit, nuts, and so on, which are good for people with diabetes and don't cause blood spikes.

>> You can avoid unnecessary additives in food that are present in many prepared varieties.

>> You can portion the sizes to what is appropriate for your meal plan.

Chapter 7 discusses in greater detail why creating a plan to make your own desserts is important to your overall health and well-being.

IN THIS CHAPTER

» Deciphering labels when shopping

» Adding diabetes-friendly dessert ingredients to your kitchen

» Assessing sweeteners

» Selecting healthful sweeteners

» Using sweeteners in place of sugar

Chapter **6**

Building a Pantry and Choosing Healthful Sweeteners

The word "pantry" conjures up images of olden times and pioneer kitchens to many people. It's perhaps one of the least trendy cooking terms, but it's time to change that. The ancient necessity of maintaining a well-stocked pantry, and fridge and freezer, for that matter, is one of the wisest ways to help keep you on your journey to good health.

This chapter explains which ingredients and sweeteners to keep on hand to not only prepare the recipes in Part 3 but also come up with your own tasty and diabetes-friendly desserts in minutes when needed.

Decoding Nutrition Labels

When you're shopping for ingredients, the nutrition label can be your friend. Nutrition fact labels are required on all packaged food in the United States and in many countries. Unfortunately, much of the information included on these labels isn't helpful to people with diabetes.

The best advice I have for you is to avoid ultraprocessed food as much as possible. For the items that you need to purchase in a package, be sure that they're low in sodium and free of trans fat. If they're high in carbs and sodium, you'll need to balance them out with low-sodium and low-carb options in the rest of your meal or what you eat the rest of the day.

Because individual needs vary, be sure to discuss your personal intake levels with your healthcare and nutrition professionals.

When you're reading a label (see Figure 6-1), focus on the following:

WARNING

>> **Ingredients:** Opt for foods with ingredients you're familiar with and can pronounce. The best options would incorporate whole grains, nuts, eggs, fruit, and small amounts of natural sweeteners.

If you can't pronounce the ingredients, don't buy the food.

>> **Sodium:** Be sure that the sodium content isn't too high (aim for less than 1,000 mg per day total sodium consumption) and be sure to discuss your personal needs with your nutrition professional.

>> **Carbohydrates:** Your nutrition professional can help you determine the proper amount of carbohydrates to consume per meal because everyone's body is different. Chapter 4 explains which carbohydrates are best to enjoy with diabetes.

In addition to the label itself, identify any healthful ingredients (see Chapter 2). This way you'll know which types of sweeteners and ingredients in general are best for people with diabetes. Avoid products with unnatural sounding ingredients and unrecognizable additives. If you're ever not sure, searching online can help you determine whether particular ingredients are safe or not.

Nutrition Facts

Serving Size 1/2 cup (140g)

Amount Per Serving

Calories 240	Calories From Fat 130

	% Daily Value *
Total Fat 15g	23%
Saturated Fat 2g	11%
Trans Fat 0g	
Cholesterol 0mg	0%
Sodium 530mg	22%
Total Carbohydrate 24g	8%
Dietary Fiber 1g	5%
Sugars 5g	
Protein 3g	

Vitamin A 15%	•	Vitamin C 60%
Calcium 2%	•	Iron 6%

* Percent Daily Values are based on a 2,000 calorie diet.

FIGURE 6-1:
Nutrition label.

Stocking Your Kitchen with Diabetes-Friendly Dessert Ingredients

Keeping a pantry — and a freezer and refrigerator — of the best ingredients for creating diabetes-friendly desserts can help you stay on track and avoid turning to unhealthful desserts to satisfy your sweet tooth. Whipping up cookies, brownies, sweet sips, cakes, puddings, and other mouthwatering desserts isn't out of reach for people with diabetes and those who prioritize their health. These sections identify what to include in your pantry, fridge, and freezer.

Supplying your pantry

When making your grocery list, make sure you have the following ingredients on hand (Chapter 2 discusses why these ingredients are healthful and nutritious):

» Butters

- Almond butter
- Unsweetened peanut butter

» Almond flour

» Alternative sweeteners (refer to the section "Identifying healthful sweeteners" later in this chapter for the 4-1-1)

- Agave nectar
- Allulose
- Coconut sugar
- Date sugar
- Dried dates
- Monk fruit sugar
- Organic vanilla coconut sugar
- Pure maple syrup
- Pure stevia
- Raw honey

» Dark chocolate

» Extra-virgin olive oil (EVOO)

» Nuts

- Almonds
- Brazil nuts
- Cashews
- Hazelnuts
- Peanuts (a legume)
- Walnuts

» Pure vanilla

- » Seeds
  - Chia seeds
  - Flaxseeds
  - Sesame seeds
  - Sunflower seeds
- » Spices
  - Cardamom
  - Cloves
  - Ginger
  - Pure cinnamon
- » Whole-grain flours
  - Barley flour
  - Oat flour
  - Whole-wheat flour
  - Whole-wheat pastry flour

Keeping your fridge stocked

Stocking your fridge is every bit as important as stocking your pantry. If you're making diabetes-friendly desserts, keep these ingredients on hand:

- » Eggs
- » Fruit
  - Apples
  - Banana
  - Berries (blackberries, blueberries, raspberries, strawberries)
  - Cherries
  - Figs
  - Kiwis
  - Lemons

- Pears

- Oranges

>> Ricotta cheese (It's great addition for giving body and texture to a recipe. Plus, it contains more protein than cream cheese and sour cream.)

>> Silken tofu (You can use silken tofu to add protein, body, and consistency to diabetes recipes instead of cheese.)

>> Whole milk

Freezing some foods

Here's what you should keep in the freezer:

>> **Frozen pre-made recipes from this book:** Chapter 7 describes how to make desserts in advance when time permits.

>> **Frozen fruit and berries:** Keeping these items on hand in fresh form when they're in season can be difficult and costly. Frozen varieties offer the same nutrients and allow them to be enjoyed any time.

>> **Frozen purees made from fresh fruit:** Puree pumpkin, apple, and banana and use them in baking when needed.

Sweetening the Pot — Sweeteners

Determining which sweetener can be best for baking and cooking diabetes-friendly foods and desserts can be confusing, even for professionals. With so many new products on the market and new research results about them, deciding which sweetener is best for you and your recipes can be difficult.

The following sections help you to tell the good from the bad and to choose the best sweeteners for your kitchen and health.

Deciphering the good from bad

Marketing terms and labels do a good job of confusing consumers at supermarkets, so knowing the difference between the terms is important. Artificial, non-healthful sweeteners get labelled under many guises and terms like "zero calorie" and "sugar free" make them sound enticing to anyone looking to purchase something that's good for them, but don't be fooled. Equip yourself with as much knowledge about sweeteners as possible so that you can enjoy desserts without worrying that they're even more harmful to you than a serving of simple carbs.

REMEMBER

Here's what you need to know: In a recent Harvard study 103,388 people, about 80 percent women with an average age of 42, recorded what they daily ate along with their medical history and health habits. According to the study, more than one-third (37 percent) used artificial sweeteners, and they consumed about 42 milligrams per day, on average — an amount roughly equal to the contents of one tabletop packet or just under a quarter-cup of diet soda. The follow-up lasted for approximately nine years, and participants were asked to fill out questionnaires and report changes in health biannually. Scientists' findings concluded that artificial sweeteners were linked to a 9 percent higher risk of any type of cardiovascular problem (including heart attacks) and an 18 percent greater risk of stroke.

Recent studies have proven that artificial sweeteners can be even more harmful than sugar itself in recipes. Even though they don't contain table sugar and may be zero-calorie, they often include more sodium, fat, and chemical substances than the traditional counterpart. The sodas, desserts, drinks, and snacks that use them aren't any safer than the regular variety. If you have diabetes or want to avoid developing it, you should avoid these items.

Look for natural sugars like those that occur naturally in foods such as fruit, vegetables, and dairy; the recipes in Part 3 use them the most.

Here I explain the difference between the terms often used.

Alternative sweeteners

They refer to both artificial and nonregular sugar sweeteners, which are alternatives to table sugar known as *sucrose*. Most table sugar is produced from sugar cane and beets. Sucrose in different forms is the sugar most people know and makes up table sugar, brown sugar, and confectioner's sugar most commonly used in baking.

The term "alternative sweetener" is popular and widely used because the word "artificial" doesn't have an appealing sound to it. For marketing purposes, companies may use the word "alternate" or "sugar free" regardless of whether the source is natural or artificial. It's up to the you, the consumer, to do the research to make sure that you're consuming the types of sweeteners that are best for you.

Many all-natural types of sweeteners use the word "alternative" sweetener to define themselves; however, make sure you read the ingredient list of the particular type you're using and to do your own research.

Artificial sugars

Artificial sugars and "sugar substitutes" — those that are chemically derived, often use the word "sweetener" — so research them before blindly trusting them.

Table sugar

Table sugar contains sucrose and is a simple carbohydrate that can cause blood sugar to rise after consuming it. Note that the amount your blood sugar rises after eating depends on many factors, including what it's paired with in the recipe, how it's prepared, and what's in the rest of your meal. Exercising after a meal can help to prevent spikes from taking place.

If you have diabetes, too much sugar can lead to poor diabetes control, which can lead to multiple health problems. Limit the overall intake of sugar and consume desserts which contain regular sugar very sparingly.

Identifying healthful sweeteners

Sugars that occur naturally in foods such as fruit, vegetables, and dairy, are the most healthful types of sweeteners and the ones used in this book. Regardless of whether a sugar or sweetening agent is natural or not, it should still be enjoyed at a minimum and in combination with foods that contain healthful fats and lean protein in order to balance out blood sugar in people with diabetes.

Here are the types of sweeteners I use in the recipes in Part 3. These sweeteners are the better choices for people with diabetes.

REMEMBER

Incorporating natural sugars alone doesn't make them good or safe for people with diabetes or prediabetes. Diabetes-friendly foods and desserts should incorporate as many not only permitted, but also good-for you foods as well. Creating balanced recipes is your key to success. Choose desserts like those in Part 3 that rely on fresh and dried fruit, dark chocolate, almonds and nuts, seeds, Greek yogurt, EVOO, and sweet spices in their preparation. These ingredients contain antioxidants that positively impact your health and are especially known to help balance blood sugar while adding flavor and essential nutrients.

Desserts that include natural sweeteners, and fruit and/or complex carbohydrates such as whole grains along with healthful sources of fat such as EVOO, nuts, seeds, and Greek yogurt, and protein such as that found in ricotta cheese, yogurt, and seeds are balanced in terms of micronutrients and won't cause blood sugar to spike.

Raw honey

Nature's ancient solution of raw honey still tops the list of the best sweeteners to use. In addition to being praised in ancient religious and medical texts, raw honey has also been proven by modern science to be the best choice for people with diabetes and everyone wanting to stay healthy. Honey is different from white or table sugar because sugar doesn't have any vitamins and minerals, whereas honey offers an array of nutrients as well as antioxidant, antimicrobial, and antibacterial properties that inhibit bacteria, fungi, and viruses. Raw honey also contains *polyphenols* (bioactive compounds that have antioxidant and anti-inflammatory properties and can also improve insulin sensitivity and promote a healthy weight).

REMEMBER

Because honey is still a source of simple carbohydrates, be sure to consume it in limited amounts and when balanced out with protein and healthy fats.

DOCTOR
SAYS

Many commercial honeys have been heated to make sure they remain liquid. Raw honeys are in their original natural state and will tend to solidify over time and in cooler temperatures. These honeys preserve the bioactive compounds which may contribute to anti-inflammatory and antioxidant properties of honey.

REMEMBER

Raw honey has been shown to increase the gut-friendly probiotic effects of plain, full-fat Greek yogurt, enabling it to offer even more healthy microflora to a person's intestines. That said, honey is still a source of carbohydrates that come from glucose and fructose, which are simple sugars. So, even though it's the "safest" and healthiest choice among sweeteners, you still want to limit your intake and to make sure that you balance the carbs in honey with healthful fats and protein in baking and desserts in order to avoid blood sugar spikes.

Pure maple syrup

When buying pure maple syrup (100 percent with no additives), make sure that it's free from added sugar, preservatives, caramel flavorings, and coloring. Pure or organic maple syrups are natural sweeteners that you can swap out 1:1 in recipes for honey or table sugar (refer to the section "Swapping Out Healthful Sweeteners in Recipes" later in this chapter).

Although maple syrup has a lower GI than other sugars, you still want to consume it in limited quantities. If you don't balance it with protein and healthful fat, consuming it can cause fluctuation in your blood sugar, so you use it in recipes that incorporate those ingredients, like the Quinoa, Cranberry, and Pecan Bars and Gingerbread Spice Squares in Chapter 10.

Pure stevia

Many different types of products utilize marketing with the name "stevia." Stevia is a sugar substitute extracted from the leaves of the *Stevia rebaudiana* plant, which is native to some parts of South America. Its leaves contain substances knowns as steviol glycosides and are between 200 and 400 times sweeter than table sugar, so a little bit goes a long way. Make sure that the stevia you purchase is pure and not mixed with other substances, which is often the case.

Organic vanilla and coconut sugar

Made from coconut sap, this sugar is derived from the dehydrated sap of the coconut palm tree and is being marketed as more nutritious with a lower GI than table sugar. Coconut sugar, unlike table sugar, offers small amounts of minerals, antioxidants, and fiber. It increases blood sugar more slowly than table sugar when consumed alone because of its inulin content.

Choose the vanilla variety because it has the additional flavor that works well in desserts. Like all other sweeteners, if you choose to use it, balance it with healthy fat and protein sources and enjoy it in limited quantities. I prefer organic vanilla and coconut sugar, but you can also use regular organic coconut sugar.

Allulose

This sweetener is relatively new on the market, and studies are still being conducted regarding its benefits. Nutritionists often tout it as a new go-to sweetener. Allulose is also known as *D-psicose* and is naturally present in only a few foods such as wheat, figs, and molasses. It tastes similar to table sugar but is only 70 percent as sweet. Allulose also provides one-tenth the calories of table sugar and doesn't appear to raise blood sugar levels or insulin levels. Some early research suggests that it may have anti-inflammatory properties, regulate blood sugar, and increase insulin sensitivity.

Date sugar and dried dates

Date sugar and dried dates can be a good, natural sweeter option for people with diabetes or prediabetes because they're natural with a low GI and high in fiber. Date sugar is a healthier alternative to refined sugar because it's free of preservatives and is a good source of potassium, magnesium, and phosphorus. Dates also promote digestion and good gut bacteria.

I first learned about the numerous health benefits from research scientists in Saudi Arabia where "5 dates a day" are recommended to "keep the doctor away" much in the same fashion as "an apple a day" is in the United States. Dates are a highly prized ingredient in the Middle East with scores of different varieties in which to choose. You can even soak dried dates in milk until they're tender and blend them in a high-speed blender to create a natural caramel.

Monk fruit sugar

Increasingly popular, monk fruit sugar is a zero-calorie, zero-carb sweetener that offers antioxidants and no harmful effects. Monk fruit looks like a small gourd and is also called *luo han guo* or *swingle.* Native to Southeast Asia, Buddhist monks in the 13th century were the first to cultivate the fruit, which explains its namesake.

Monk fruit spoils rather quickly. Traditionally, people used dried monk fruit in herbal medicines. The fruit's extract contains substances called *mogrosides*, which are intensely sweet —150 to 200 times sweeter than table sugar. It's sometimes sold in combination with other sugars or sweeteners to balance out the intensity so be sure to read the labels.

Agave nectar

Although some people have turned to agave nectar as a general swap out for sugar because it has a lower GI, the jury is still out on its effects, so use it sparingly. Agave contains higher levels of fructose than table sugar and most other sweeteners. Because the body releases less insulin after fructose consumption, blood glucose levels could remain higher after consuming agave nectar than it would after consuming table sugar.

REMEMBER

Agave is 1.5 sweeter than table sugar, so if you're replacing it in a recipe, you can divide the amount of table sugar by 1.5 to find the correct measurement. Even though agave nectar can be enjoyed in lower amounts in recipes or as part of a meal that's balanced with protein and healthful fat, don't make it your main, go-to swap out for diabetes-friendly desserts.

Molasses

Because it's a natural product, some nutritionists recommend it and molasses is often believed to be a healthful choice and is used in diabetes-friendly recipes, but I try to limit it. Even though it's free from artificial ingredients, it can be harmful to people with diabetes and can cause weight gain. Molasses may be a good alternative to refined sugar for most people if they consume it in moderation, but consuming too much of any added sugar can have adverse effects, particularly harmful to those with diabetes.

A BIT OF SUGAR HISTORY

Sugar cane, which the Persians brought to Egypt, is a type of perennial grass that has been cultivated in the Middle East since antiquity. Still today in the southern Egyptian cities of Luxor and Aswan, for example, sugar cane is harvested and processed in heavy duty juicers to make a fresh juice that people enjoy on the street and in cafes during hot days on the Nile.

In ancient times sugar was so expensive that it was mainly used in recipes created as offerings for the gods. In wealthy ancient Egypt it was also used in the royal bakeries. Not until centuries later was it introduced into Europe as an ingredient that only the noble classes could afford. Up until a few hundred years ago, French apothecaries sold sugar by the teaspoon as a medicine to combat melancholy. The poorer classes had to make do with honey and cheaper forms of sweeteners, like molasses when possible.

Nowadays sugar has become so inexpensive, processed, and overused that many people are addicted to it just like one would be addicted to other types of harmful drugs. Sodas and artificial-sweetener-laden—bottled salad dressings, sauces, and most commercially prepared foods have added sweeteners such as corn syrup for cheap flavor and their ability to help products be shelf stable.

Tip: If you want to be healthy, avoid sodas and commercially prepared packaged foods. If you do eat them on a regular basis, swapping out healthier alternatives for them alone can make a significant difference in your health and enable you to indulge in better, wholesome dessert options like the recipes in Part 3 on a regular basis.

Swapping Out Healthful Sweeteners in Recipes

Becoming comfortable with the more healthful sweeteners is important. What's more important is being able to swap out unhealthy sweeteners and know how to use them in recipes so that you can create both delicious and healthful desserts.

REMEMBER

For someone with diabetes, switching sweeteners alone won't make a dessert diabetes-friendly. Using a sweetener is more than just replacing an unhealthy one with a healthful one. You also need to ensure that the recipe has a good balance of macronutrients (see Chapter 4 for more discussion). That means the following:

>> **Fat:** A healthful fat component such as almonds, nuts, seeds, EVOO

>> **Protein:** Some protein such as plain full-fat Greek yogurt, ricotta cheese, and/or nuts

>> **Carbohydrate:** Quality carbohydrates like whole grains instead of white flour whenever possible

The recipes in Part 3 take these factors into consideration. In addition, eating a balanced yet especially low in simple carb meal and getting exercise throughout the day will make eating the desserts in this book better for you.

TIP

Keep in mind that many American and European desserts consist of copious amounts of sugar. Royal courts created many historical recipes because they wanted to demonstrate that they could afford then-expensive sugar. You can almost always reduce the amount of table sugar in traditional recipes without noticing it. For example, if I see a cake recipe with more than 1 cup of table sugar, I usually reduce it to 1 cup when trying out the recipe.

Table 6-1 shows what healthful sweetener to swap out for table sugar in recipes to make them diabetes-friendly:

REMEMBER

This table is a rough guide and individually baked items vary depending on the other ingredients in the recipe. You may have to experiment a few times to perfect your favorite recipe into a diabetes-friendly version, but it will be worth the effort.

REMEMBER

I try to limit table sugar as much as possible when making diabetes-friendly desserts. In some lighter cakes and in limited quantities, it's okay to consume it, but raw honey, ripe banana, and vanilla and coconut sugar are my preferred substitutes.

REMEMBER

The sweeteners in Table 6-1 cost a considerable amount more than table sugar. Although the cost can be a deterrent, keep in mind that you should be consuming less sweeteners in the first place. What's more important is the quality of the sweetener compared to the quantity that matters most to your health. If blood sugar spikes are a concern to you, be sure to keep your medicine/insulin administration logged along with daily meals and times of each. Speak with your health-care team to help you determine the best plan for you.

TABLE 6-1 **Substituting Table Sugar with Healthful Sweeteners**

Healthful Sweetener	Swap-out Instructions for Table Sugar	Best Used in These Recipes	Miscellaneous
Raw honey	1:1 ratio	Sweet breads, more rustic fruit cakes, drinks, cookies, brownies, and bars.	Don't swap it out in a light, airy cake such as a sponge cake, angel food cake, or chiffon, birthday-style cake.
Pure maple syrup (make sure it's pure)	1:1 ratio	Sweet breads, more rustic fruit cakes, drinks, cookies, brownies, and bars.	Imparts its own unique and beloved flavor and lends a nice aroma to plain, vanilla-scented sweets and desserts and those that feature fruit like pumpkin, apples, and blueberries.
Pure stevia (make sure it's pure with no erythritol)	Replace 1 cup sugar with 1 teaspoon pure stevia.	Has an anise or licorice aftertaste, so pair pure stevia in recipes that would benefit from that flavor.	Sweetness is between 200 and 400 times sweeter than table sugar. Keep in mind that depending upon recipe you may need to add ripe banana or applesauce or another ingredient to make up for the smaller quantity.
Organic vanilla and coconut sugar	1:1 ratio Usually provides a slightly darker color in recipe	Light textured recipes such as chiffon cakes, angel food cakes, and sponge cakes that need a light textured sugar and a similar flavor to sugar.	Raises blood sugar more slowly than table sugar. However, because it can still cause a slight increase in blood sugar, be sure to pair it in dessert recipes that have healthful proteins such as eggs, nuts, Greek yogurt, and/or ricotta cheese.
Allulose	Use 1⅓ cup pure allulose for every cup of sugar	Recipes with dried fruit or those that have other sweet-tasting ingredients like cinnamon, vanilla, and fresh fruit.	
Date sugar and dried dates (especially Medjool dates)	1:1 ratio	Blend dried dates soaked in water or milk to drinks, heavier cakes, sweet breads, and cookies.	Adds a caramel-like richness.
Monk fruit sugar	About 150 to 200 times sweeter than table sugar, so a teaspoon is enough	Recipes that include pure vanilla, cinnamon, or sweet fruit.	Tastes sweet but can have a bitter aftertaste.

Healthful Sweetener	Swap-out Instructions for Table Sugar	Best Used in These Recipes	Miscellaneous
Ripe banana	½ cup mashed (very ripe) banana for each 1 cup sugar	Recipes for smoothies, sweet breads, cakes, cookies, brownies, and bars that would also benefit from the banana flavor.	As soon as bananas start to get brown spots on the outside, their levels of sweetness increase and adding them to recipes significantly reduces the need for other sugars.
Agave nectar	Divide the amount of table sugar by 1.5 to find the correct measurement of agave.	More plain recipes so that it doesn't overwhelm the flavor or the darker varieties in more full-flavored recipes such as a dense fruit cake or a dark chocolate dessert.	Has its own flavor that can be caramel-like.
Molasses	1:1 ratio	Works in sweet breads, muffins, and rustic American-style baked goods	Molasses is high in carbohydrates and doesn't quickly break down into glucose, making it slightly safer than table sugar for people with diabetes.

Chapter 7

Fitting Homemade Desserts into Your Schedule

A lack of time is what prevents many people from cooking at home. Baking from home seems to be even more of a luxury for most people. Just like with cooking, however, being able to control the quality of ingredients when baking or making desserts is a real benefit — especially for people managing their blood sugar levels.

This chapter explores how to make the most of your time so you can create your own desserts and enjoy them without the guilt.

Analyzing Your Schedule to Include Baking

If you're interested in keeping yourself or someone else you know on the right nutrition track, finding the time to make food from scratch is a top priority. The food that you consume, combined with your mindset, attitude, physical activity, and your emotions are the strongest players in your overall health. By choosing quality, homemade desserts over purchased varieties you can ensure that you're getting wholesome ingredients without eliminating sweet treats from your diet.

The following sections discuss how you can create a baking schedule.

Getting started

Here's what you need to do to plan ahead and make baking a part of your schedule:

>> **Start with a weekly calendar.** Purchase a planner or create your own.

>> **Write in each activity that you do each day.** Include work, household activities, exercise, socialization, errands, sleep, administrative tasks, and so on.

>> **Note pockets in your schedule that don't have anything planned.** Decide which of these activities you can do to shop, plan, and prep desserts in advance and write them in.

>> **Repeat the same process for an entire month.** After you've written down everything, continue the same schedule for a month so that it becomes a habit.

>> **If you have a pocket or two of a few hours each week, you can create your own food/desserts in them.** For example, if you have a few hours on a Saturday or Sunday free, this can be your designated time to make desserts that help you stay on track with your eating plan and health goals.

Figure 7-1 shows an example of how you can keep a calendar and plan out your meals and desserts.

If you find that you have 2 hours per week to dedicate to homemade dessert making, you can accomplish a lot, not rely on purchasing desserts, plus you can enjoy yourself in the process. If you only have a few hours a month, you can still make great desserts, taking advantage of the strategies in the section "Making Desserts in Advance" later in this chapter.

Fitting baking into your schedule

Nowadays people's schedules are busier than ever. Navigating harried work weeks, running kids around with afterschool activities, driving in congested traffic, and maintaining a household are all necessary and consuming activities that can't be changed. By switching up one of the variable schedule items, such as movie time, TV, social media, and dining out every now and then with baking time, you can fit it in and make time for it.

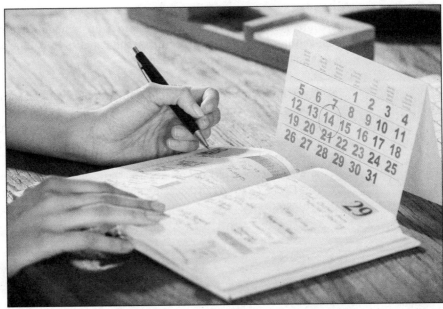

FIGURE 7-1:
Use a calendar to plan your meals and desserts for the week (and even month).

Andrey Popov/Adobe Stock Photos

SPENDING MORE TIME IN THE KITCHEN

It's often assumed that people in the past weren't as busy, and they had lives that weren't as demanding, and for that reason they had time to bake and make homemade desserts. But nothing could be further from the truth. Although life may have been simpler a century ago, being a homemaker was highly challenging. Women had to wash and iron all their laundry by hand. Without electricity and modern plumbing, even heating a stove was a major, tiresome product.

Getting ingredients was certainly more challenging, and cars weren't widely used yet. If people in those days could make things from scratch, I like to think I can easily do it, thanks to all the modern conveniences available today. Don't be discouraged; you get out of the kitchen what you put into it. By putting a bit of effort in, you'll reap the rewards in terms of health and taste. Hopefully, you'll even find some joy in the process.

Making your own desserts or trying to avoid making your own may sound frivolous if you've been diagnosed with diabetes, but that's not true. Nearly everyone craves desserts and will indulge in them from time to time. Imagining a life without ever eating a dessert is a sentence that few people, if anyone, would be able to handle. By taking control of the desserts along with the regular foods that you eat you can satisfy your desires (which prevents overeating and unhealthful binges) and regulate your blood glucose levels, which differs from the outdated "diet" model of avoiding all tasty foods in order to be healthy and enables you to enjoy positive nutrition in the long term.

Here are some ways to fit baking into your schedule (refer to the section "Reinventing Baking Day: Recognizing the Benefits to Baking with Others" later in this chapter for more information:

>> **If you have children, swap out another family event or activity for baking.** For example, a lot of people enjoy game or movie nights with kids. Once a month, try making a baking play date with the family. This night not only helps developing healthy eating habits and forming a useful skill, but it also strengthens the family bond. Allow your kids to get excited about baking and let them help pick out recipes. You can involve your kids when baking (see Figure 7-2); you can delegate simple tasks such as measuring or mixing the ingredients.

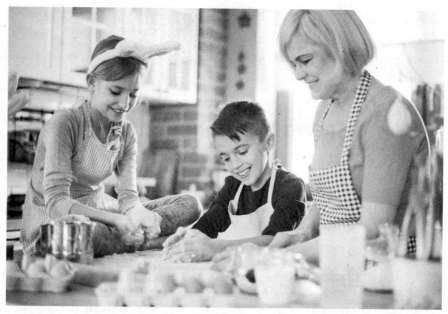

FIGURE 7-2:
You can bond with your kids or grandkids by baking together.

gpointstudio/Adobe Stock Photos

>> **If you live with a partner, use baking time to create your own traditions and reconnect with one another.** Take turns picking your favorite recipes.

>> **Involve your friends.** Friends can swap a coffee date or a lunch or restaurant out with time in the kitchen. Socialization is a key component to living well with or without diabetes.

>> **Make time for baking, even if you're single.** Baking alone can be rewarding and balancing and recenter you. Swap out some movie/TV, social media, or other another regular activity for baking.

Making desserts on your own may seem like a challenge, but it can turn out to be one of your favorite activities. If you're not an avid cook or baker already, pledge to take the challenge. Decide that you want to create the best tasting good-for-you desserts possible and enjoy yourself in the process. In my *Mediterranean Lifestyle For Dummies* (John Wiley & Sons, Inc.) book, I write about the joy of cooking and the pleasure principle — how the activities we enjoy most are the best for it.

Believe it or not, you can learn to love cooking and baking. Psychologists believe that cooking and baking are both therapeutic because they cause behavioral activation, a type of therapy that alleviates depression, anxiety and ADHD by increasing goal-oriented behavior and preventing procrastination. The sense of control used in cooking and baking are mentally empowering and require constant focused attention, which is affectionately called *tasty meditation.*

Creating a plan to make desserts

After you decide the time to make desserts in your schedule, start to develop your plan. Here are some tips that can help:

>> **Earmark or make copies of the recipes in this book that you want to make and notice the time it takes to make them.** When making grocery lists, refer to them and add the ingredients of what you want to bake.

>> **Be sure to have all ingredients at hand.** A grocery list or ordering food prior to when you plan to bake will help. Chapter 6 includes a list you can use.

>> **Before you begin baking or cooking, be sure to have all the ingredients prepped and measured out.** Referred to as the French term *mise en place,* this strategy can save you time when you're actually mixing ingredients. It makes the baking process run more smoothly. Mise en place also includes oiling all pans and baking sheets so everything is ready to go.

>> **Store the desserts properly so that they'll be ready when needed.** If freezing, be sure to allow enough thawing time before serving.

DOCTOR SAYS

According to Dr. Simon Poole in our *Diabetes Meal Planning & Nutrition For Dummies,* Second Edition, "Having a plan in advance equips you to resist the powerful biological, psychological, and social influences that lead to overconsumption and consumption of the wrong foods. When your plan is consistent with healthy eating for diabetes management, you can not only leave the stress of thinking about food behind while you're eating out, but you can also truly enjoy and feel good about what you're eating."

Making Desserts in Advance

Make-ahead desserts are a host's best friend. In fact, they're the first items I make when preparing a menu because I purposely choose desserts that I can prepare and freeze. When I'm entertaining, all I need to do is pull them out of the freezer, thaw them, and serve. If you only have a bit of time per month to make desserts in advance, you can still benefit from them all month long.

REMEMBER

Here are some make-ahead desserts that live up to their name:

- » **Brownies:** Brownies are quick and easy to make and can be frozen for up to a month! Check out Chapter 10 for some recipes.

- » **Squares:** You can make squares and bars several days ahead and freeze them. Head to Chapter 10.

- » **Cookies and biscotti:** They last several days at room temp and can be frozen. Refer to Chapter 11 more recipes.

- » **Spoon desserts:** Most puddings, trifles, tiramisu, and such, need to chill several hours in the refrigerator so they're always better made the day before. Check out the recipes in Chapter 12.

- » **Frozen desserts:** They need time to freeze, so make them in advance. Chapter 14 has some tasty options.

- » **Tarts and pies:** You can bake tarts and pies a day or two in advance and refrigerated until serving. Refer to Chapter 15 for diabetes-friendly recipes.

- » **Cakes:** With the exception of the Upside-Down Kiwi Cake in Chapter 17, you can make all the recipes in advance and freeze them for up to a month.

TIP

To plan ahead and make desserts in advance, check out the other recipes in Part 3 and decide which ones you like the most and whether or not you need to store them overnight, for longer periods, or a combination of both. For example, if you only have 2 hours to make desserts each week or month, I suggest making three of the desserts from the preceding list during each session to freeze.

Whipping Together Last-Minute Desserts

If you have unexpected guests or are looking for a nutritious dessert to satisfy a craving in lieu of storebought versions, never fear! You can create something quickly that's nutritious and tasty in less time than it takes to go to the grocery store or order out.

Just because they only take a few minutes to make doesn't mean that last-minute desserts are less impressive or satisfying. Consider the following recipes to save the day:

>> Fresh Fruit Kabobs, Mixed Berry Compote, Cantaloupe in White Balsamic Vinegar (refer to Chapter 9)

>> Chocolate Oatmeal No-Bake Cookies (see Chapter 11)

>> Chocolate Almond Pudding, Mixed Berry and Mascarpone Parfaits, Almond and Cherry Clafoutis (flip to Chapter 12)

>> Date, Almond, and Cocoa Balls, Stuffed Figs dipped in Chocolate (see Chapter 13)

>> All the sweet drinks in Chapter 16

TIP

You can't make desserts at the last minute if you don't have the ingredients on hand. Be sure to keep fresh fruit, frozen berries, oats, dark cocoa, almonds, plain Greek yogurt, dried dates, dried figs, and dark chocolate in your fridge and pantry along with ingredients for any of the special recipes mentioned in the preceding list (that way you can turn to them whenever needed).

TIP

If you're attending a meal at someone's home, going for a visit, or participating in a potluck or an event when you're asked to bring a dish, I suggest you take a dessert. Most events have some type of healthful food being offered, but party desserts tend to be overly sugary and full of fat. By bringing a dessert such as the preceding recipes, you're contributing something sweet that everyone can enjoy without derailing your nutrition plan.

Reinventing Baking Day: Recognizing the Benefits to Baking with Others

During much of history, when homemaking was a profession consisting of necessary activities to sustain a family that have since been industrialized, women partook in baking days. From antiquity all the way through the beginning of the 20th century, a certain day of the week was dedicated to baking bread, biscuits, and sweet treats that a family would consume throughout the week.

In less industrialized parts of the world, baking days are still practiced. In some areas people bake their items in communal ovens and work together, creating both a communal and a ceremonial aspect to the ritual of baking.

Although today's society obviously doesn't *need* to bake for survival or out of necessity anymore and you can easily enjoy baked goods from around the world with the click of a finger, baking your own foods and making a habit out of it can provide nutritional and mental benefits.

Baking can also be a pleasurable form of therapy. In a 2016 study published in the *Journal of Positive Psychology*, the experience of 12 mental health service users who engaged in a baking study were analyzed. The results found that baking has many recognizable benefits for service users. Researchers followed people around in their daily activities for two weeks and discovered that when the research subjects performed seemingly ordinary tasks like cooking and baking, the subjects felt "more enthusiastic about their pursuits the next day."

Psychologists are also now using cooking and/or baking as a form of behavioral therapy. Tasks like weighing and measuring ingredients, which require a good deal of focus, can help to relieve stress in the same way that meditation does.

REMEMBER

Here are some benefits to baking:

>> **Provides stress relief:** It can also reduce stress hormones.

>> **Improves sleep and immune system:** Through relaxation and stress reduction, baking can help you to sleep better, which in turn improves your immune system.

>> **Lowers blood pressure:** The therapeutic properties of baking include the ability to create calmness, which in turn lowers blood pressure.

>> **Enhances creativity:** By providing a space to experiment with flavors, aromas, and textures, baking improves creativity.

>> **Boosts mood:** Because it forces you to be present in the moment, baking can improve mood.

>> **Stimulates all five senses which improves mental health:** People rely so heavily on all their senses when baking and cooking. Dopamine, often referred to as the *reward chemical,* which promotes happiness, is enhanced by completing tasks, eating food, and celebrating little wins — all part of baking.

>> **Strengthens relationships when done communally:** Like other shared activities, completing baking projects with others strengthens bonds.

>> **Increases self confidence levels:** Baking provides both a challenging and a rewarding activity that requires patience and skill. This helps to build confidence and create a sense of pride in the baker.

Are you convinced that baking is a worthwhile activity yet? If so, you can improve its efficacy when indulging in a regular basis. You may want to get friends or family involved. A baking partner, like an exercise partner, can help to keep you on track. Baking can also be a fun joint activity that helps to create stronger bonds.

REMEMBER

Reclaiming the wholistic benefits and interpreting them in modern terms for your physical and emotional health can be extremely rewarding. My baking days started with my maternal grandmother and my paternal grandfather. Going to their homes and preparing baked goods was the highlight of my youth. Those sessions included quality time, life lessons, and unsolicited therapy, teaching me the skills and love of baking that I take forward into my daily life and profession. I try to keep the baking day tradition alive weekly, which usually works out to Sunday with my current schedule. When I can't bake, because I have to travel or work, I notice that concentrating becomes more difficult for me, and I don't feel as creative. If I go too long without baking, I have to stop and spend time baking in order to re-center myself. I'm grateful to have this free tool and source of inspiration to be able to tap into when needed. I hope that others can embrace baking's beauty and power as well.

3

Preparing Diabetes-Friendly Desserts: The Recipes

IN THIS PART . . .

Discover how to make diabetes-friendly base recipes.

Figure out how to create fruit-based desserts, brownies, bars, and cookies.

Create spoon desserts, puddings, truffles, and fruit-based sweet treats.

Cool down with gelato, ice cream, frozen desserts, and sweet drinks.

Master how to make tarts, pies, and cakes.

Chapter **8**

Introducing Base Recipes to Your Kitchen

RECIPES IN THIS CHAPTER

⏱ **Homemade Pie Crust**

⏱ **Basic Tart Crust**

⏱ **Vanilla Cream Custard**

⏱ **Dark Chocolate Ganache**

⏱ **Light Fruit "Ganache"**

Understanding a few basics in the kitchen can ensure your recipes turn out just right. In addition, they help you to plan, save time and money, and ensure that you're eating fresh, wholesome ingredients. For this reason, professional pastry chefs learn the basics as building blocks for more complicated recipes. After you learn them, you'll be able to create not only the classics, but also mouthwatering new recipes.

This chapter explains how to make flaky crusts, creamy custards, and rich, decadent ganache from scratch. I also introduce variations to increase your dessert repertoire.

Baking Crusts

A good crust is the key to a great pie, crostata (Italian-style tarte), tarte (thinner pastry without a top layer), and quiche (unsweetened pastry with savory filling), but the convenience of store-bought versions has led people to believe that they're hard to make. Many storebought versions, however, contain additives and other ingredients that people with diabetes should avoid.

Making your own wholesome crusts enables you to whip up delicious and diabetes-friendly desserts in no time. With a few techniques under your sleeve and the proper ingredients, you can have the tools you need to make a restaurant-worthy creation.

A BRIEF HISTORY OF BAKING CRUSTS

Elaborate bakeries in Ancient Egypt dating back to the Old Kingdom showed baked goods being made in large quantities and created the first version of what is now known as pie crust. In fact, ancient Egyptian *fateer,* which is comprised of layers of thin, sweet or savory filled pastry is still enjoyed today.

The ancient Greeks also used pie pastry in their diets. The ancient Romans used pastry dough to create the predecessor to modern cheesecake (their filling was savory). By the Middle Ages, pies were commonplace in many areas of the world.

In Great Britain the word "pie" referred to fish or meat encased in pastry. Queen Elizabeth first enjoyed cherry pie — and it became a staple in the British court and has been ever since. The English brought their love of pies to America, which of course, created their own spin on the beloved treat.

Homemade Pie Crust

PREP TIME: 5 MIN	COOK TIME: 20-30 MIN	YIELD: 8 SERVINGS

INGREDIENTS

1½ cups (168g) almond flour

1 tablespoon (21g) raw honey

¼ teaspoon (1.2g) sea salt

1 tablespoon (13.3g) Amy Riolo Selections or other EVOO

1 large egg

DIRECTIONS

1 In a medium bowl with a wooden spoon, stir together the almond flour, honey, and sea salt. Stir in the EVOO and egg until the dough comes together and resembles coarse crumbs.

2 Turn out into a 9-inch glass or ceramic pie plate. Press firmly with your fingers into the bottom and along the sides of the pie plate. Use a flat-bottomed glass to even out the bottom and prick the bottom with a fork.

3 If baking unfilled, heat the oven to 325 degrees F (160 degrees C) and bake until the edges are golden brown, about 20 minutes. To bake a filled pie, bake the unfilled crust 10 to 12 minutes and let the pie crust cool before adding the fillings. After it's filled, bake for an additional 10 to 15 minutes, or until desired doneness is achieved.

TIP: When baking a filled pie for the second time, cover the edges in foil to avoid overbrowning. You can also use this same dough to fill smaller pie shells to make individual pies.

NOTE: I specifically chose the combination of almond flour and olive oil for this pie crust because they taste great, have fantastic texture, and are two of the most nutritious ingredients that someone with diabetes could consume. You can bake this (unfilled) pie crust in advance, store it in the refrigerator overnight, and fill it the next day. Be sure to allow a few hours for the filling to set.

VARY IT! You may swap out whole-wheat flour, or finely crumbled cookies instead of the almond flour and melted butter for the olive oil. Make it chocolate by adding ¼ dark cocoa powder to the almond flour mixture.

PER SERVING: *Calories 153 (From Fat 115); Fat 13g (Saturated 1g); Cholesterol 26mg; Sodium 68mg; Carbohydrate 7g (Dietary Fiber 3g); Protein 5g; Sugars 3g.*

🍅 Basic Tart Crust

PREP TIME: 10 MIN | COOK TIME: 20 MIN | YIELD: 12 SERVINGS

INGREDIENTS

¾ cup (127.5g) quinoa flour

¼ cup (50g) date sugar

1 teaspoon (2.6g) ground cinnamon

⅓ cup (41g) finely chopped walnuts

3 tablespoons (42.5g) cold, unsalted butter, cut into small cubes, plus extra for greasing pan

DIRECTIONS

1 Mix the flour, sugar, cinnamon, and walnuts in a medium bowl.

2 Using the back of a fork or a pastry cutter, incorporate the butter into the mixture a few pieces at a time until a dough is formed (pieces of butter should be exposed). If dough is too loose, add in a tablespoon of very cold water at a time, and mix until it forms a dough.

3 Grease a 9-inch fluted tart pan with a removable bottom with butter. Press the dough into the prepared pan, ensuring to cover the bottom and sides evenly.

4 Freeze the tart shell for 30 minutes. Then, preheat oven to 425 degrees F (220 degrees C). Bake 10 minutes. Reduce the oven setting to 350 degrees (180 degrees C). Add the filling and bake until the filling is set, about 15 to 20 minutes. Cool 1 hour on a wire rack. Refrigerate if not serving immediately or fill with your favorite tart ingredients.

TIP: Premade shells come in handy for desserts and quiches. If using for a savory recipe, omit the sugar.

NOTE: You can purchase quinoa flour from the supermarket or make your own by grinding quinoa in a food processor until it's fine, and has a flour-like consistency.

VARY IT! Substitute almond flour, coconut flour, whole-wheat flour, or a combination of flours for the quinoa flour.

PER SERVING: *Calories 102 (From Fat 50); Fat 6g (Saturated 2g); Cholesterol 8mg; Sodium 1mg; Carbohydrate 12g (Dietary Fiber 1g); Protein 2g; Sugars 4g.*

Whipping Up Custard

Homemade custards are great basics to have on hand when making desserts. A *custard* is a dessert made of eggs, sugar, and milk, either baked, boiled, or frozen. They can be used to fill pie or tart shells, eaten on their own or with fruit, or layered in sophisticated desserts. In terms of cooking methods, custards can be stirred, steamed, or baked. Custards made without eggs but with the addition of a thickening agent are considered puddings.

The classic custards include

>> **Crème Anglaise:** It translates to "English cream" in French and is a pouring custard, or a thin custard, with a rich and silky feel. Because of its consistency, it makes a wonderful sauce but can't be used as a filling because it's too thin and will simply run out of the pie or tart crust. Bread puddings often use Crème Anglaise as a base and/or garnishing sauce.

>> **Pastry cream:** Also referred to as *crème patissiere*, this cream is a thicker custard that's used to fill different desserts such as choux pastry, profiteroles, cream puffs, eclairs, tarts, and cakes. French pastry cream is usually thickened with cornstarch while the Italian version uses flour.

Meanwhile, here are some variations to custard:

>> **Baked custard:** Heated milk tempered with eggs (or egg yolks) and baked in the oven to make the runny custard.

>> **Baked custard pie filling:** Made by mixing usually milk or cream, sugar, eggs, and flavoring and then poured into an unbaked or pre-baked pie shell and baked until the custard is set.

>> **Bavarois:** Crème Anglaise with gelatin and whipped cream folded in. This custard is then set in fluted molds and refrigerated before serving.

>> **Crème brulee:** Baked custard with caramelized sugar on top.

>> **Cremeux:** Crème Anglaise mixed with dark or white chocolate and allowed to set.

>> **Diplomat cream:** Also referred to as *crème diplomat*, pastry cream that has whipped cream folded into it and is also used for a filling of many desserts.

>> **Mousseline cream:** Also referred to as *crème mousseline*, pastry cream with butter added in for an increasingly rich consistency.

Vanilla Cream Custard

PREP TIME: 5 MIN	COOK TIME: 15 MIN	YIELD: 8 SERVINGS

INGREDIENTS

2 cups (473mL) whole milk

1 teaspoon (4.2g) pure vanilla

4 eggs yolks

½ cup (100g) date sugar

4 tablespoons (31g) all-purpose flour

DIRECTIONS

1 Pour the milk into a saucepan. Add the vanilla and bring to a boil over medium heat.

2 In a medium bowl, beat the egg yolks in a bowl with the date sugar. Then, with a whisk, incorporate the flour, whisking continuously.

3 After the milk begins to boil, remove it from the heat and slowly add the egg, sugar, and flour mixture, whisking as you go. The resulting mixture should be soft and creamy.

4 Transfer the mixture to the stove over medium heat. Stir continuously until the cream becomes dense and coats the back of a spoon, about 10 to 15 minutes.

5 Transfer the cream to a bowl and cover with plastic wrap and let it cool in the refrigerator. Be sure to cover the bowl well so that a film doesn't form on the surface of the cream.

TIP: Make the custard a day ahead of time to make prep easier.

NOTE: This recipe is for a classic Italian pastry cream, which is the base of many desserts and can be enjoyed on its own, in a pie or tart, or as a filling in more complicated pastries.

VARY IT! Add ¼ cup (31g) of dark cocoa powder in with the vanilla in Step 1 to make a chocolate custard. You may also add lemon or other citrus zest and the flavorings of your choice.

PER SERVING: Calories 134 (From Fat 38); Fat 4g (Saturated 2g); Cholesterol 111mg; Sodium 31mg; Carbohydrate 19g (Dietary Fiber 0g); Protein 4g; Sugars 16g.

Making Ganache

Ganache is an emulsion of solid chocolate and a liquid, usually cream, milk, or fruit pulp. It can be used as a glaze, icing, sauce, or filling for pastries, and provides a decadent, lush mouthfeel that pleases the tastebuds.

Types of ganache include

» **Dark chocolate ganache:** 1:1 ratio of chocolate to cream, milk, or fruit puree

» **Milk chocolate ganache:** 1.5:1 ratio of chocolate to cream, milk, or fruit puree

» **White chocolate:** 2.5:1 ratio of chocolate to cream, milk, or fruit puree

TIP

To cut down on the fat content of the classic ganache recipe, I suggest substituting unsweetened fruit puree instead of cream. You can also use whole milk in place of heavy cream, although it will produce a slightly thinner result. Dark chocolate (the higher the percentage the better) is a good choice, when consumed in small amounts, for people with diabetes because it can be beneficial in balancing blood sugar levels (refer to the Dark Chocolate Ganache recipe in this section).

Dark Chocolate Ganache

PREP TIME: 5 MIN	COOK TIME: 15 MIN	YIELD: 12 SERVINGS

INGREDIENTS

¾ cup (177mL) heavy cream

¾ cup (99g) 70 percent or higher dark chocolate, chopped

DIRECTIONS

1 Place a medium saucepan over a double boiler. Pour in the heavy cream and the chocolate pieces.

2 Heat the double boiler on high heat and stir continuously. As the chocolate melts, switch to a whisk and continue stirring until you create a thick smooth chocolate sauce, then set aside to cool until preferred temperature is reached.

3 Store the leftover ganache in an airtight container in the refrigerator.

TIP: To make the ganache more quickly, you can skip the double boiler and place the cream and chocolate in a saucepan directly over a medium flame. Be sure to stir constantly and don't let the mixture boil in order to emulsify it properly.

NOTE: A little bit of chocolate ganache goes a long way. You can use it to decorate cakes, pies, ice cream, and tortes.

VARY IT! Substitute ¾ of your favorite (sugar-free) fruit puree for the heavy cream in this recipe for a healthier and fruity-flavored ganache.

PER SERVING: *Calories 101 (From Fat 81); Fat 9g (Saturated 5g); Cholesterol 21mg; Sodium 7mg; Carbohydrate 4g (Dietary Fiber 1g); Protein 1g; Sugars 2g.*

Light Fruit "Ganache"

| PREP TIME: 5 MIN | COOK TIME: 15 MIN | YIELD: 12 SERVINGS |

INGREDIENTS

¾ cup (177mL) whole milk

¾ cup (174g) pureed fresh fruit such as berries, mango, or cooked pears

DIRECTIONS

1 Place a medium saucepan over a double boiler. Pour in the milk and the pureed fruit.

2 Heat the double boiler on high heat and stir continuously. As the ingredients combine, switch to a whisk and continue stirring until you create a thick smooth sauce, then set aside to cool until preferred temperature is reached.

3 Store the leftover "ganache" in an airtight container in the refrigerator.

TIP: Use this mixture as a filling for cakes or pies and on ice cream.

PER SERVING: *Calories 14 (From Fat 5); Fat 1g (Saturated 0g); Cholesterol 2mg; Sodium 7mg; Carbohydrate 2g (Dietary Fiber 0g); Protein 1g; Sugars 2g.*

Chapter **9**

Focusing on Fruit-Based Desserts

RECIPES IN THIS CHAPTER

- 🍎 **Watermelon, Cantaloupe, Kiwi, Feta, and Mint Mosaic**
- 🍎 **Fresh Fruit Kabobs**
- 🍎 **Cantaloupe in White Balsamic Vinegar**
- 🍎 **Baked Spice & Almond Stuffed Apples**
- 🍎 **Broiled Figs & Balsamic Reduction**
- 🍎 **Mixed Berry Compote**
- 🍎 **Kiwi and Raspberry Trees with Honey**
- 🍎 **Summer Berry and Fresh Fig Salad**
- 🍎 **Watermelon "Cake"**
- 🍎 **Turkish-Stuffed Apricots**
- 🍎 **Broiled Pineapple with Yogurt and Honey**

F ruit is often on the tip of many peoples' tongues when discussing forbidden foods for people with diabetes. Many individuals with diabetes diagnoses completely cut fruit out of their life because they believe that it will cause their blood sugar to spike. The truth of the matter, however, is that fruit can and should be a part of a diabetes-friendly diet and is a better choice than heavier, sugar-, and processed-flour laden treats.

This chapter explores how you can incorporate fruit into your lifestyle in order to satisfy your sweet tooth and keep your blood glucose balanced at the same time.

Transforming Fruit into Dessert

Per Mediterranean diet guidelines, you should be consuming 9 to 12 portions of fresh fruits and vegetables per day. Unfortunately many people fall short. Leafy greens, cruciferous, and a wide

- Poached Pears with Vanilla and Cardamom Cream
- Cherries with Goat Cheese and Pistachios
- Roasted Plums with Mascarpone Cheese
- Avocado, Yogurt, and Mango Salad
- Seasonal Italian Fruit Platter
- Grape, Goat Cheese, and Almond Skewers

variety of rainbow-colored vegetables should play a major role in meals for people with diabetes. And if you're trying to stay healthy and eat desserts, which I bet you are because you're reading this book, then you want to eat fruit, which can make delicious snacks and desserts while helping you increase your daily intake of fresh produce.

All carbohydrates contain sugars and are a necessary and nutrient-rich part of a healthy and balanced diet. Parts 1 and 2 discuss the best types of carbohydrates to eat, especially for people with prediabetes and diabetes. When adding sugars, evidence is beginning to emerge to suggest that for most people unprocessed or *raw*, which retains natural antioxidant, anti-inflammatory, and antimicrobial compounds might be better at controlling blood glucose and insulin response than other added sugars.

The high-quality carbs and natural sugars found in fruit are much better for you compared to those found in processed foods. In addition, fresh fruit contains antioxidants and polyphenols, which are beneficial to your health. (Refer to Chapters 2 and 3 where I discuss the benefits to eating fruit in your desserts.)

The following desserts in this section are the most healthful in the book and the ones that you should eat on a regular basis:

» **Watermelon, Cantaloupe, Kiwi, Feta, and Mint Mosaic:** A beautiful and nutritious sweet treat that you can also start your day with

» **Fresh Fruit Kabobs:** Perfect for parties and outdoor gatherings — even kids love it

» **Cantaloupe in White Balsamic Vinegar:** An Italian summertime classic that adds elegance to any meal

» **Baked Spice & Almond Stuffed Apples:** A satisfying fall dessert

» **Broiled Figs & Balsamic Reduction:** Easy to make and nutritious to eat

» **Mixed Berry Compote:** Delicious on its own or as homemade pie filling

» **Kiwi and Raspberry Trees with Honey:** A festive addition to holiday dessert and breakfast tables

» **Summer Berry and Fresh Fig Salad:** A delightful way to end a meal European style

» **Watermelon "Cake":** A delicious alternative to a traditional cake

Watermelon, Cantaloupe, Kiwi, Feta, and Mint Mosaic

PREP TIME: 30 MIN | YIELD: 4 SERVINGS

INGREDIENTS

½ pound (227g) of watermelon (without rind)

½ pound (227g) of cantaloupe (without rind)

½ pound (227g) kiwifruit (approximately 4)

8 ounces (227g) block plain feta cheese (not crumbled)

1 bunch fresh mint leaves, whole

DIRECTIONS

1 Cube the fruit and cheese into equal-sized 1-inch (2.5 cm) pieces and place one piece of watermelon, cantaloupe, kiwi, and cheese on a plate in a row, alternating the fruit and cheese pieces.

2 Stick toothpicks in the middle of each piece of fruit on the bottom layer. Continue layering different fruits and cheese on top of each (for example, place cantaloupe on top of watermelon, kiwi on top of cantaloupe, cheese on top of kiwi, and watermelon on top of cheese).

3 Continue layering until you have at least three rows on top creating a cube-like appearance. Garnish with spearmint sprigs. Refrigerate until serving.

TIP: Precut the fruit a day in advance to save time assembling. Even though this recipe takes a few minutes to assemble, the effort is worth it because it makes a beautiful edible centerpiece for the table.

NOTE: This recipe includes feta cheese because it's a low-calorie protein choice. It also has the second lowest salt content among cheeses and contains probiotics that can help improve gut and digestion. Seek authentic feta made from sheep and goat milk cheese that has a wide range of vitamins beneficial to people with diabetes.

VARY IT! All you need to make this beautiful mosaic are two kinds of fruit. You can use just watermelon and cantaloupe, honey dew and watermelon, or kiwi with melon, if desired.

PER SERVING: Calories 223 (From Fat 113); Fat 13g (Saturated 9g); Cholesterol 50mg; Sodium 646mg; Carbohydrate 20g (Dietary Fiber 3g); Protein 10g; Sugars 15g.

🍑 Fresh Fruit Kabobs

PREP TIME: 10 MIN | **YIELD: 5 SERVINGS**

INGREDIENTS

10 strawberries, hulled

10 (1-inch) (2.54cm) cubes cantaloupe

10 (1-inch) (2.54cm) cubes fresh pineapple

3 kiwi, peeled and sliced

20 red raspberries

1 cup (227g) plain Greek yogurt

1 teaspoon (7g) honey

4 tablespoons (28g) ground flaxseeds

DIRECTIONS

1   If using wooden or bamboo skewers, remove all the splinters by rolling two skewers together in your hands or rubbing them over each other as if you're sharpening a knife.

2   Thread a strawberry onto a skewer. Then thread the cantaloupe, pineapple, and kiwi, and finish the skewer with 2 raspberries on the pointed end. Make sure to push the raspberries up high so they don't slip off the skewer. Repeat with the remaining skewers.

3   Combine the yogurt, honey, and flaxseeds in a small serving bowl. Place the bowl on a serving platter and surround with fruit kabobs. Serve immediately or store in the refrigerator overnight until serving.

TIP: Slice the kiwi in half and scoop out the flesh with a spoon before slicing.

NOTE: The addition of yogurt and flaxseeds provide glucose-balancing protein and healthful fats to the recipe.

NOTE: Use ten 5-to 6-inch wooden or metal skewers.

VARY IT! Use your favorite seasonal fruits when making this recipe. Peaches, apricots, plums, and other berries all make great choices.

PER SERVING *(2 kabobs): Calories 126 (From Fat 33); Fat 4g (Saturated 1g); Cholesterol 5mg; Sodium 22mg; Carbohydrate 19g (Dietary Fiber 4g); Protein 7g; Sugars 11g.*

Cantaloupe in White Balsamic Vinegar

PREP TIME: 15 MIN, PLUS OVERNIGHT CHILLING	YIELD: 6 SERVINGS

INGREDIENTS

1 cantaloupe, washed and halved

⅓ cup (79mL) Amy Riolo Selections White Balsamic or other quality balsamic vinegar

½ teaspoon (2.4g) sea salt

½ cup (61.5g) shelled pistachios, ground

DIRECTIONS

1 Use a melon baller to scoop out balls of melon (or cut into 1-inch pieces) and place into a large bowl. Pour vinegar over the cantaloupe, sprinkle with sea salt, and mix to combine. Cover the bowl and refrigerate overnight or for at least six hours.

2 To serve, scoop equal portions of melon into 6 ice cream bowls. Sprinkle with pistachios and serve.

TIP: In Italy, balsamic vinegar is often used to macerate and coax the natural sweet flavors out of fruit. Be sure to choose balsamic vinegars that are traditionally aged and free from caramel and sugar. Amy Riolo Selections White Balsamic vinegar has an especially sweet flavor (without any added ingredients) because it's made with only Trebbiano grapes and aged in barrels in the same way that traditional balsamic is.

NOTE: Several studies have been conducted on the benefits of consuming balsamic vinegar with high glycemic foods to reduce blood sugar.

VARY IT! Strawberries and balsamic vinegar are a classic Italian combination that can be served alone or as a topping for ice cream, frozen yogurt, or puddings.

PER SERVING: *Calories 101 (From Fat 43); Fat 5g (Saturated 1g); Cholesterol 0mg; Sodium 174mg; Carbohydrate 13g (Dietary Fiber 2g); Protein 3g; Sugars 10g.*

Baked Spice & Almond Stuffed Apples

PREP TIME: 15 MIN	COOK TIME: 30 MIN	YIELD: 6 SERVINGS

INGREDIENTS

3 tablespoons (43g) Amy Riolo Selections or other EVOO

2 tablespoons (42g) honey

1 teaspoon (2.6g) ground cinnamon

½ teaspoon (1.3g) ground cloves

¼ cup (21g) old-fashioned whole rolled oats

¼ cup (21g) ground almonds

6 large apples (use whatever variety you prefer), rinsed and patted dry

DIRECTIONS

1 Preheat the oven to 425 degrees F (220 degrees C). To make the filling, combine the EVOO, honey, cinnamon, cloves, oats, and almonds in a medium bowl and mix with a wooden spoon to combine.

2 Using a sharp paring knife and a spoon or an apple corer, core the apples. Cut around the core, about halfway or three-quarters down into the apple.

3 Place the cored apples in a 9-inch baking pan, cake pan, or pie dish. Spoon the filling into each apple and top off. Pour warm water into the pan around the apples to cover up to an inch of the bottom of the apples (the water helps prevent the apples from drying out and burning).

4 Bake for 30 minutes or until the apples appear slightly soft. Bake longer for softer baked apples. The time depends on how firm your apples were and how soft you want them to be. When finished, remove the apples from the oven and baste the outside of the apples with juices from the pan. Serve immediately.

NOTE: This recipe includes anti-inflammatory spices as well as the anti-inflammatory and healthful fat in EVOO along with protein and healthful fats in almonds that balance out the natural sugars in the recipe.

VARY IT! Pears can be halved and filled with the same mixture. When peaches and plums are in season, they can be swapped out for the apples too.

PER SERVING: *Calories 232 (From Fat 84); Fat 9g (Saturated 1g); Cholesterol 0mg; Sodium 3mg; Carbohydrate 40g (Dietary Fiber 6g); Protein 2g; Sugars 29g.*

Broiled Figs & Balsamic Reduction

PREP TIME: 5 MIN	COOK TIME: 4 MIN	YIELD: 4 SERVINGS

INGREDIENTS

12 dried figs, stems peeled, soaked overnight in water to cover

12 almonds

2 whole black peppercorns

1 cinnamon stick

¼ cup (64g) Amy Riolo Selections White Balsamic or other quality balsamic vinegar

2 tablespoons (28g) mascarpone cheese

½ cup (113g) plain Greek yogurt

1 tablespoon (21g) honey

1 teaspoon (4.2g) vanilla

DIRECTIONS

1 Heat the broiler to high. Drain the figs and make a slit on one side. Stuff the insert with an almond and then place onto a baking sheet under broiler for 3 to 4 minutes or until the figs are plumped and tender.

2 Bring the peppercorns, cinnamon, and balsamic vinegar to a boil over high heat in a small saucepan. Reduce the heat and cook for 5 minutes or until it's reduced by two-thirds.

3 Remove from the heat and set aside. Combine the mascarpone, yogurt, honey, and vanilla in a small bowl and mix well to combine.

4 To serve, place three figs on each plate. Top with ¼ of the cheese mixture and drizzle some balsamic reduction over the top.

TIP: You can soak and stuff the almonds a few days in advance and store them in the refrigerator.

NOTE: Figs are high in fiber and are fat-free, cholesterol-free, and sodium-free. Stuffing them with almonds is a tradition in my ancestral homeland of Calabria, Italy. The almonds, yogurt, and cheese balance the natural sugars in the recipe.

PER SERVING: *Calories 174 (From Fat 62); Fat 7g (Saturated 4g); Cholesterol 10mg; Sodium 20mg; Carbohydrate 25g (Dietary Fiber 3g); Protein 5g; Sugars 20g.*

☺ Mixed Berry Compote

| PREP TIME: 5 MIN | COOK TIME: 5 MIN | YIELD: 4 SERVINGS |

INGREDIENTS

½ cup (74g) blueberries

¼ cup (36g) strawberries, trimmed and quartered

¼ cup (36g) blackberries

¼ cup (36g) red raspberries

1 tablespoon (8g) cornstarch dissolved in ¼ cup (60ml) water

1 cinnamon stick

¼ cup (85g) honey

1 cup (134g) macadamia nuts, finely chopped

DIRECTIONS

1   Combine the blueberries, strawberries, blackberries, and raspberries in a medium saucepan. Add the cornstarch mixture, cinnamon stick, and honey.

2   Bring to a boil over high heat, reduce the heat to medium, stir slowly, and continue to cook 3 to 5 minutes until the mixture becomes thick like a pie filling.

3   Stir in the macadamia nuts. Remove from the heat and allow to cool. Discard the cinnamon stick. Allow to cool to room temperature and serve. Store the remaining mixture in an airtight container in the refrigerator for up to a week or the freezer for up to a month.

TIP: This mixture can be eaten alone or used to top toast or yogurt, or as a nutritious, pie filling alternative.

NOTE: The nuts and cinnamon balance out the natural sugars in the fruits.

VARY IT! Swap macadamia nuts for almonds. If you have a nut allergy, omit the macadamia nuts and serve the ¼ of the mixture over a bed of ¼ cup (61g) plain Greek yogurt, cottage cheese, or ricotta cheese. If fresh berries aren't in season, swap out frozen.

PER SERVING: *Calories 333 (From Fat 231); Fat 26g (Saturated 4g); Cholesterol 0mg; Sodium 90mg; Carbohydrate 29g (Dietary Fiber 4g); Protein 3g; Sugars 22g.*

Kiwi and Raspberry Trees with Honey

PREP TIME: 15 MIN | YIELD: 4 SERVINGS

INGREDIENTS

4 kiwifruit peeled (save skin), and sliced

2 tablespoons (23g) pomegranate arils

2 tablespoons (15g) red raspberries

1 slice pineapple

1 teaspoon (7g) honey

DIRECTIONS

1 Arrange the kiwi slices on a plate in the shape of Christmas tree. Sprinkle with the pomegranate arils to look like decorations.

2 Place the pineapple slice on a cutting board and use a small star cookie cutter to cut out a star. Place on top of the tree.

3 Place the raspberries in various places around the tree to resemble ornaments.

4 Drizzle with honey. Use the remaining kiwi skin to create a tree trunk.

TIP: This festive dish is fun to serve at Christmas time because it's shaped like an evergreen tree. It can be a nutritious dessert or a creative addition to a brunch table.

NOTE: Make this dish ahead of time by preparing the whole recipe (except the addition of the honey). Add the honey at the time of serving. If you aren't eating this recipe immediately after a meal or with other foods that contain protein and healthful fat, be sure to enjoy it with a handful of raw almonds, Greek yogurt, peanut butter, or cheese to balance the sugar levels.

NOTE: Refer to the color insert for a photo of this recipe.

PER SERVING: *Calories 68 (From Fat 4); Fat 0g (Saturated 0g); Cholesterol 0mg; Sodium 3mg; Carbohydrate 17g (Dietary Fiber 3g); Protein 1g; Sugars 11g.*

Summer Berry and Fresh Fig Salad

PREP TIME: 10 MIN PLUS OVERNIGHT CHILLING	YIELD: 4 SERVINGS

INGREDIENTS

1 cup (5 small or 200g) fresh figs, trimmed and quartered

½ cup (62g) raspberries

½ cup (72g) strawberries, thinly sliced

½ cup (74g) blueberries

¼ cup (85g) honey

Juice of half a lemon

¼ cup (23g) finely chopped fresh mint, plus 4 whole mint leaves

1 cup (246g) whipped ricotta cheese

DIRECTIONS

1 Combine all the fruit in a large salad bowl. Mix the honey, lemon juice, and mint together in a small bowl. Drizzle the honey mixture over the fruit and mix gently to combine.

2 Cover the bowl and store in the refrigerator for a minimum of 5 hours or maximum of overnight.

3 Transfer to individual bowls before serving. Garnish with whipped ricotta and a mint leaf, if desired.

TIP: This salad can pass for a dessert or snack and can even follow a traditional green salad in a meal.

NOTE: Use seasonal fruit in this recipe. Many types and species of fruit grow throughout the different seasons around the globe so you can vary this salad, depending on the time of the year.

NOTE: If you can't find whipped ricotta, you can whip it yourself by placing the ricotta in the bowl of a standing mixer with a whisk attachment or in a bowl with hand mixers and whip for a few minutes until light and fluffy.

VARY IT! When watermelon is in season, use it in place of figs and swap the ricotta for whipped feta.

PER SERVING: *Calories 237 (From Fat 76); Fat 8g (Saturated 5g); Cholesterol 31mg; Sodium 55mg; Carbohydrate 36g (Dietary Fiber 4g); Protein 8g; Sugars 29g.*

🍅 Watermelon "Cake"

PREP TIME: 30 MIN	YIELD: 8 SERVINGS

INGREDIENTS

1 seedless watermelon

1½ cups (222g) berries of your choice (blueberries, red raspberries, blackberries)

1 kiwifruit

½ cup (45g) fresh mint, divided

2 cups (453g) plain Greek yogurt

2 tablespoons (42g) honey

1 teaspoon (4.2g) vanilla

DIRECTIONS

1 Halve the watermelon vertically down the center. Using a 9-inch round cake pan as a guide, slice a circle out of the center of one of the watermelon sides and trim off the rind. Shape it into a perfect circle by removing all the white rind.

2 Using a 6-inch round cake pan or a 6-inch circular piece of paper as a guide, cut a 6-inch layer that's 4 inches deep out of the other side. With the leftover watermelon, carve out a 3-inch round slice that's also 4 inches deep.

3 Peel the kiwi and cut into 4 thick slices. Use a small cookie cutter or a cutout from a piece of paper to shape them into stars. Place the largest layer of watermelon on a serving platter and insert a few toothpicks halfway in the middle. Add the 6-inch layer, pressing down on the toothpicks so that they adhere. Using the same technique with the toothpicks, layer the 3-inch piece on top.

4 Scatter berries and kiwi stars around the sides and top of the watermelon, placing one star on the top. Scatter half of the mint leaves round the watermelon cake. Refrigerate until serving. Combine the remaining mint, yogurt, honey, and vanilla in a small bowl. Mix well to incorporate the ingredients, cover, and chill until serving. When ready to serve, slice the cake into 8 equal size pieces and top with berries and a few tablespoons of the yogurt mixture.

NOTE: Refer to the color insert for a photo of this recipe.

PER SERVING: *Calories 270 (From Fat 13); Fat 1g (Saturated 0g); Cholesterol 6mg; Sodium 54mg; Carbohydrate 53g (Dietary Fiber 3g); Protein 17g; Sugars 40g.*

Preparing Creamy Fruit and Dairy Desserts

Sweet is one of the basic tastes, just like sour and salty, and craving sweet foods is normal. The difference between sweetness and the other tastes, however, is that it's the first flavor infants perceive when they drink their mothers' milk. Because breastmilk is sweet, infants immediately correlate it with feelings of nourishment, satisfaction, safety, and comfort. Sweets, especially creamy ones, can pick you up when you're down and that's why consuming them often comforts you in the short term.

DOCTOR SAYS

Fruit is the go-to daily dessert in many parts of the world. Dr. Simon Poole recommends that combining fresh fruit with dairy for dessert is a great way to enjoy natural sweetness while increasing the fiber, vitamin, mineral, and antioxidant servings in your daily diet. When paired with a few healthful fats such as dairy and nuts, eating fresh fruit enables you to satisfy your sweet tooth while keeping your blood glucose levels in check.

Some fruits have a higher glycemic load (GL) than others, and every person may have a different blood glucose response to one fruit or another. Monitor these effects and find out which fruit is best for you.

The recipes in this section include the following:

- **»** **Turkish-Stuffed Apricots:** A sweet and spicy recipe that dates back to Ottoman times

- **»** **Broiled Pineapple with Yogurt and Honey:** A cool and refreshing dessert loaded with health benefits

- **»** **Poached Pears with Vanilla and Cardamom Cream:** A fall classic enriched with the intoxicating sweet aromas of vanilla and cardamom

- **»** **Cherries with Goat Cheese and Pistachios:** An unexpected pairing

- **»** **Roasted Plums with Mascarpone Cheese:** A decadent treat that will have you forgetting that it's good for you

- **»** **Avocado, Yogurt, and Mango Salad:** A unique way to enjoy favorite fruits

- **»** **Seasonal Italian Fruit Platter:** A traditional Italian way to end a weekday meal or serve after a sweeter dessert during a holiday meal

- **»** **Grape, Goat Cheese, and Almond Skewers:** A fun addition to a buffet

🍅 Turkish-Stuffed Apricots

| PREP TIME: 15 MIN | YIELD: 4 SERVINGS |

INGREDIENTS

1 cup (227g) plain Greek yogurt

1 teaspoon (2g)
ground cardamom

3 tablespoons (63g)
honey, divided

1 tablespoon (13.5g) Amy Riolo
Selections or other EVOO

1 cup (130g) dried no-sugar-
added apricots, soaked in
water overnight

Juice and zest 1 orange

2 tablespoons (15g) raw
pistachios, finely chopped

DIRECTIONS

1 Dry the apricots and make a slit in the middle to open them
(leaving the base intact), the same way that you'd slice a bun
to fill it but without cutting through the base.

2 In a medium bowl, combine the yogurt and cardamom, stirring until incorporated. Stir in a tablespoon of honey and the
EVOO. Then place the yogurt mixture into a pastry bag with a
wide tip or into a sealable plastic bag with the tip cut off in
order to fill the apricots. Pipe the yogurt mixture into the
apricots being sure to fill completely to the edges.

3 Dip the exposed yogurt into the pistachios and arrange onto
a serving platter.

4 In a small saucepan, bring the remaining 2 tablespoons honey,
orange juice, and zest to a boil over high heat. Reduce the heat
to low and allow to simmer for 5 to 10 minutes or until the
mixture becomes thick and syrupy. Drizzle over the pistachios. Allow to cool slightly and serve.

TIP: This decadent no-cook/bake dessert that dates to Ottoman times traditionally uses cream as a filling instead of yogurt. I replace the cream for
yogurt and add citrus juice and zest to make it more appropriate for
blood sugar balancing.

NOTE: Cardamom is rich in antioxidants, particularly compounds called
cineole and limonene, which may have anti-inflammatory and digestive
benefits. It also contains minerals like potassium and magnesium, supporting heart health.

VARY IT! Use dates, raisins, dried figs, and your favorite nuts instead of
apricots and pistachios.

PER SERVING: Calories 264 (From Fat 53); Fat 6g (Saturated 1g);
Cholesterol 6mg; Sodium 62mg; Carbohydrate 41g (Dietary Fiber 3g);
Protein 15g; Sugars 32g.

Broiled Pineapple with Yogurt and Honey

PREP TIME: 5 MIN	COOK TIME: 3 MIN	YIELD: 4 SERVINGS

INGREDIENTS

8 fresh pineapple rings, or chunks, if preferred

3 tablespoons (63g) honey

½ cup (113g) plain Greek yogurt

1 teaspoon (2.6g) cinnamon

1 tablespoon (5.7g) finely chopped fresh mint

DIRECTIONS

1 Preheat the broiler. Place the pineapple on a baking sheet and watching carefully, broil it for 2 to 3 minutes or until golden. Remove from the oven, drizzle with 1 tablespoon (21g) honey, and set aside.

2 Combine the honey with yogurt and cinnamon and whisk until you achieve a smooth cream.

3 To serve, place 2 of the pineapple rings on individual dessert plates. Top each plate with ¼ of the yogurt mixture, and garnish with fresh mint.

TIP: Pineapple is a good source of vitamin C and manganese, contributing to immune health and bone formation. It contains bromelain, an enzyme with anti-inflammatory properties that may aid in digestion. Cinnamon contains cinnamaldehyde, a compound with antioxidant and anti-inflammatory properties. It may help regulate blood sugar levels and contribute to heart health.

NOTE: You can prepare the pineapple rings on a preheated grill or grill pan.

VARY IT! Fresh peach and apricot halves can also be prepared in the same manner as the pineapple.

PER SERVING: *Calories 144 (From Fat 4); Fat 0g (Saturated 0g); Cholesterol 3mg; Sodium 25mg; Carbohydrate 31g (Dietary Fiber 2g); Protein 7g; Sugars 24g.*

Poached Pears with Vanilla and Cardamom Cream

PREP TIME: 5 MIN	COOK TIME: 20 MIN	YIELD: 4 SERVINGS

INGREDIENTS

4 Bosc pears, peeled

2 tablespoons (30.5g) lemon juice

5 cardamom pods

4 tablespoons (84g) honey, divided

1 cup (246g) whole milk ricotta

1 teaspoon (2g) ground cardamom

1 teaspoon (4.2g) vanilla

DIRECTIONS

1 Place the pears in a medium saucepan and cover with water. Add the lemon juice, cardamom, and 2 tablespoons honey. Bring to boil over high heat, reduce the heat to medium low, and simmer, about 20 minutes or until the pears are tender. Turn off the heat and drain pears.

2 Mix the ricotta, cardamom, vanilla, and remaining 2 tablespoons honey together and place in a small bowl.

3 Spoon 4 equal portions of ricotta cream onto 4 dessert plates and use the back of a spoon to spread around into a thick circle. When the pears are cool enough to handle, stand them upright in the middle of the ricotta. If the pears fall over, slice off the bottoms to make them stand firmly. Serve immediately.

TIP: This is a simple and elegant dessert that can also be served for breakfast.

NOTE: Pears are a low GI food, which can help control blood sugar and lower your chances of type 2 diabetes and stroke.

VARY IT! Swap apples for the pears. You can use a nut butter for the base instead of ricotta.

PER SERVING: Calories 263 (From Fat 74); Fat 8g (Saturated 5g); Cholesterol 31mg; Sodium 54mg; Carbohydrate 43g (Dietary Fiber 5g); Protein 8g; Sugars 32g.

Cherries with Goat Cheese and Pistachios

PREP TIME: 10 MIN	YIELD: 4 SERVINGS

INGREDIENTS

1 cup (138g) cherries, pitted whole

8 ounces (227g) goat cheese log

3 ounces (85g) pistachios

1 tablespoon (21g) honey

DIRECTIONS

1 Divide the cherries onto 4 dessert plates. Place 2 ounces of goat cheese onto each plate. Add 1 ounce of pistachios to each plate. Drizzle the honey over the goat cheese and serve.

TIP: Fruit, nut, and cheese platters are popular European desserts that also make great snacks.

NOTE: The combination of low GI cherries, which are a good source of carbohydrates along with the protein and healthful fats in goat cheese and pistachios, make this dish a balanced choice that will satisfy your sweet tooth while keeping blood sugar levels in check.

VARY IT! Substitute apples, pears, or fresh figs for the cherries and walnuts or almonds for the pistachios.

PER SERVING: *Calories 364 (From Fat 236); Fat 26g (Saturated 13g); Cholesterol 44mg; Sodium 235mg; Carbohydrate 17g (Dietary Fiber 3g); Protein 18g; Sugars 11g.*

⏾ Roasted Plums with Mascarpone Cheese

PREP TIME: 10 MIN	COOK TIME: 25 MIN	YIELD: 4 SERVINGS

INGREDIENTS

2 tablespoons (27g) Amy Riolo Selections or other EVOO, divided

4 ripe plums, pitted and halved

4 teaspoons (16.8g) date sugar

¾ cup (170g) plain Greek yogurt

¼ cup (56g) mascarpone

2 tablespoons (2.5g) finely chopped fresh basil

2 teaspoons (14g) honey, divided

DIRECTIONS

1 Preheat the oven to 400 degrees F (200 degrees C). Oil a large baking dish with ½ teaspoon (6.5g) olive oil and place inside the plums, cut side up, and sprinkle 1 teaspoon (4.2g) date sugar over each half of a plum. Bake, uncovered, for 25 minutes.

2 While the plums are baking, stir together the yogurt, mascarpone, basil, remaining 1½ tablespoons (21.5g) EVOO, and 1 teaspoon (7g) honey.

3 Spoon half of the yogurt mixture onto the bottom of each of 4 plates or a large serving platter.

4 When the plums are finished baking, remove them from the oven and place 2 halves over the yogurt on each plate. Fill the holes with the yogurt mixture, drizzle the remaining honey on each, and serve warm.

TIP: After completing Step 4, spoon the remaining yogurt mixture into a pastry bag fitted with a star tip and fill the plum that way for an elegant presentation.

NOTE: Make this recipe when plums are in season. Plums are a rich source of fiber and are a low GI fruit, making them an ideal fruit for people with diabetes and heart disease. Refer to the color insert for a photo of this recipe.

VARY IT! Use peaches instead of plums.

PER SERVING: Calories 207 (From Fat 133); Fat 15g (Saturated 7g); Cholesterol 25mg; Sodium 19mg; Carbohydrate 16g (Dietary Fiber 1g); Protein 6g; Sugars 14g.

Avocado, Yogurt, and Mango Salad

PREP TIME: 15MIN	YIELD: 4 SERVINGS

INGREDIENTS

2 avocados

1 mango

1 cup (227g) plain Greek yogurt

Juice and zest of 1 lime

1 tablespoon (13.5g) Amy Riolo Selections or other EVOO

2 tablespoons (42g) honey

DIRECTIONS

1 Slice the avocados in half, remove the pit and skin, and dice. Place into a large bowl. Slice the mango, remove the pit, scoop out the flesh, and cut the fruit into cubes (twice the size of the avocado). Place into the same bowl and top with lime juice. Toss to coat.

2 In a small bowl, combine the Greek yogurt, lime zest, EVOO, and honey and mix well to combine. Spoon the yogurt onto the bottom of 4 salad plates. Top each plate with ¼ of the fruit mixture and serve immediately.

TIP: To save time purchase pre-cubed mango from the supermarket.

NOTE: Avocados are a low GI fruit with a good source of healthful fats and fiber, which make them a good option for people with diabetes. Figure 9-1 shows how to prepare them.

VARY IT! Swap out oranges, mandarins, or clementines for mango.

PER SERVING: Calories 282 (From Fat 126); Fat 14g (Saturated 2g); Cholesterol 6mg; Sodium 52mg; Carbohydrate 29g (Dietary Fiber 6g); Protein 15g; Sugars 17g.

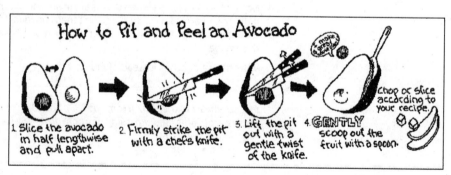

FIGURE 9-1: Preparing an avocado.

How to Pit and Peel an Avocado

1. Slice the avocado in half lengthwise and pull apart.
2. Firmly strike the pit with a chef's knife.
3. Lift the pit out with a gentle twist of the knife.
4. GENTLY scoop out the fruit with a spoon.
Chop or slice according to your recipe.

© John Wiley & Sons, Inc.

🍅 Seasonal Italian Fruit Platter

PREP TIME: 5 MIN	YIELD: 4 SERVINGS

INGREDIENTS

1 bunch red grapes

8 fresh figs, halved

2 plums, sliced

1 cup (125g) walnuts

4 ounces (113g) Parmigiano-Reggiano cheese, sliced into thin pieces

4 teaspoons (28g) honey

DIRECTIONS

1 Arrange the grapes, figs, and plums on a large serving platter. Place the walnuts in a small ramekin and set on one end of the platter. Arrange the Parmigiano slices in the middle and drizzle with honey.

TIP: Parmigiano-Reggiano cheese is a rich source of calcium and protein, supporting bone health and muscle function. It also contains vitamin B12, contributing to nerve function, and phosphorus, supporting energy metabolism. The aging process enhances its umami flavor and makes it easier to digest for people with lactose sensitivity.

NOTE: You can make this platter in advance and drizzle the honey over the Parmigiano before serving.

VARY IT! The fruits used in this recipe are usually ripe in late summer-early autumn in Italy, but you can use whichever combination of fruit is seasonal in your area when preparing it.

PER SERVING: *Calories 426 (From Fat 235); Fat 26g (Saturated 6g); Cholesterol 19mg; Sodium 457mg; Carbohydrate 36g (Dietary Fiber 5g); Protein 19g; Sugars 28g.*

☙ Grape, Goat Cheese, and Almond Skewers

PREP TIME: 20 MIN	YIELD: 8 SERVINGS

INGREDIENTS

1 pound seedless red grapes (48 exactly)

2 ounces (57g) goat cheese

3 tablespoons (46g) milk

½ cup (71g) blanched almonds, coarsely ground, plus extra for garnish

1 orange, for serving

DIRECTIONS

1 Remove 48 grapes from the stem and wash well. In a small bowl, combine the goat cheese and milk and mix well until a creamy, icing–like consistency is formed and then transfer to a plate.

2 Place the almonds on another plate. Thread 6 grapes onto each skewer leaving at least an inch border from the point end. Roll each one into the goat cheese mixture by using a brush or your fingers to make a thin, even coat on all sides of grapes. Dip the skewer into the almonds and turn to coat. Shake off any excess almonds and set the skewer on a plate. Continue until all eight skewers are complete.

3 Cut off the bottom of an orange to make it flat. Stick the skewers point–side into the orange to look like a bouquet.

TIP: Wash the grapes, soak the skewers, and make the goat cheese mixture a day in advance for efficiency. The Spanish culture has the tradition of the "12 uvas" or 12 grapes eaten at midnight on New Year's in order to ensure good luck for each of the 12 months of the year. I like to serve this recipe with 12 grapes instead of 6 on New Year's Eve for that reason.

NOTE: In addition to being a low GI fruit, grapes have an abundance of antioxidants that have the ability to regulate insulin and glucose metabolism, and to reduce oxidative stress induced in this disease.

NOTE: Refer to the color insert for a photo of this recipe.

PER SERVING: *Calories 97 (From Fat 60); Fat 7g (Saturated 2g); Cholesterol 6mg; Sodium 32mg; Carbohydrate 7g (Dietary Fiber 2g); Protein 4g; Sugars 5g.*

Chapter **10**

Making Brownies and Bars

RECIPES IN THIS CHAPTER

- Dark Chocolate & Extra-Virgin Olive Oil Brownies
- Date, Dark Chocolate, and Cashew Bars
- Ricotta, Chocolate, and Orange Brownies
- Strawberry-Studded Blondies
- Blackberry Lemon Bars
- Orange and Almond Bars
- Blueberry and Lemon Oatmeal Bars
- Quinoa, Cranberry, and Pecan Bars
- Gingerbread Spice Squares

The mere mention of brownies and sweet bars leaves many people swooning — and for good reason! These beloved treats are normally loaded with butter, plain flour, and lots of sweet chocolate. Their chewy texture and sweet, decadent taste is easy to fall in love with. For people with diabetes, however, brownies and bars make the traditional recipe off-limits.

This chapter explores how you can make brownies and bars in both nutritious and delicious fashion. These recipes are designed to help you to rekindle your relationship with the classic desserts while keeping your glucose in check at the same time.

Make any of these recipes in advance, and they're perfect for entertaining. Double these recipes and freeze the second batch for when you have guests or need to give a special gift.

Be sure to peruse the recipes before preparing them to see which ones appeal to you so you can complement the meal that you're eating. For example, the higher-protein, lower-carb desserts can follow a typical diabetes-friendly meal. If you're planning to indulge in one of the higher-carb, sweeter desserts, consume a meal that's low in carbs and sugar.

Indulging in Chocolate Brownies and Bars

Like many people, for many years I had a single standard brownie recipe that I used repeatedly. But brownies are one of my most requested items to prepare as a chef. When I'm working overseas, especially in Italy and other places in the Mediterranean, I often get requests to share my brownie recipe and to prepare them for events. I wanted to create a version or two that would satisfy people's sweet tooth, and at the same time still be true to my Mediterranean diet and philosophy, so I started switching up the ingredients. I've been making brownies with good quality extra-virgin olive oil (EVOO) for years. I love the rich texture and additional flavor that the EVOO provides.

The recipes in this section combine a wide array of ingredients that are beneficial to people with diabetes. In addition to EVOO, I use dark chocolate, fresh fruit, monk fruit as a sweetener, almond flour, almond butter, flaxseeds, and other nutritious foods to provide a healthful and tasty experience.

You can find these recipes in this section:

>> **Dark Chocolate & Extra-Virgin Olive Oil Brownies:** A decadent combination rich in powerful antioxidants and flavor.

>> **Date, Dark Chocolate, and Cashew Bars:** This no-bake dessert is basically homemade energy bars, a healthier alternative to the store-bought version, that can be kept on hand for traveling, post-workout snacks, or a nutritious breakfast on the go.

>> **Ricotta, Chocolate, and Orange Brownies:** Creamy ricotta cheese and citrus-infused chocolate brownies are an elevated twist on the classic.

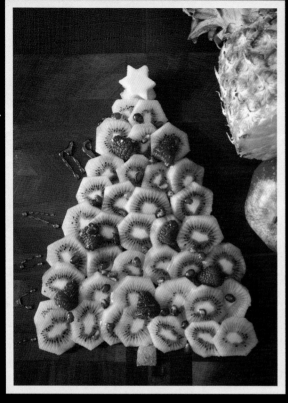

Serve this festive Kiwi and Raspberry Trees with Honey recipe from Chapter 9 at breakfast or as an easy dessert during the holiday season.

This show-stopping Watermelon "Cake" from Chapter 9 is perfect for warm weather celebrations.

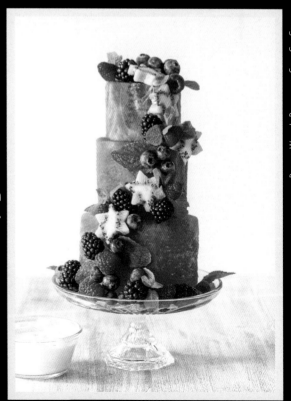

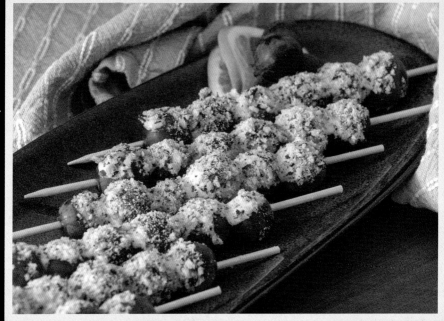

Enjoy this Mediterranean-inspired Grape, Goat Cheese, and Almond Skewers recipe from Chapter 9 at the next game-day buffet.

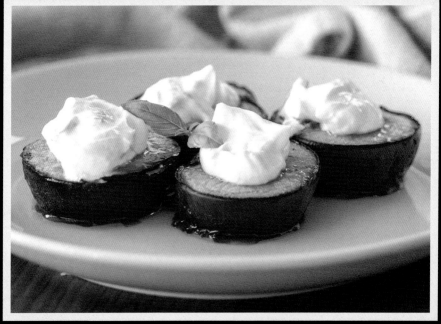

Juicy, sweet Roasted Plums with Mascarpone Cheese from Chapter 9 are proof that fruit and cheese are the perfect way to end a meal.

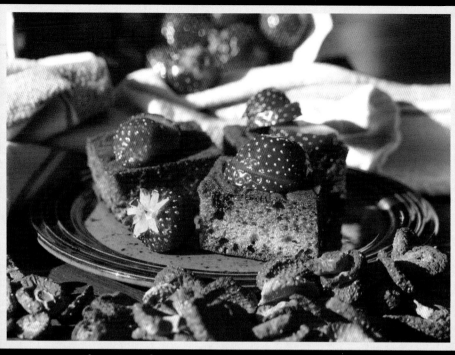

These Strawberry-Studded Blondies from Chapter 10
are a favorite of kids and adults alike!

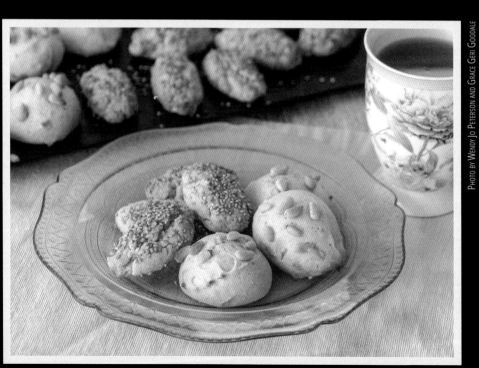

These Moroccan Sesame Cookies and Italian Pine Nut Cookies from Chapter 11
make perfect partners for a cup of tea, coffee, or espresso.

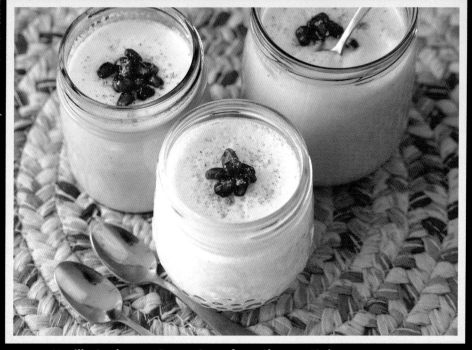

Vanilla Cardamom Panna Cotta from Chapter 12 is a creamy way to end a meal Italian style.

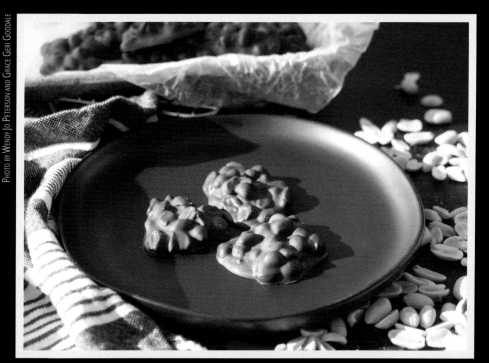

Swap out store-bought chocolate peanut candy for these healthful and delicious Chocolate Peanut Clusters in Chapter 13.

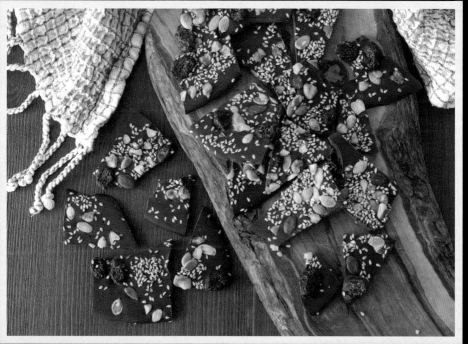

Chocolate Swirl Bark from Chapter 13 gives a sweet
and nutritious finale to any meal.

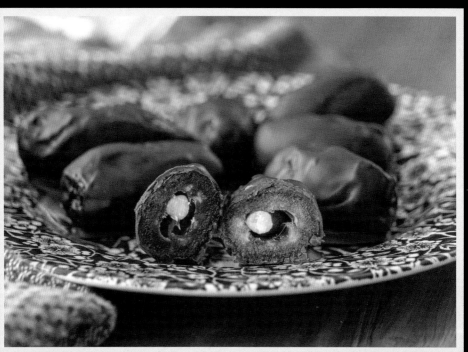

Chocolate-Covered Stuffed Dates from Chapter 13 are a decadent
and nutrient-dense candy alternative.

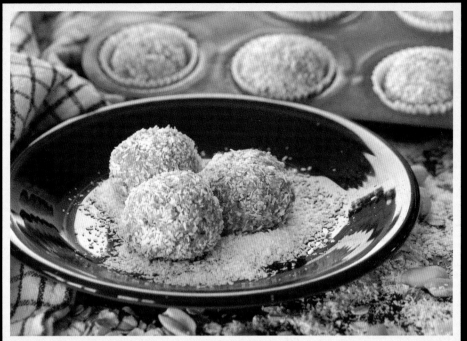

Peanut Butter and Coconut Bombs from Chapter 13 are a fun, festive, and nutritious finale to any meal.

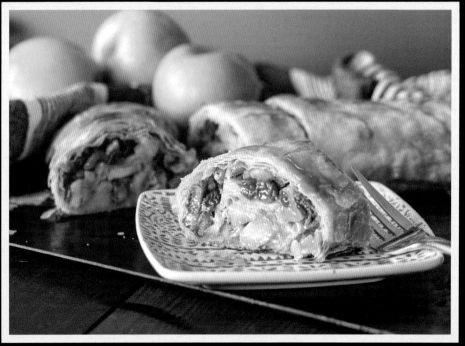

Try this Apple, Raisin, and Nut Strudel from Chapter 15 when you're looking for a tasty, classic, and healthful way to end a meal.

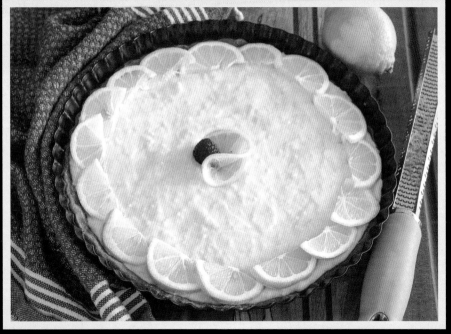

This swoon-worthy Creamy Lemon Crostata from Chapter 15 is ideal for special occasions.

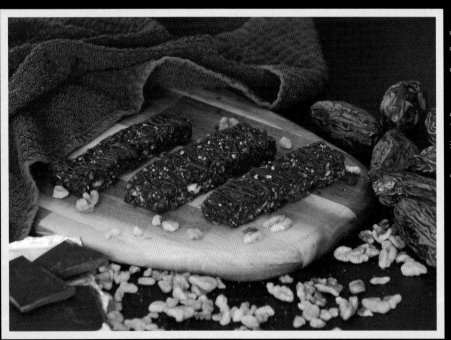

The Date, Dark Chocolate, and Cashew Bars recipe from Chapter 10 can be served as a decadent dessert or as tasty energy bars.

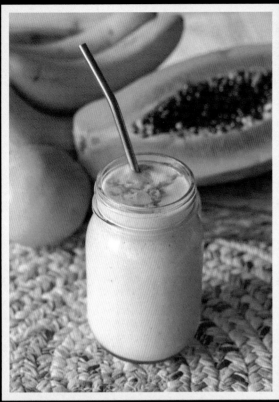

This Papaya, Banana, and Orange Smoothie from Chapter 16 can be a pre-or post-workout drink.

Warm up with this sweet Hot Spiced Chocolate drink from Chapter 16.

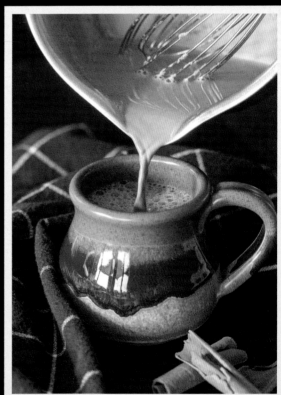

🍅 Dark Chocolate & Extra-Virgin Olive Oil Brownies

PREP TIME: 10 MIN	COOK TIME: 25 MIN	YIELD: 16 SERVINGS

INGREDIENTS

½ cup (108g) plus 1 teaspoon (4.5g) Amy Riolo Selections or other EVOO

¾ cup (94g) unbleached all-purpose flour

⅓ cup (28g) cocoa powder

1 teaspoon (4.6g) baking powder

½ cup (122g) unsweetened applesauce

1 teaspoon (3g) powdered pure stevia extract

3 large eggs

1 teaspoon (5g) cold brewed coffee or espresso

2 teaspoons (8.4g) vanilla extract

4.75 ounces (135 grams) dark chocolate (80 percent or higher), cut into small pieces

1 cup (120g) coarsely chopped walnuts or pecans, divided

DIRECTIONS

1 Preheat the oven to 350 degrees F (180 degrees C). Line an 8-x-8-inch baking pan with parchment paper, extending over the edges to form handles. Coat the liner with 1 teaspoon (4.5g) EVOO.

2 In a small bowl, combine the flour, cocoa powder, and baking powder. Set aside. In a medium bowl, using an electric mixer on low speed (or by hand with a large spoon), combine the remaining EVOO, applesauce, stevia, eggs, espresso, and vanilla. Add flour mixture a bit at a time, stirring until dry ingredients are absorbed. Stir in ½ cup each chocolate pieces and chopped nuts.

3 Spread the brownie batter in the prepared pan. Sprinkle the remaining chocolate and nuts on top of the batter. Bake for 25 to 30 minutes, or until a toothpick inserted into the center comes out with fudgy crumbs. Cool the brownies in the pan. When cool, lift them out of pan onto a cutting board. Peel away the liner and cut the brownies into squares. Store them in an airtight container.

NOTE: Refer to the front cover for a photo of this recipe.

PER SERVING: *Calories 205 (From Fat 151); Fat 17g (Saturated 4g); Cholesterol 40mg; Sodium 46mg; Carbohydrate 12g (Dietary Fiber 2g); Protein 4g; Sugars 3g.*

Date, Dark Chocolate, and Cashew Bars

PREP TIME: 15 MIN PLUS 1 HR CHILLING TIME	YIELD: 12 SERVINGS

INGREDIENTS

2 cups (300g) Medjool dates, pitted and chopped

¼ cup (54g) Amy Riolo Selections or other EVOO

2¾ cups (375g) raw cashews (unsalted)

¾ cup (65g) cocoa powder

¼ teaspoon (1.2g) sea salt

½ cup (40g) unsweetened shredded coconut

2 tablespoons (26g) vanilla extract

2 tablespoons (29g) cold coffee or espresso

DIRECTIONS

1 Line an 11½-x-4½ inches (29-x-12 cm) loaf pan with parchment paper (with the excess hanging over the sides). Combine the chopped dates, EVOO, cashews, cocoa powder, and sea salt in a food processor. Pulse and process all the ingredients together until the texture is coarse.

2 Add the shredded coconut, pulse a few times, and add the vanilla extract, with a tablespoon of coffee at a time until it reaches a dry but moist dough consistency. Scrape the dough mixture into the lined pan, pressing evenly with a rubber spatula.

3 Chill for at least an hour. To serve, lift the bars out of the pan with the parchment paper. Slice into 12 (1-inch; 2.5cm) thick pieces.

NOTE: If the dates aren't very soft, soak them in water overnight or for at least an hour before serving. See the color insert for a photo of this recipe.

TIP: For more of a coffee flavor, add an extra tablespoon of cold coffee or espresso

VARY IT! Substitute water or orange juice for the coffee and almonds for the cashews.

PER SERVING: *Calories 322 (From Fat 191); Fat 21g (Saturated 5g); Cholesterol 0mg; Sodium 46mg; Carbohydrate 32g (Dietary Fiber 5g); Protein 8g; Sugars 18g.*

Ricotta, Chocolate, and Orange Brownies

PREP TIME: 10 MIN	COOK TIME: 30 MIN	YIELD: 16 SERVINGS

INGREDIENTS

8 ounces (227g) dark chocolate (80 percent or higher) cut into small pieces, divided

1 cup (246g) whole milk ricotta cheese

2 eggs

¼ teaspoon (.6g) 100 percent pure monk fruit extract

Grated zest and juice of 1 orange

1 teaspoon (4.2g) vanilla extract

⅓ cup (28g) dark cacao powder

1½ cups (168g) almond flour

¼ cup (57g) plain Greek yogurt

½ teaspoon (2.3g) baking powder

¼ teaspoon (1.2g) sea salt

DIRECTIONS

1 Preheat the oven to 350 degrees F (180 degrees C) and line an 8-x-8-inch square baking dish with parchment paper.

2 Microwave 4 ounces unsweetened chocolate in a large, microwave safe bowl at 30 second intervals until melted, stirring after each interval. Let cool slightly. Add the ricotta cheese, egg, monk fruit, orange juice and zest, vanilla extract, cocoa powder, almond flour, Greek yogurt, baking powder, and sea salt. Mix until combined and then stir in the remaining chocolate pieces. Spread onto a baking dish and bake for 30 minutes, or until the brownies are set but still slightly wobbly. Allow to cool completely, cut into squares, and serve.

TIP: Be sure to choose pure monk fruit without additives in your recipes.

NOTE: Monk fruit has been used as a sweetener for centuries, and it's recently become easier to find in grocery stores around the globe. Pure monk fruit is 300 times sweeter than sugar but doesn't cause spikes in blood sugar.

VARY IT! Substitute ¼ cup coconut flour for the almond flour.

PER SERVING: *Calories 193 (From Fat 128); Fat 14g (Saturated 5g); Cholesterol 35mg; Sodium 72mg; Carbohydrate 11g (Dietary Fiber 3g); Protein 7g; Sugars 4g.*

Savoring Fruit-Studded Brownies and Bars

The culinary combination of fruit and chocolate in brownies is hard to beat. Plus, fresh and dried fruit add additional flavor, texture, and depth to baked goods while upping the nutrient quotient. No matter whether you love sweet strawberries, ripe blackberries, zesty oranges, or crisp blueberries, these recipes help you transform fruit into rich and gooey goodness.

It's hard to believe that despite people's deep-rooted love affair with brownies and blondies, they've only been around for a little more than a century. Fannie Farmer is credited with creating the first blondie recipe when she baked her cookie recipe in a rectangular pan and published it in the 1896 edition of *The Boston Cooking-School Cookbook.*

In the next decade various types of brownies appeared in print, and ten years later Farmer published an updated version of her book with both brownies and blondies in it. Nowadays both brownies and blondies are among the most popular American desserts in the world.

Sweet bars, on the other hand, come in many forms. Some recipes are basically large sheet cakes or slab cakes that are a bit denser than a regular chiffon-style cake used for birthdays, so they're called bars. Other bar recipes are nutrient-dense homemade energy bars that can also be enjoyed as sweet treats. Best of all, some bars don't require baking! These easy-to-make, mouthwatering recipes are sure to become fan favorites in your household.

You can enjoy the following recipes in this section:

>> **Strawberry-Studded Blondies:** A delicious summer square that travels well

>> **Blackberry Lemon Bars:** Beautiful and delicious bites that take advantage of summer's bounty

>> **Orange and Almond Bars:** A delicious and nutritious sweet treat to enjoy on the go

>> **Blueberry and Lemon Oatmeal Bars:** Classic flavors combined for the perfect warm-weather dessert or breakfast bar

🍓 Strawberry-Studded Blondies

INGREDIENTS

½ cup (108g) plus 1 teaspoon (4.5g) Amy Riolo Selections or other EVOO, divided

½ cup (56g) almond flour

½ teaspoon (2.4g) sea salt

1 teaspoon (4.6g) baking powder

3 eggs

2 teaspoons (8.4g) vanilla extract

½ cup (59g) pure monk fruit

1 cup (24g) dried strawberries without added sugar, chopped

1½ cups (248g) chopped fresh strawberries

DIRECTIONS

1 Heat the oven to 350 degrees F (180 degrees C). Line an 8-x-8-inch baking dish with parchment paper and coat the paper on the bottom and sides with 1 teaspoon (4.5g) olive oil.

2 In a medium bowl mix together the flour, sea salt, and baking powder. In another bowl mix together the eggs, vanilla, and monk fruit.

3 Add the flour mixture to the wet ingredients. Using a spoon, stir the mixture until everything is combined. Fold in the strawberries and pour the batter into the dish. Use a spatula to spread the mixture evenly.

4 Bake for 30 to 40 minutes. Test with a toothpick to see if they're finished (they're done when the toothpick comes out clean). After they cool, remove them from the baking dish and cut into 12 squares. Store in an airtight container for 2 days or in the refrigerator for up to 5 days.

TIP: The batter in this recipe will seem thick, but don't worry. It's okay.

NOTE: Refer to the color insert for a photo of this recipe.

VARY IT! Swap the almond flour for whole-wheat or gluten-free flour and the berries for your favorite fruit.

PER SERVING: *Calories 144 (From Fat 117); Fat 13g (Saturated 2g); Cholesterol 53mg; Sodium 137mg; Carbohydrate 5g (Dietary Fiber 1g); Protein 3g; Sugars 3g.*

Blackberry Lemon Bars

INGREDIENTS

¾ cup (162g) plus 1 teaspoon (4.5g) Amy Riolo Selections or other EVOO, divided

¼ teaspoon (.6g) pure monk fruit

½ teaspoon (2.4g) sea salt

1 tablespoon (13g) vanilla extract

2 cups (250g) unbleached all-purpose flour

1 teaspoon (2.6g) ground cinnamon

Zest and juice of 1 lemon

1½ cups (216g) fresh blackberries, rinsed and patted dry

½ cup (54.5g) chopped pecans

DIRECTIONS

1 Preheat the oven to 350 degrees F (180 degrees C). Line an 8-x-8-inch baking pan with parchment paper with over-hanging edges and coat with EVOO. Stir ¾ cup EVOO and monk fruit together. Stir in the sea salt and vanilla. Mix in the flour, cinnamon, and lemon zest, stir just until combined.

2 Using your fingers, pat ⅔ of the dough into the bottom of the pan.

3 Spread the blackberries and pecans out across the dough, drizzle with lemon juice. Break up the remaining dough into scattered pieces on top to create an open crust. Scatter pieces of the dough over the blueberries and pecans in a random fashion. Bake for about 30 to 40 minutes until just beginning to get golden around the edges and cool on a rack.

TIP: Be sure to use fresh, in season blackberries.

NOTE: In Step 2, the dough should be soft and sticky, so do your best to cover the entire surface of the bottom; you don't need to compact the dough, just lightly pat it down.

NOTE: The combination of EVOO, nuts, and fruit make it balanced in terms of macronutrients so that you can eat it after a meal or on its own.

PER SERVING: *Calories 323 (From Fat 209); Fat 23g (Saturated 3g); Cholesterol 0mg; Sodium 105mg; Carbohydrate 25g (Dietary Fiber 3g); Protein 4g; Sugars 2g.*

Orange and Almond Bars

PREP TIME: 10 MIN PLUS	30 MIN FREEZING	YIELD: 10 SERVINGS

INGREDIENTS

3 oranges, zested and peeled

¼ cup (59mL) maple syrup

1 teaspoon (4.2g) vanilla extract

1 tablespoon (16g) almond butter

1 cup (112g) ground flaxseeds

2 cups (224g) almond flour

¼ teaspoon (1.2g) sea salt

DIRECTIONS

1 In a blender combine the oranges and blend until smooth. Then strain the juice into a large mixing bowl. Combine the maple syrup, vanilla, and almond butter into the orange juice and mix well.

2 Stir in the flaxseeds, almond flour, and sea salt into the wet ingredients and mix well with a wooden spoon until you have a solid dough.

3 Line an 8-x-8-inch baking pan with parchment paper with overhanging edges and coat with EVOO. Spoon the batter onto the prepared pan. Then, grease your palms to avoid the dough sticking. Spread the dough evenly in the bowl and place the bowl in the freezer for 30 minutes. Take out the bars and slice them into 10 pieces.

TIP: This no-bake bar recipe is great for taking on picnics and traveling.

NOTE: This recipe lasts up to a week in a sealed container in the refrigerator.

VARY IT! Swap almond butter for peanut butter and almond flour for all-purpose or gluten-free flour.

PER SERVING: *Calories 235 (From Fat 152); Fat 17g (Saturated 1g); Cholesterol 0mg; Sodium 58mg; Carbohydrate 17g (Dietary Fiber 7g); Protein 7g; Sugars 9g.*

Blueberry and Lemon Oatmeal Bars

PREP TIME: 10 MIN	COOK TIME: 20 MIN	YIELD: 12 SERVINGS

INGREDIENTS

¾ cup (162g) Amy Riolo Selections or other EVOO

1 teaspoon (4.2g) pure vanilla

1 teaspoon (2.6g) cinnamon

1¼ teaspoon (.62g) pure monk fruit extract, divided

2 cups (224g) almond flour

7 large eggs

5 lemons, zested and juiced

1 cup (81g) steel cut oatmeal

1 cup (148g) fresh blueberries, rinsed and dried

DIRECTIONS

1 Preheat the oven to 350 degrees F (180 degrees C). Line a 9-x-13 baking dish with parchment paper. Stir ¾ cup EVOO, vanilla, cinnamon, and ¼ teaspoon monk fruit together with a mixer. Add the almond flour and mix until a crumbly dough forms. Press the dough into the prepared dish and bake for 18 to 20 minutes or until firm.

2 Prepare the filling in a large bowl by whisking the eggs together, adding 1 teaspoon monk fruit. Whisk until it's fully dissolved. Mix in the lemon zest and lemon juice.

3 Add the oatmeal and mix well to combine. Fold the blueberries into the batter. Pour the filling over the shortbread crust. Place in the oven and bake for 30 to 35 minutes, rotating halfway through. Remove from the oven and let cool for 1 hour before serving or refrigerating. Dust with powdered sugar just before serving and enjoy!

VARY IT! Replace oatmeal with almond flour and blueberries with raspberries.

PER SERVING: *Calories 311 (From Fat 239); Fat 27g (Saturated 4g); Cholesterol 123mg; Sodium 42mg; Carbohydrate 12g (Dietary Fiber 4g); Protein 9g; Sugars 3g.*

Whipping Up Whole-Grain Goodness Bars and Squares

Sweet bars and squares are a good dessert to incorporate whole grains. Because they often include dense flavors that can stand up to the nuttiness in whole grains, the use of whole-wheat and nut flours not only add more nutrition to the recipes in this section, but they also add more flavor.

REMEMBER

You may also want to swap out whole grains for all-purpose flour in some of your own favorite recipes. Here are a few things to keep in mind when baking with whole grains instead of all-purpose flour:

>> Whole-wheat pastry flour is a good choice for baked goods, but it isn't the only type of whole grain available. Spelt, einkorn, and rye also make good choices.

>> When you substitute whole-grain flour (except for spelt, quinoa, oatmeal, and einkorn) into an all-purpose flour recipe, you usually need to increase the liquid by a few tablespoons. Doing so compensates for the extra absorptive bran and germ in the whole-grain flour ensuring the proper amount of moisture in the recipe.

>> Cake, cookie, and pie crust recipes usually have liquid in the form of water, milk, or vanilla extract. You can add a bit more of those liquids to achieve the desired texture when baking with whole grains.

REMEMBER

One of these recipes uses molasses as a sweetener. Molasses doesn't quickly break down into glucose, which makes it a better choice than plain sugar for people with diabetes. However, it's high in carbohydrates, so it should be consumed with moderation and, if eaten as dessert, should follow a low-carb meal.

Try the following recipes:

>> **Quinoa, Cranberry, and Pecan Bars:** A nutritious and tasty alternative to store-bought protein bars that will satisfy your sweet tooth

>> **Gingerbread Spice Squares:** A comforting classic to enjoy during winter holidays

🍅 Quinoa, Cranberry, and Pecan Bars

PREP TIME: 10 MIN, PLUS 1 HR CHILLING | YIELD: 12 SERVINGS

INGREDIENTS

1 teaspoon (4.5g) EVOO

1 cup (99g) pecans, roughly chopped

⅓ cup (43g) pepitas

⅔ cup (30.4g) dried cranberries

1¾ cups (297.5g) quinoa, ground into a powder

1 teaspoon orange zest

½ teaspoon (1.3g) ground cinnamon

1 cup (250g) creamy unsalted almond butter

½ cup (170g) honey

1½ teaspoons (6.3g) vanilla extract

DIRECTIONS

1 Line a 9-x-9-inch baking dish with parchment paper and coat the paper on the bottom and sides with EVOO. In a medium skillet over medium heat, toast the pecans and pepitas until they're fragrant, about 2 to 3 minutes. Transfer them to a food processor. Add the cranberries and process for about 10 seconds, until the nuts and cranberries are chopped, or chop by hand on a cutting board.

2 In a large mixing bowl, combine the contents of the food processor with the quinoa, orange zest, and cinnamon. Mix well to combine. In a medium mixing bowl, combine the almond butter, honey, and vanilla and mix until well blended. Pour the liquid ingredients into the dry ingredients. Use a mixer or a wooden spoon to mix them together until the two are evenly combined.

3 Transfer the mixture to the prepared pan. Use a spoon to arrange the mixture fairly evenly in the pan. Pack the mixture down as firmly and evenly as possible. Cover the pan and refrigerate for at least one hour, or preferably overnight. When you're ready to slice, lift the bars out of the pan by grabbing both pieces of parchment paper on opposite corners. Use a sharp knife to slice the bars into 1-inch strips and then slice them in half through the middle.

PER SERVING: *Calories 355 (From Fat 197); Fat 22g (Saturated 2g); Cholesterol 0mg; Sodium 6mg; Carbohydrate 35g (Dietary Fiber 4g); Protein 9g; Sugars 12g.*

Gingerbread Spice Squares

INGREDIENTS

½ cup (108g) plus 1 teaspoon (4.5g) Amy Riolo Selections or other EVOO, divided

2⅓ cups (280g) spelt or whole-wheat pastry flour

1½ teaspoons (6.9g) baking powder

1 teaspoon (1.8g) ground ginger

1 teaspoon (2.6g) ground cinnamon

½ teaspoon (2.3g) baking soda

¼ teaspoon (1.2g) sea salt

¼ teaspoon (.52g) ground cloves

¼ teaspoon (.55g) nutmeg

¼ cup (85g) honey

1¼ cups (296mL) cold water

⅔ cup (222g) full-flavor molasses

2 eggs, lightly beaten

Confectioners' sugar for dusting

DIRECTIONS

1 Preheat oven to 350 degrees F (180 degrees C). Lightly coat a 13-x-9-x-2-inch baking pan with 1 teaspoon (4.5g) EVOO; set aside. In a medium bowl, stir together the flour, baking powder, ginger, cinnamon, baking soda, sea salt, cloves, and nutmeg; set aside.

2 In a large bowl, whisk together ½ cup (108g) EVOO and honey until combined. Add the cold water, molasses, and eggs; whisk until combined. Add the flour mixture and stir until smooth and incorporated. Pour into baking pan.

3 Bake for 40 to 45 minutes or until a toothpick inserted near the center comes out clean. Cool completely on a wire rack. Sift confectioners' sugar if desired.

PER SERVING: *Calories 150 (From Fat 58); Fat 6g (Saturated 1g); Cholesterol 21mg; Sodium 104mg; Carbohydrate 22g (Dietary Fiber 2g); Protein 3g; Sugars 10g.*

Chapter **11**

Enjoying Cookies

RECIPES IN THIS CHAPTER

- **Chocolate Chip Almond Butter Cookies**
- **Chocolate, Pistachio, and Cranberry Biscotti**
- **Lemon and Walnut Biscotti**
- **Hazelnut Cookies**
- **Pistachio Macaroons**
- **Tuscan Cantucci**
- **Almond Orange Biscotti**
- **Moroccan Sesame Cookies**
- **Honey Citrus Cookies**
- **Carrot Cookie Bites**
- **Meringues**
- **Italian Pine Nut Cookies**
- **Oatmeal Cookies**
- **Chocolate Oatmeal No-Bake Cookies**
- **Oatmeal Cranberry Cookies**

Cookies are popular all over the globe. Whether they're enjoyed at dessert, for breakfast, during a coffee break, or at teatime, cookies are a fun way to brighten your day. This chapter combines healthful ingredients like nuts, olive oil, dark chocolate, and oats to create diabetes-friendly versions that the whole family will crave. In this chapter you discover the different types of cookies and enjoy recipes that are as fun to make as they are delicious to eat.

Making Cookies: The Basic How-To Techniques

Here are a few different cookie-making techniques that you may want to become acquainted with. Cookies are broadly classified according to how they are formed:

» **Drop cookies:** They're made from a soft dough that is dropped by spoonfuls (rounded or freeform) onto a baking sheet. They spread out during baking.

>> **Refrigerator/icebox cookies:** They're made from a stiff dough that is refrigerated so it becomes even stiffer. The dough is typically shaped into cylinders that are sliced into round cookies before baking.

>> **Molded cookies:** They're made from a stiffer dough that's molded into balls or cookie shapes by hand before baking. Sometimes an actual cookie mold is used to form the cookies into specific shapes.

>> **Rolled cookies:** They're made from a stiff dough that is rolled out and cut into shapes. Check out the recipe for Moroccan Sesame Cookies.

>> **Pressed cookies:** They're made from soft dough that's extruded from a cookie press into various decorative shapes before baking.

>> **Bar cookies:** They consist of batter or other ingredients that are poured or pressed into a pan (sometimes in multiple layers) and cut into cookie-size pieces after baking. Brownies and cereal bars are examples of bar cookies. You can find these recipes in Chapter 10.

>> **Sandwich cookies:** They're rolled or pressed cookies that are assembled as a sandwich and filled with jam, marshmallow, or chocolate.

>> **Confectionery cookies:** These cookies are decorated with royal icing. Their overall aesthetic appeal and sugar content makes them more like candy than cookie.

>> **Piped cookies:** They have very loose batters that are piped out of a pastry bag and onto a lined baking sheet in specific shapes. Refer to the Italian Pine Nut Cookies recipe in this chapter.

A QUICK LOOK AT COOKIE HISTORY

Cookies have been around since antiquity. The earliest versions were similar to Italian biscotti but were drier and less sweet. In Egypt, a toasty version of anise biscotti called rusk has been around for millennia. Since the Romans conquered and occupied Egypt for its wheat, more than likely they also got their beloved biscotti recipe there, which they used to carry on trading ships. As wheat and sugar became more plentiful, cookies became more and more prominent and extravagant.

The first cookie recipe appeared in a book by Apicius (the Roman philosopher and first known cookbook author), and it consisted of this: "A thick paste of fine wheat flour that was boiled and spread out on a plate, allowed to harden, and then fried and topped with honey and pepper." Another Roman mixture consisting of flour, water, sugar, and spices was cut into pieces and fried.

By the seventh century, sugar was less expensive and more widely available in Persia, which is when cookies became commonplace in the Middle East. Arab cookery also boasted molded cookie recipes as early as the ninth century. These recipes, including shortbread cookies called *ghrayebeh* in Arabic and *montecados* in Spanish, made their way from the Arab world to Muslim Spain and eventually were dispersed throughout Europe. By the 14th century, they were available in all levels of European society, and every place from royal palaces to street vendors served them.

A variety of cookies evolved and flourished in the Middle Ages, including gingerbread. Ginger was brought to Europe from India via Arab traders. In the 1600s in France, meringue cookies including savoy cookies, were made with egg whites, sugar, and flour. Lisbon biscuits, Naples biscuits, and Spanish biscuits, based on the same ingredients and baking style, became popular as control of the Southern European countries volleyed back and forth between various empires.

Baking skills reached new heights during the Renaissance in Italy, when Catherine de Medici married King Henri IV of France and brought her bakers from Florence with her to Paris. Many Italian recipes (like amaretti) were morphed into French recipes like macarons. They, along with many others, were altered and became part of the French repertoire. The English word for cookie comes from the Dutch word *koekje*, which means "little cake"; it's believed to have been brought to the United States via the Dutch.

In the 18th and 19th centuries, the prices of sugar and flour dropped in Europe. Chemical leavening agents like baking soda were also developed, which led to more widespread cookie making. With the Industrial Revolution, manufactured cookies appeared on the scene. Since that time, the homemade cookie has been a real treat — and a labor of love.

Baking Cookies with Chocolate

Given the worldwide popularity of chocolate cookies, one would think that they've been around forever. But that's not the case: The cocoa tree originated in the Amazon around 4,000 BCE and the Maya and Aztecs used chocolate as a drink, currency, and aphrodisiac. In the 16th century chocolate became popular in Spain and spread throughout Europe. In 1828 cocoa powder was developed and in 1910 the first chocolate bar. In the 20th century, baking, especially cookies with chocolate, became a trend and nowadays it's commonplace.

REMEMBER

In addition to its addictive, decadent flavor, baking with chocolate, especially dark chocolate with more than 85 percent cocoa content, can be especially beneficial to people with diabetes for these reasons:

>> Dark chocolate contains *polyphenols* (plant compounds that have antioxidant and anti-inflammatory properties and may help lower blood sugar levels) that may improve *insulin sensitivity* (how well insulin works in the body). This, in turn, may help control blood sugar levels from spiking.

>> Dark chocolate may help lower blood pressure.

>> Dark chocolate contains bioactive compounds that may help reduce inflammation, which can increase the risk of complications with type 2 diabetes.

>> Dark chocolate's *flavanols* (plant-based compounds that act as antioxidants) may inhibit the growth of harmful bacteria in the gut.

Here are the recipes you can find in this section:

>> **Chocolate Chip Almond Butter Cookies:** This perennial favorite is an updated, healthier, and tastier version of classic chocolate chip cookies.

>> **Chocolate, Pistachio, and Cranberry Biscotti:** These twice-baked Italian cookies are so delicious that no one will guess that they're actually nutritious.

Chocolate Chip Almond Butter Cookies

PREP TIME: 15 MIN	COOK TIME: 10 MIN	YIELD: 2 DOZEN

INGREDIENTS

½ cup (56g) almond flour

¼ cup (22g) unsweetened cocoa powder

⅔ cup (103g) rolled oats ground into a powder (use gluten-free if needed)

1 teaspoon (4.6g) baking powder

½ teaspoon (2.3g) baking soda

¼ teaspoon (1.2g) sea salt

⅔ cup (165g) unsweetened almond butter

⅓ cup (60g) date sugar

2 large eggs

1 teaspoon (4g) vanilla extract

2 teaspoons (10g) cold espresso or coffee

⅔ cup (111g) dark chocolate chips

DIRECTIONS

1 Heat the oven to 375 degrees F (190 degrees C). Line two baking sheets with parchment paper. Whisk together the almond flour, cocoa, and oats in a large mixing bowl with the baking powder, baking soda, and sea salt. Set aside.

2 With a wooden spoon, combine the almond butter, date sugar, eggs, vanilla, and espresso in another medium bowl and mix thoroughly to combine. Transfer the wet mixture to the bowl with the dry mixture and stir together until fully combined. Add the chocolate chips and stir until combined.

3 Scoop the dough into 24 equal-sized balls, about 1 heaping tablespoon, and set about 2 inches (5cm) apart onto the baking sheets. Gently press the dough balls down with your fingers to flatten them slightly. Bake for 9 to 10 minutes or until the tops start to turn slightly golden brown. Remove from the oven and cool before transferring to a wire rack. Store in an airtight container on the counter for up to 5 days or freeze for up to 3 months.

PER SERVING *(2 cookies): Calories 230 (From Fat 134); Fat 15g (Saturated 3g); Cholesterol 35mg; Sodium 207mg; Carbohydrate 21g (Dietary Fiber 4g); Protein 6g; Sugars 10g.*

Chocolate, Pistachio, and Cranberry Biscotti

PREP TIME: 10 MIN PLUS 30 MIN RESTING	COOK TIME: 50 MIN	YIELD: 3 DOZEN

INGREDIENTS

3 cups (360g) spelt flour

2 teaspoons (9.2g) baking powder

½ teaspoon (2.4g) sea salt

½ cup (96g) date sugar

6 large eggs

2 tablespoons (27g) Amy Riolo Selections or other EVOO

2 teaspoons (8.4g) almond extract

1 teaspoon (4.2g) vanilla extract

¾ cup (96g) raw unsalted pistachios, shelled

¾ cup (35g) dried unsweetened cranberries

½ cup (84g) dark chocolate chips

DIRECTIONS

1 Preheat the oven to 350 degrees F (175 degrees C). Line two large baking sheets with parchment paper or silicone mats. Whisk the flour, baking powder, and sea salt in a medium bowl until combined. Beat together the sugar, eggs, EVOO, and almond and vanilla extracts in a large bowl until blended. Add the flour mixture and beat until smooth. Stir in the pistachios, cranberries, and chocolate chips.

2 Drop heaping teaspoonfuls of dough in two (12-x-3-inch) logs that are at least 3 inches apart on the baking sheets. Use your fingertips to press down and form even shaped logs. Bake the cookies for 30 minutes, remove from the oven, and let cool for about 30 minutes more.

3 Reduce the oven temp to 325 degrees F (165 degrees C). Transfer the logs to a cutting board. With a serrated knife, cut each log into ½-inch (1.25 cm) thick slices. Stand the biscotti upright in 3 rows on a baking sheet and return to the oven. Bake for 20 minutes or until golden. Allow to cool and store in an airtight container at room temperature for up to a week or freeze for a few months.

PER SERVING (2 cookies): Calories 193 (From Fat 63); Fat 7g (Saturated 2g); Cholesterol 70mg; Sodium 147mg; Carbohydrate 26g (Dietary Fiber 4g); Protein 5g; Sugars 8g.

Enjoying Nutty Cookies

Cookies with nuts have been popular since the Middle Ages. Nowadays they can be eaten on a regular day and are always appreciated at holiday time.

Nuts are great additions to diabetes–friendly cookies because of the following:

>> They add flavor, texture, and depth.

>> They provide healthful fat and minerals such as magnesium.

>> The protein content helps to balance the glycemic load of the recipe.

>> The nuts make cookies more filling so you can eat less and still be satisfied.

When you're looking for a nutritious cookie that will satisfy your sweet tooth, turn to one of the following recipes:

>> **Lemon and Walnut Biscotti:** You can enjoy this classic recipe with espresso or tea.

>> **Hazelnut Cookies:** This unique northern Italian gluten-free recipe is great for the holidays or whenever the mood strikes.

>> **Pistachio Macaroons:** This gluten-free favorite is perfect for Passover.

>> **Tuscan Cantucci:** If you've never made biscotti before, don't be intimidated. Because of their crisp, twice-baked exterior, they last for weeks.

>> **Almond Orange Biscotti:** One of my family's recipes, it hails from Calabria, Italy where oranges and almonds abound. I inherited my love of baking from my great-grandmother who always included citrus and almonds in her baking.

TIP

You can eat any of them after dinner, at an afternoon coffee or tea break, or at breakfast time. Whenever you choose to make them, make extras for gifts.

Lemon and Walnut Biscotti

PREP TIME: 15 MIN	COOK TIME: 45 MIN PLUS COOLING TIME	YIELD: 14 SERVINGS

INGREDIENTS

2¼ cups (171g) walnut flour

½ cup (96g) date sugar

2 teaspoons (9g) baking powder

¼ teaspoon (1.2g) sea salt

4 large eggs

2 tablespoons (42g) honey

2 tablespoons (31g) lemon juice

2 tablespoons (12g) lemon zest

1 teaspoon (4.2g) vanilla extract

1 teaspoon (4g) lemon extract

½ cup (50g) walnuts, toasted and sliced in half

DIRECTIONS

1 Preheat the oven to 375 degrees F (190 degrees C). Line a baking sheet with parchment paper or silicon mats. Stir the flour, sugar, baking powder, and sea salt in a large bowl with a wooden spoon to combine.

2 In another large bowl, combine the eggs, honey, lemon juice and zest, vanilla and lemon extracts, and mix well to combine.

3 Pour the egg mixture into the flour mixture. When done mixing, stir in the opposite direction to make sure that all ingredients have been incorporated. If the dough is too thick, add water, a tablespoon at a time, until it's the consistency of a chocolate-chip cookie batter.

4 Stir in the walnuts. Drop dough onto baking sheet to form two 14-x-4-inch logs that are spaced 2 to 3 inches (5 to 7.5 cm) apart.

5 Wet your fingertips and smooth out the logs into even shapes. Bake for 20 to 25 minutes until the logs are golden. Remove from the oven and allow to cool 10 minutes.

6 Reduce the oven to 325 degrees F (160 degrees C). Carefully transfer the logs to a work surface and, using a serrated knife, cut them into ½-inch (1.25 cm)-thick slices. Re-line the baking sheet and arrange the slices on the sheet. Bake again for 10 minutes, or until golden. Cool completely and store in an airtight container. Serve with espresso or coffee for dunking.

TIP: You can purchase walnut flour or make it by placing walnuts in a food processor and pulsing on and off until they're ground into a very fine, dust-like consistency.

VARY IT! You can substitute lemons for oranges and walnuts for unsalted pistachios. If you can't eat nuts, replace the same amount with unsweetened dried fruit, such as figs or dates, or chopped dark (90 percent) chocolate.

NOTE: In addition to their flavor, the walnuts and walnut flour add healthful fats, protein, and minerals that help to balance the sugar in this recipe. The eggs provide an additional protein boost as well.

PER SERVING *(1 cookie): Calories 164 (From Fat 106); Fat 12g (Saturated 1g); Cholesterol 60mg; Sodium 124mg; Carbohydrate 11g (Dietary Fiber 2g); Protein 4g; Sugars 9g.*

A BIT ABOUT BISCOTTI

In the Italian language, all cookies are called *biscotti*. So to an Italian speaker a chocolate chip cookie and an oatmeal cookie would be considered a kind of biscotti. Around the world, however, the word "biscotti" is used to describe only the twice-baked Italian variety. The twice-baked version was the ancient predecessor to today's modern cookies. They're also great to enjoy because they last a long time and travel well.

Italians don't necessarily consider biscotti a dessert, but rather an after-dinner treat to be enjoyed by dipping into espresso or a bit of sweet wine. They can also do double-duty at breakfast when they're dipped into a cappuccino or caffe latte. Some people enjoy them with a mid-afternoon espresso as a pick-me-up. Whatever you make, store in an airtight container. Whenever you decide to enjoy them, they'll satisfy your sweet tooth and add a bit of Italian flair to your day!

🍅 Hazelnut Cookies

PREP TIME: 15 MIN	COOK TIME: 25 MIN	YIELD: 10 SERVINGS

INGREDIENTS

1½ cups (203g) whole hazelnuts plus 10 halved nuts, divided

¾ cup (90g) confectioners' sugar

⅛ teaspoon (.6g) sea salt

1 large egg white, lightly beaten

2 teaspoons (8.4g) pure vanilla extract

1 teaspoon (7g) honey

DIRECTIONS

1 Heat the oven to 350 degrees F (175 degrees C). Spread the hazelnuts on a large-rimmed baking sheet and toast for about 12 minutes, until the nuts are fragrant and the skins blister. Transfer the hazelnuts to a kitchen towel and close it to cover. Allow the nuts to cool, then rub them together to remove their skins.

2 In a food processor, pulse the hazelnuts with the confectioners' sugar and sea salt until finely chopped. Scrape the hazelnut mixture into a medium bowl. Stir in the egg white, vanilla, and honey.

3 Line a baking sheet with parchment paper. Roll teaspoon-size mounds of the hazelnut dough into rough circles (they needn't be perfectly round). Place onto the prepared baking sheet 1 inch (2.5 cm) apart and place a halved hazelnut into the center. Press down slightly.

4 Bake the cookies in the center of the oven for about 10 to 14 minutes, or until browned in a few spots. Let the cookies cool on the baking sheet before serving.

NOTE: These cookies originally come from the northern Italian province of Piedmont, where they're known as *brutti ma buoni* or "ugly but good" cookies. In Piedmont, bakers have their own variations; they often use the same ingredients but change the number of chopped nuts. For example, some people like to use half chopped hazelnuts and half whole hazelnuts.

VARY IT! You can substitute almonds for the hazelnuts.

TIP: In Step 4, you can change the baking time to about 13 minutes for chewy cookies or 15 minutes for slightly crisp cookies.

PER SERVING (1 cookie): Calories 256 (From Fat 187); Fat 21g (Saturated 2g); Cholesterol 0mg; Sodium 29mg; Carbohydrate 15g (Dietary Fiber 3g); Protein 5g; Sugars 11g.

Pistachio Macaroons

PREP TIME: 15 MIN	COOK TIME: 25 MIN PLUS 2 HRS RESTING	YIELD: 12 SERVINGS

INGREDIENTS

8 ounces (120g) shelled, unsalted pistachios

½ cup (96g) coconut sugar

Pinch of sea salt

2 large egg whites

1 teaspoon (4.2g) pure vanilla extract

1 teaspoon (2.5g) confectioners' sugar

DIRECTIONS

1 In a food processor combine the pistachios, coconut sugar, and sea salt. Grind them together until you reach a fine, flour-like consistency.

2 In a medium bowl using beaters on high speed or in the bowl of a standing mixer fitted with the whisk attachment, beat the egg whites and vanilla until stiff peaks form, being careful not to overbeat until the egg whites are dry. With a spatula, carefully fold in the pistachios.

3 Line a baking sheet with parchment paper or silicone mats. Use 2 teaspoons or soup spoons to form walnut-sized pieces of the pistachio mixture and shape into a ball with a slightly pointy top.

4 Place on the baking sheets and allow to sit for 2 hours. Sift confectioners' sugar over the top. Heat the oven to 300 degrees F (150 degrees C) and bake the macaroons for about 20 to 25 minutes or until they begin to turn golden. Remove and allow to cool.

TIP: You can skip the 2 hour resting time if you're in a hurry, but the cookies won't have the characteristic chewy texture of macaroons.

NOTE: I have cut the amount of sugar in the traditional recipe in half for this version. I find that it's still sweet enough. Pistachios are a healthful fat and add protein to this recipe. They're also rich in dietary fiber and unsaturated fatty acids, which are known to positively impact glucose regulation and cardiovascular health.

VARY IT! Blanched almonds are used to make traditional macaroons. Simply swap out blanched almonds for pistachios and almond extract for the vanilla in this recipe to make the traditional variety.

PER SERVING (2 cookies): Calories 183 (From Fat 83); Fat 9g (Saturated 1g); Cholesterol 0mg; Sodium 119mg; Carbohydrate 6g (Dietary Fiber 2g); Protein 5g; Sugars 2g.

Tuscan Cantucci

PREP TIME: 15 MIN	COOK TIME: 35 MIN PLUS 10 MIN RESTING	YIELD: 28 SERVINGS

INGREDIENTS

2 ¼ cups (281g) unbleached, all-purpose flour

¾ cup (144g) plus 1 tablespoon (12g) date sugar

2 teaspoons (9g) baking powder

¾ teaspoon (3.6g) sea salt

4 large eggs

2 tablespoons (42g) honey

2 tablespoons (31g) lemon juice

1 tablespoon (6g) lemon zest

2 teaspoons (8.4g) vanilla extract

1 teaspoon (4.2g) almond extract

1 cup (145g) blanched whole almonds, toasted

DIRECTIONS

1 Heat the oven to 375 degrees F (190 degrees C). Line a large baking sheet with parchment paper or silicone mats. Stir the flour, ¾ cup date sugar, baking powder, and sea salt in a large bowl to combine.

2 In a separate bowl, combine the eggs, honey, lemon juice, lemon zest, and vanilla and almond extract and mix well. Pour the egg mixture into the flour mixture and stir until incorporated. Stir in the almonds.

3 Drop the dough onto a baking sheet to make two 14-x-4-inch logs spaced 2 to 3 inches apart. Wet your fingertips and smooth out the logs to even shapes. Sprinkle logs with remaining tablespoon of sugar. Bake for 20 or 25 minutes, or until the logs are golden. Remove and rest on the baking sheet for 10 minutes.

4 Reduce the oven to 325 degrees F (160 degrees C). Carefully transfer the logs to a work surface and, using a serrated knife, cut them into ½-inch (1.25 cm)-thick slices. Arrange them on their sides on a clean baking sheet lined with parchment and bake for about 10 minutes, or until they're golden. Cool completely.

PER SERVING *(2 cookies): Calories 213 (From Fat 62); Fat 7g (Saturated 1g); Cholesterol 60mg; Sodium 193mg; Carbohydrate 30g (Dietary Fiber 4g); Protein 6g; Sugars 13g.*

Almond Orange Biscotti

PREP TIME: 15 MIN	COOK TIME: 45 MIN PLUS RESTING	YIELD: 14 SERVINGS

INGREDIENTS

2¼ cups (252g) almond flour

½ cup (96g) date sugar

2 teaspoons (9g) baking powder

¼ teaspoon (1.2g) sea salt

4 large eggs

2 tablespoons (42g) honey

2 tablespoons (31g) orange juice

2 tablespoons (12g) orange zest

1 teaspoon (4.2g) vanilla extract

1 teaspoon (4.2g) almond extract

½ cup (73g) whole almonds, toasted and roughly chopped

DIRECTIONS

1 Preheat the oven to 375 degrees F (190 degrees C). Line a baking sheet with parchment paper or silicone mats. Stir the flour, date sugar, baking powder, and sea salt in a large bowl with a wooden spoon to combine.

2 In another large bowl, combine the eggs, honey, orange juice and zest, vanilla and almond extracts, and mix well to combine. Pour the egg mixture into the flour mixture. When done mixing, stir in the opposite direction to make sure that all ingredients have been incorporated. Stir in the almonds. Drop the dough onto baking sheet to form two 14-x-4-inch logs that are spaced 2 to 3 inches (5 to 7.5 cm) apart.

3 Wet your fingertips and smooth out the logs into even shapes. Bake for 20 to 25 minutes until the logs are golden. Remove and allow to cool 10 minutes. Reduce the oven to 325 degrees F (160 degrees C). Carefully transfer the logs to a work surface, and using a serrated knife, cut them into ½-inch (1.25 cm)-thick slices. Re-line the baking sheet and arrange the slices. Bake again for 10 minutes, or until golden. Cool completely and store in an airtight container.

PER SERVING (1 cookie): Calories 195 (From Fat 117); Fat 13g (Saturated 1g); Cholesterol 60mg; Sodium 125mg; Carbohydrate 14g (Dietary Fiber 4g); Protein 7g; Sugars 10g.

Traveling the World: Classic Cookies from around the Globe

Cookies are popular in most cultures. What makes them unique is not only the ingredients they use, but also when they're served. Americans tend to think of cookies (especially because American varieties tend to be very high in sugar and fat) as dessert, but Mediterranean cultures usually serve cookies with tea or coffee in the afternoon or along with breakfast because they provide an energy boost earlier in the day.

You can find these healthful recipes in this section:

>> **Moroccan Sesame Cookies:** These cookies are a healthier version of the traditional recipe that uses butter and vegetable oil instead of EVOO, which has anti-inflammatory properties and helps to reduce the glycemic load of carbohydrates, helping to prevent blood sugar from spiking.

>> **Honey Citrus Cookies:** These fragrant cookies have an old-fashioned aroma; they're perfect for serving during the holidays and cooler months.

>> **Carrot Cookie Bites:** If you love carrot cake, these cookies are a nutritious and delicious alternative.

>> **Meringues:** Meringues are a classic treat low in fat with a light, airy texture. Because of the sugar content, don't eat these cookies on an empty stomach; you can enjoy 1 or 2 after a balanced, low-carb meal on occasion.

>> **Italian Pine Nut Cookies:** These cookies were popular at weddings when I was growing up. Nowadays, they're easy to find in pastry shops and people tend to enjoy them more often.

REMEMBER

You can make each of these cookies in advance, store them in an airtight container, and keep frozen for up to a few months before serving. They're wonderful to have on hand in case company comes or you need a last-minute host gift.

☙ Moroccan Sesame Cookies

PREP TIME: 20 MIN	COOK TIME: 20 MIN	YIELD: 24 COOKIES

INGREDIENTS

1¾ cups (219g) unbleached all-purpose flour, plus extra for work surface

¼ cup (28g) almond flour

½ cup (75g) sesame seeds, unhulled, divided

⅓ cup (60g) coconut sugar

1½ teaspoons (7g) baking powder

Pinch of sea salt

⅓ cup (71g) Amy Riolo Selections or other EVOO

1 teaspoon (4.2g) rose water

⅓ cup (78mL) whole milk

2 teaspoons (8.4g) pure vanilla extract

DIRECTIONS

1 Preheat oven to 375 degrees F (190 degrees C). Line two baking sheets with parchment paper or silicone mats.

2 Combine the flour, almond flour, ¼ cup sesame seeds, coconut sugar, baking powder, and sea salt in a large bowl. Stir in the EVOO and mix well.

3 Combine the rose water, milk and vanilla in a small bowl and stir into the large bowl. Mix the ingredients well to form a dough and turn the dough out onto a lightly floured work surface.

4 Pour the remaining ¼ cup sesame seeds onto a plate. Break off 1-inch (2.5 cm) pieces of dough and roll them to create finger shapes.

5 Place on the baking sheets and flatten the top of the cookies slightly with a finger. Bake for 18 to 20 minutes, or until very light golden. Store cookies in an airtight container at room temperature for one week or in the freezer for up to one month.

NOTE: Refer to the color insert for a photo of this recipe; pair it with Moroccan mint tea.

VARY IT: Replace almond flour with oat flour if you're allergic to nuts.

PER SERVING: *Calories 96 (From Fat 47); Fat 5g (Saturated 1g); Cholesterol 0mg; Sodium 43mg; Carbohydrate 11g (Dietary Fiber 1g); Protein 2g; Sugars 3g.*

♨ Honey Citrus Cookies

PREP TIME: 15 MIN	COOK TIME: 15 MIN	YIELD: 18 SERVINGS

INGREDIENTS

2 eggs

⅓ cup (112g) honey

Juice and zest of 1 orange

¾ cup (90g) whole-wheat flour

2 teaspoons (8.4g) pure vanilla

1 teaspoon (4.6g)
baking powder

½ cup (108g) Amy Riolo
Selections or other EVOO

DIRECTIONS

1 Heat the oven to 400 degrees F (205 degrees C).

2 Combine the eggs, honey, and orange juice and zest in a medium bowl with a wooden spoon. Add the flour, vanilla, and baking powder. Mix well to combine. Stir in the EVOO and continue to mix well.

3 Spoon the dough into a pastry bag fitted with a 1-inch (2.5 cm) round tip or a large plastic storage bag with the tip cut off. Twist the ends to seal the bag and force all of the batter to one end.

4 Pressing down, pipe the cookies that are 2½ inches (6.5 cm) long and 1-inch (2.5 cm) wide. Bake until golden, approximately 15 minutes. Allow to cool and serve.

TIP: You can also spoon the dough in equal size portions instead of piping it.

NOTE: These were once traditional homemade breakfast cookies that were made before the invention of commercially packaged biscotti eaten at breakfast. The EVOO helps to reduce the glycemic load.

VARY IT! For a gluten-free version, swap out wheat flour with almond flour or your favorite gluten-free flour.

PER SERVING: *Calories 100 (From Fat 60); Fat 7g (Saturated 1g); Cholesterol 24mg; Sodium 36mg; Carbohydrate 9g (Dietary Fiber 1g); Protein 1g; Sugars 6g.*

Carrot Cookie Bites

PREP TIME: 15 MIN | COOK TIME: 20 MIN | YIELD: 60 COOKIES

INGREDIENTS

2 eggs, lightly beaten

½ cup (128g) almond butter

¼ cup (54g) Amy Riolo Selections or other EVOO

½ cup (161g) maple syrup

1 teaspoon (4.2g) pure vanilla extract

1 cup (162g) oat flour

1 cup (156g) old-fashioned oats

½ cup (56g) almond flour

1 teaspoon (4.6g) baking powder

¼ teaspoon (1.2g) sea salt

2 teaspoons (5g) cinnamon

½ teaspoon (1g) cloves

1 cup (110g) grated carrots

⅓ cup (36g) chopped pecans

DIRECTIONS

1   Preheat your oven to 350 degrees F (175 degrees C). Line 2 large baking sheets with parchment paper. In a large bowl, whisk together the eggs, almond butter, EVOO, maple syrup, and vanilla until smooth and uniform. Add the oat flour, oats, almond flour, baking powder, sea salt, cinnamon, and cloves and mix to combine.

2   Stir in the carrots and pecans. Using a small ice cream scoop, transfer 1 tablespoon of the batter onto the baking sheets. Bake for 15 to 20 minutes. Allow to cool on the baking sheets.

TIP: Gather and measure all your ingredients to make the recipe more quickly. You can make the batter a day in advance and bake the cookies the following day.

NOTE: A few of these cookie bites make a great breakfast on the go.

VARY IT! Use a medium-sized ice cream scooper filled with 3 tablespoons of batter to make a large cookie.

PER SERVING *(2 cookies): Calories 125 (From Fat 66); Fat 7g (Saturated 1g); Cholesterol 14mg; Sodium 60mg; Carbohydrate 13g (Dietary Fiber 2g); Protein 3g; Sugars 4g.*

☺ Meringues

PREP TIME: 15 MIN | **COOK TIME: 2 HRS 20 MIN** | **YIELD: 80 COOKIES**

INGREDIENTS

4 large egg whites room temperature

½ teaspoon (1.5g) cream of tartar

⅛ teaspoon (.6g) sea salt

½ cup (100g) date sugar

1 teaspoon (4.2g) vanilla extract

DIRECTIONS

1 Preheat the oven to 225 degrees F (105 degrees C) and line a large baking sheet (or two regular-sized baking sheets — make sure they'll fit in your oven together) with parchment paper. Set aside.

2 Combine the egg whites, cream of tartar, and sea salt in a large bowl. Using an electric mixer or a stand mixer fitted with the whisk attachment, mix on low until the mixture becomes foamy. Increase to high.

3 With the mixer on high, gradually add the date sugar, about 1 tablespoon at a time, stirring after each addition until sugar is dissolved, about 15 to 20 seconds between each addition. Beat until the mixture is thick and shiny and has increased in volume and stiff peaks form. Stir in the vanilla.

4 Fit a large disposable piping bag with a large tip or snip the edge of the piping bag for a "kiss" formation and transfer the meringue to the piping bag and pipe onto the baking sheets, spacing them at about ¼-inch (⅔ cm) apart. Bake for 1 hour. Turn off the oven as soon as the baking time has passed and don't open the oven. Allow the cookies to cool completely in the oven (1 to 2 hours) before removing.

NOTE: Meringue cookies should be crisp and can be stored in an airtight container. Keep away from heat and moisture because they can soften meringues. You can freeze the meringues for up to a few months.

TIP: Be sure to use a very clean, grease-free bowl and beaters in order for the egg whites to mix properly.

PER SERVING *(2 cookies): Calories 12 (From Fat 0); Fat 0g (Saturated 0g); Cholesterol 0mg; Sodium 11mg; Carbohydrate 3g (Dietary Fiber 0g); Protein 0g; Sugars 3g.*

🍅 Italian Pine Nut Cookies

PREP TIME: 15 MIN	COOK TIME: 12 TO 14 MIN	YIELD: 36 COOKIES

INGREDIENTS

¾ cup (144g) organic coconut and vanilla sugar

¼ cup (85g) honey

¼ teaspoon (1.2g) sea salt

3 large eggs

2¼ cups (281g) all-purpose flour

½ teaspoon (2.3g) baking powder

2 teaspoons (8.4g) almond extract

6 tablespoons (50g) pine nuts

1 teaspoon (2.5g) confectioners' sugar, if desired, for garnish

DIRECTIONS

1 Place the sugar, honey, sea salt, and eggs in a bowl. Beat the mixture with an electric mixer until the eggs are foamy.

2 Fold in the flour, baking powder, and almond extract. The batter should be the consistency of chocolate chip cookie dough. If it's too thin, add a little more flour, 1 tablespoon at a time, until it reaches the right consistency.

3 Line 2 baking sheets with parchment paper. Drop rounded teaspoons full of dough about 2 inches apart on the baking sheets. Sprinkle each cookie with 6 to 8 pine nuts and bake for 12 to 14 minutes, until light golden brown.

4 Remove the cookies from the oven. Dust the confectioners' sugar on the tops. Allow to cool in the baking sheet and serve.

TIP: Many people like to make large batches and keep them on hand for unexpected guests. You can serve these cookies at breakfast time, tea-time, or snack time. They can be frozen for several months in airtight containers and thawed before enjoying.

NOTE: Because this recipe contains sugar, eat these cookies along with or after a meal that includes a healthful source of protein. Refer to the color insert for a photo of this recipe.

VARY IT! Swap all-purpose flour for almond flour.

PER SERVING (2 cookies): Calories 133 (From Fat 26); Fat 3g (Saturated 0g); Cholesterol 35mg; Sodium 52mg; Carbohydrate 24g (Dietary Fiber 1g); Protein 3g; Sugars 12g.

Adding Oatmeal Cookies to Your Repertoire

Oatmeal cookies originated from Scottish oatcakes and transitioned from porridge to baked goods in Victorian times. The first recorded oatmeal cookie recipes appeared in the late 1800s, with Fannie Merritt Farmer popularizing the oatmeal raisin cookie.

Some studies reveal that oatmeal has the following health benefits:

>> Oatmeal's fiber and protein content helps you feel fuller longer and slows the release of blood glucose.

>> Oatmeal contains *beta-glucan,* a soluble fiber that can lower bad LDL cholesterol and reduce the risk of heart disease.

>> The beta-glucan also can activate white blood cells and boost your immune system.

>> Oatmeal is high in selenium and zinc, which can help prevent illnesses.

>> Oatmeal's soluble fiber can help control blood sugar.

>> Oatmeal's high fiber content can help regulate your digestion and bowels and can help relieve constipation.

Kids and adults alike love oatmeal cookies. Try these recipes whenever the mood strikes:

>> **Oatmeal Cookies:** The combination of wholesome almond flour, oats, and EVOO boost the fiber, protein, and healthy fat quotient in this recipe.

>> **Chocolate Oatmeal No-Bake Cookies:** The whole family will love this kid-friendly favorite!

>> **Oatmeal Cranberry Cookies**: These classic cookies can do double-duty as well as on-the-go breakfast.

⊙ Oatmeal Cookies

PREP TIME: 10 MIN	COOK TIME: 10 MIN	YIELD: 22 SERVINGS

INGREDIENTS

1 cup (112g) almond flour

½ teaspoon (2.4g) sea salt

1 teaspoon (4.6g) baking powder

¼ teaspoon (.65g) cinnamon

2 large eggs

1 teaspoon (4.2g) vanilla extract

¾ cup (162g) Amy Riolo Selections or other EVOO

½ cup (96g) coconut sugar

3 cups (468g) old fashioned oats

½ cup (84g) dark chocolate chips

DIRECTIONS

1 Preheat the oven to 375 degrees F (190 degrees C). In a medium bowl whisk together the dry ingredients and set aside.

2 In a large bowl whisk together the eggs and the vanilla extract. Then whisk in the EVOO until incorporated. Add the coconut sugar and whisk until well incorporated.

3 Mix in the dry ingredients and then fold in the oats and the chocolate chips with a wooden spoon or strong rubber spatula. Mix until all the ingredients are well combined.

4 Using a small 1-to-2 tablespoon scoop, scoop the cookies on two parchment-lined baking sheets. Flatten the cookies to ½-inch thick with a rubber spatula.

5 Bake the cookies for about 8 to 10 minutes until the edges are slightly brown and crispy. Remove and allow to cool before moving them to a cooling rack.

TIP: Place blanched almonds in the food processor and pulse them until fine to make your own flour.

VARY IT: You can use all-purpose flour in place of almond flour.

PER SERVING: *Calories 219 (From Fat 117); Fat 13g (Saturated 2g); Cholesterol 19mg; Sodium 72mg; Carbohydrate 22g (Dietary Fiber 3g); Protein 5g; Sugars 7g.*

Chocolate Oatmeal No-Bake Cookies

PREP TIME: 15 MIN | COOK TIME: 5 MIN | YIELD: 24 SERVINGS

INGREDIENTS

¼ cup (54g) Amy Riolo Selections or other EVOO

½ cup (100g) sugar

½ cup (122g) milk

4 tablespoons (22g) dark cocoa

½ cup (128g) creamy, no-sugar-added peanut butter

2 teaspoons (8.4g) vanilla

3 cups (468g) quick cooking oats

DIRECTIONS

1 Add the first four ingredients into a 4-quart saucepan. Bring to a rolling boil and hold for 1 minute. Remove from the heat.

2 Add the peanut butter into the hot mixture and stir until melted. Add the vanilla.

3 Mix in the oats until they're completely coated. If mixture doesn't stick together, add more milk, 1 tablespoon at a time. Drop the cookies by tablespoonfuls onto a parchment-lined baking sheet. Cool until set in the refrigerator.

TIP: Store these cookies between sheets of wax paper in the refrigerator or in the freezer.

TIP: Make sure you buy erythritol-free, preferably fresh peanut butter, if possible.

VARY IT! You can use almond butter instead of peanut butter.

PER SERVING: Calories 152 (From Fat 61); Fat 7g (Saturated 1g); Cholesterol 0mg; Sodium 27mg; Carbohydrate 19g (Dietary Fiber 3g); Protein 5g; Sugars 5g.

Oatmeal Cranberry Cookies

PREP TIME: 10 MIN	COOK TIME: 10 MIN	YIELD: 22 SERVINGS

INGREDIENTS

1 cup (162g) oat flour

½ teaspoon (2.4g) sea salt

1 teaspoon (4.6g)
baking powder

¼ teaspoon (.65) cinnamon

2 large eggs

1 teaspoon (4.2g) vanilla extract

¾ cup (162g) Amy Riolo
Selections or other EVOO

½ cup (96g) organic
coconut sugar

3 cups (468g) old
fashioned oats

1 cup (46g) unsweetened dried
cranberries

DIRECTIONS

1 Preheat the oven to 375 degrees F (190 degrees C). In a medium bowl whisk together the flour, sea salt, baking powder, and cinnamon. Set aside.

2 In a large bowl whisk together the eggs and the vanilla extract. Then whisk in the EVOO until incorporated. Add the coconut sugar and whisk again until well incorporated.

3 Mix in the dry ingredients and then fold in the oats and the chocolate chips with a wooden spoon or strong rubber spatula. Mix until all the ingredients are well combined.

4 Using a small 1-to-2 tablespoon scoop, scoop the cookies on two parchment-lined baking sheets. Flatten the cookies to ½-inch thick with a rubber spatula.

5 Bake the cookies for about 8 to 10 minutes until the edges are slightly brown and crispy. Remove and allow to cool before moving them to a cooling rack.

VARY IT! You can substitute almond flour for the oat flour.

PER SERVING: *Calories 207 (From Fat 90); Fat 10g (Saturated 2g); Cholesterol 19mg; Sodium 74mg; Carbohydrate 25g (Dietary Fiber 3g); Protein 5g; Sugars 5g.*

Chapter **12**

Preparing Spoon Desserts and Puddings

RECIPES IN THIS CHAPTER

🍮 **Vanilla Cardamom Panna Cotta**

🍮 **Chocolate Almond Pudding**

🍮 **Cherry Chocolate Bread Pudding**

🍮 **Chocolate Orange Rice Pudding**

🍮 **Vanilla Pudding with Berries**

B ecause they don't require advanced baking skills, spoon desserts and puddings have historically been popular with home cooks. They're also featured on many restaurant menus because they can be made by regular chefs and enable restaurants to feature delicious desserts without the need to hire a separate pastry chef to make them.

In this chapter, I explain how to make classics like panna cotta, an array of puddings, crisps, cobblers, parfaits, and trifles that will satisfy your sweet tooth and impress your guests without causing your blood sugar to spike.

⏱ Sweet Holiday Couscous

⏱ Yogurt Custard with Apricots and Pistachios

⏱ Citrus and Cinnamon Rice Pudding

⏱ Wheat Berry Pomegranate Pudding with Pistachios

⏱ Blueberry Cream Cobbler

⏱ Sweet Peach Cobbler

⏱ Apple Cinnamon Crisp

⏱ Strawberry Basil Crisp

⏱ Passionfruit Tiramisu

⏱ Strawberry Shortcake

⏱ Pumpkin Gingerbread Trifle

⏱ Mixed Berry and Mascarpone Parfaits

⏱ Ricotta and Berry Cheesecake Torte

⏱ Almond and Cherry Clafoutis

Making Panna Cotta and Puddings

Panna cotta means cooked cream in Italian and is a type of custard that's thickened with gelatin. Extremely popular in Italian restaurants, this dessert will add sophistication to your repertoire.

This section presents the following recipes for you to try:

» **Vanilla Cardamom Panna Cotta:** A creamy Italian classic elevated with a hint of cooling cardamom

» **Chocolate Almond Pudding:** A delicious and nutritious pudding that's as tasty as it is good for you

» **Cherry Chocolate Bread Pudding:** A decadent crowd-pleaser

» **Chocolate Orange Rice Pudding:** A favorite with kids and adults alike

» **Vanilla Pudding with Berries:** A new way of enjoying pudding alone or as a pie filling

» **Sweet Holiday Couscous:** A delicious and nutritious sweet treat that you can enjoy anytime

» **Yogurt Custard with Apricots and Pistachios:** A light and refreshing Turkish-inspired pudding for breakfast

» **Citrus and Cinnamon Rice Pudding:** Classic rice pudding with Mediterranean flavors

» **Wheat Berry Pomegranate Pudding with Pistachios:** Hearty dessert based on a Middle Eastern recipe and great for breakfast

There's a perfect spoon dessert for each occasion and time of year. Best of all, they can be made in advance and served cold when needed.

Vanilla Cardamom Panna Cotta

PREP TIME: 10 MIN	COOK TIME: 10 MIN PLUS COOLING TIME	YIELD: 6 SERVINGS

INGREDIENTS

1½ cups (354mL) whole milk

10 cardamom pods crushed, seeds only

½ cup (100g) coconut sugar

1½ gelatin sheets, soaked in cold water to cover (5 minutes), and drained

1½ (420g) cups plain Greek yogurt, strained in a colander one hour before using

2 teaspoons (8.4g) pure vanilla

½ teaspoon (1g) ground cardamom

DIRECTIONS

1 Place the milk, cardamom seeds, and sugar in a saucepan and bring almost to a boil over medium heat.

2 Remove from the heat. Strain and squeeze any excess water from the gelatin sheets and stir them in. Whisk well to combine so the mixture doesn't curdle.

3 Add the yogurt and vanilla, whisking vigorously, and mix well to incorporate.

4 Place the panna cotta into a glass or ceramic container. Cover and refrigerate for at least one hour.

5 Sprinkle with cardamom and berries, if desired, and serve!

TIP: This recipe combines milk and yogurt for added depth of flavor and balanced macronutrients, but traditional recipes were made with just fresh cream alone. You can try it both ways and decide which one you prefer. Greek yogurt contains inulin that helps to regulate blood sugar.

NOTE: You can prepare the panna cotta in individual ramekins and unmold and serve them at the table or make and chill them in wine glasses or other decorative glasses.

VARY IT! You can add a few tablespoons of cocoa to the milk to make a chocolate panna cotta. I often substitute ½ cup (118mL) of the milk for coffee to make a Turkish coffee–inspired version.

PER SERVING: Calories 184 (From Fat 23); Fat 3g (Saturated 1g); Cholesterol 12mg; Sodium 75mg; Carbohydrate 24g (Dietary Fiber 0g); Protein 15g; Sugars 20g.

☕ Chocolate Almond Pudding

PREP TIME: 5 MIN	COOK TIME: OVERNIGHT CHILLING	YIELD: 4 SERVINGS

INGREDIENTS

½ cup (43g) cocoa powder

¾ teaspoon (3.6g) sea salt

1 cup (177g) chia seeds

½ cup (168g) organic agave nectar

2⅔ cups (232mL) unsweetened almond milk

1 teaspoon (4.2g) pure vanilla

½ cup (69g) almonds sliced

2 ounces (57g) dark chocolate, 90 percent, shaved, for garnish

DIRECTIONS

1 In a medium mixing bowl, whisk together the cocoa powder and sea salt. Mix in the chia seeds and agave nectar.

2 Pour in the almond milk and vanilla and stir until combined well.

3 Pour into 4 pudding dishes or small dessert bowls.

4 Cover and refrigerate for at least an hour or preferably overnight.

5 Garnish each with ¼ of the almond flakes and shaved dark chocolate and serve.

TIP: The longer this pudding sits, the thicker and smoother it will become.

NOTE: Both the Aztec and Mayan civilizations used cacao and chia seeds in their diets for their medicinal purposes. The use of chia seeds in this recipe acts as a thickener, replacing the need for corn or potato starch while adding protein, healthful fats, protein, iron, magnesium, phosphorous, and zinc.

VARY IT! Swap out almond milk for soy, rice, or regular milk.

PER SERVING: *Calories 566 (From Fat 284); Fat 32g (Saturated 6g); Cholesterol 0mg; Sodium 365mg; Carbohydrate 68g (Dietary Fiber 24g); Protein 14g; Sugars 37g.*

⬤ Cherry Chocolate Bread Pudding

PREP TIME: 5 MIN	COOK TIME: 50 MIN	YIELD: 6 SERVINGS

INGREDIENTS

7 large eggs

2 large egg whites

1¾ cups (414mL) whole milk

½ cup (96g) date sugar

½ cup (43g) unsweetened cocoa powder

½ cup (84g) dark chocolate chips

1 tablespoon (13g) pure vanilla extract

1 medium ripe banana, mashed

4 cups day-old whole-wheat bread cubes (½-inch, 1.27cm)

1 teaspoon (4.5g) Amy Riolo Selections or other EVOO

1 cup (46g) dried pitted unsweetened cherries

DIRECTIONS

1 Preheat the oven to 350 degrees F (175 degrees C). Whisk the eggs and egg whites in a large bowl. Whisk in the milk, date sugar, cocoa powder, chocolate chips, and vanilla until combined. Add the banana and stir until incorporated. Add the bread and stir until combined.

2 Let stand for 30 minutes, turning and pressing the bread into the liquid a few times to help it absorb the custard mixture.

3 Coat a shallow 2-quart baking dish (or 6 individual ramekins) with the EVOO.

4 Stir the cherries into the pudding and transfer them into the prepared dish. Bake for 40 to 50 minutes for baking dish or approximately 30 minutes for the ramekins or until the top of pudding is golden. Let cool for 15 minutes before serving.

NOTE: The mashed banana adds natural sweetness and texture while the date sugar adds flavor and helps to prevent blood sugar from spiking. Eggs and egg whites add protein, making this a balanced dessert that could also do double-duty as a decadent breakfast once in a while.

PER SERVING: *Calories 379 (From Fat 133); Fat 15g (Saturated 6g); Cholesterol 254mg; Sodium 226mg; Carbohydrate 48g (Dietary Fiber 9g); Protein 15g; Sugars 30g.*

Chocolate Orange Rice Pudding

PREP TIME: 5 MIN	COOK TIME: 45 MIN	YIELD: 4 SERVINGS

INGREDIENTS

⅔ cup (132g) Calrose rice, Egyptian rice, Arborio rice, or short grain rice

3¼ cups (768mL) whole milk

¼ cup (21.5g) unsweetened cocoa

Zest of 1 grated orange, plus additional for garnish

¼ cup (59mL) freshly squeezed orange juice

⅔ cup (127g) date sugar

1 teaspoon (4.2g) pure vanilla extract

DIRECTIONS

1 Rinse the rice and drain well. Pour the milk into a medium saucepan. Add the drained rice, cocoa, orange zest and juice, and date sugar. Stir with a wooden spoon and bring to a boil over medium-high heat.

2 As soon as the mixture boils, reduce the heat to low, stir, and cover. Simmer for 40 minutes, stirring occasionally, until the rice is tender and the liquid is absorbed.

3 Allow the pudding to cool at room temperature. Pour into a serving bowl to serve.

TIP: Make this pudding in advance when entertaining.

NOTE: Any short or medium grain starchy rice works in this recipe. Because this recipe contains rice, fruit juice, and date sugar, be sure to enjoy this recipe after a meal that contains lean protein and greens without simple carbohydrates.

VARY IT! Swap out the orange juice and zest for lemon and exclude the cocoa to make lemon pudding.

PER SERVING: *Calories 394 (From Fat 66); Fat 7g (Saturated 4g); Cholesterol 20mg; Sodium 87mg; Carbohydrate 67g (Dietary Fiber 8g); Protein 10g; Sugars 38g.*

Vanilla Pudding with Berries

PREP TIME: 5 MIN	COOK TIME: 10 MIN	YIELD: 4 SERVINGS

INGREDIENTS

3¾ cup (887mL) whole milk, almond, or rice milk

3 tablespoons (24g) cornstarch dissolved in ¼ cup (61g) milk

⅓ cup (112g), plus 1 tablespoon (21g) honey, divided

1 teaspoon (4.2g) vanilla

1 cup (148g) mixed blueberries, blackberries, and raspberries

1 tablespoon (16g) Amy Riolo Selections White Balsamic or your favorite balsamic vinegar

DIRECTIONS

1 Place the milk in a medium saucepan and bring to a simmer over medium heat. Stir in the honey.

2 Increase the heat to medium high and whisk continuously, ensuring that it doesn't stick to the bottom or sides of the pan or scald, until the milk thickens.

3 Whisking continuously, cook until the pudding coats the back of a spoon. Remove from the heat and allow to cool.

4 Mix the berries with the tablespoon of honey and white balsamic vinegar. Stir and allow to cool until the desired temperature is reached.

5 When the pudding is cool enough to eat, pour it into a serving bowl or 4 smaller bowls, top with berries, and serve warm, or cool overnight in the refrigerator.

TIP: This type of milk pudding is a popular Middle Eastern ingredient also used to fill phyllo pastries.

NOTE: A high protein version of this recipe isn't available, so consume it after a meal that consists of lean protein and nonstarchy vegetables.

VARY IT! Add ¼ cup cocoa to turn this into a chocolate pudding.

PER SERVING: Calories 301 (From Fat 73); Fat 8g (Saturated 5g); Cholesterol 24mg; Sodium 108mg; Carbohydrate 51g (Dietary Fiber 1g); Protein 8g; Sugars 45g.

☙ Sweet Holiday Couscous

PREP TIME: 5 MIN	COOK TIME: 10 MIN PLUS 5 HR CHILLING	YIELD: 6 SERVINGS

INGREDIENTS

2½ cups (590mL) whole milk, divided

⅔ cup (114g) whole-wheat couscous

½ cup (96g) plus 1 tablespoon (12g) date sugar, divided

⅛ teaspoon (.6g) sea salt

1 cup (145g) blanched whole almonds

4 tablespoons (32g) cornstarch, dissolved in ¼ cup (59mL) milk

½ cup (61.5g) raw, unsalted pistachios, shelled, and ground

1 teaspoon (2.6g) cinnamon, for topping

DIRECTIONS

1 Preheat the oven to 375 degrees F (190 degrees C). Bring ½ cup (118mL) milk to a boil over high heat. Turn off the heat and stir in the couscous, 1 tablespoon date sugar, and sea salt. Cover and allow to stand for 10 minutes.

2 In the meantime, place the almonds on a cookie sheet and toast for 5 to 10 minutes, until slightly golden. Allow to cool and finely grind in a food processor. Remove the lid from the couscous, fluff with a fork, and stir in the almonds. Spoon the mixture into a 9-inch glass or ceramic baking dish.

3 In a medium saucepan, combine the cornstarch mixture, 2 cups milk, and the remaining date sugar over medium heat. Stir slowly and constantly with a wooden spoon or whisk, in the same direction, being sure to scrape down the sides and bottom of the pan with each stir. Cook the mixture until it thickens, about 20 minutes. Pudding is done when it coats the back of a spoon and its volume has been reduced by about half.

4 Stir the pistachios into the pudding and spread the pudding on top of the couscous. Sprinkle with cinnamon. Allow to cool, cover with plastic wrap, and refrigerate for 5 hours or until chilled.

NOTE: The combination of proteins and healthful fats in the nuts and milk balance the sugar.

VARY IT! Swap out rice for couscous.

PER SERVING: *Calories 434 (From Fat 186); Fat 21g (Saturated 4g); Cholesterol 11mg; Sodium 96mg; Carbohydrate 48g (Dietary Fiber 8g); Protein 13g; Sugars 23g.*

Yogurt Custard with Apricots and Pistachios

PREP TIME: 5 MIN	COOK TIME: 15 MIN	YIELD: 4 SERVINGS

INGREDIENTS

2 cups (200g) plain, full-fat Greek yogurt

1 teaspoon (4.2g) vanilla extract

1 teaspoon (4.2g) almond extract

4 tablespoons (32g) cornstarch dissolved in 2 tablespoons (31g) skim milk

2 tablespoons (15.6g) cinnamon

3 tablespoons (63g) pure, organic agave nectar

4 tablespoons (31g) ground pistachios

8 unsweetened apricots, chopped

DIRECTIONS

1 Combine the yogurt, vanilla and almond extract, cornstarch mixture, cinnamon, and agave nectar in a medium saucepan. Bring the mixture to boil over medium-high heat while stirring slowly and constantly with a wooden spoon.

2 Allow the mixture to boil for 2 minutes, reduce the heat to low, and stir slowly for 10 minutes or until the mixture has thickened and coats the back of a spoon.

3 Remove the mixture from the stove and cover the top of the actual custard with wax paper to prevent a skin from forming. When the custard is cool, spoon it into small dessert bowls or cups and garnish with a sprinkling of pistachios and apricots.

NOTE: Make this recipe in advance to serve at brunch or dessert buffets.

VARY IT! Swap out pistachios and apricots for almonds and figs or pecans and cherries.

PER SERVING: *Calories 244 (From Fat 32); Fat 4g (Saturated 0g); Cholesterol 0mg; Sodium 51mg; Carbohydrate 42g (Dietary Fiber 4g); Protein 12g; Sugars 32g.*

🍑 Citrus and Cinnamon Rice Pudding

PREP TIME: 5 MIN	COOK TIME: 1 HR	YIELD: 4 SERVINGS

INGREDIENTS

⅔ cup (123g) Arborio rice

3¼ cups (768mL) whole milk

1 cinnamon stick

Grated zest of 1 lemon

¼ cup (62.5mL) freshly squeezed lemon juice

⅔ cup (127g) date sugar

DIRECTIONS

1 Rinse the rice and drain well. Pour the milk into a medium saucepan. Add the drained rice, cinnamon stick, lemon zest, lemon juice, and sugar. Stir with a wooden spoon and bring to a boil over medium–high heat.

2 As soon as the mixture boils, reduce the heat to low, stir, and cover.

3 Simmer for an hour, stirring occasionally, until the rice is tender and the liquid is absorbed. Remove and discard the cinnamon stick. Allow the pudding to cool at room temperature and pour into a serving bowl.

TIP: You can use any short- or medium-grain starchy rice; Egyptian and Calrose rice work well in this recipe too.

NOTE: Don't be intimidated by the lengthy cooking time. You can leave this recipe on the stove while you're doing other things at home. As the rice cooks and releases its starches slowly, the pudding thickens and the result is very creamy.

VARY IT! Add ¼ cup (25g) cocoa powder and omit the lemon to make a chocolate rice pudding.

PER SERVING: *Calories 297 (From Fat 59); Fat 7g (Saturated 4g); Cholesterol 20mg; Sodium 85mg; Carbohydrate 46g (Dietary Fiber 5g); Protein 7g; Sugars 37g.*

Wheat Berry Pomegranate Pudding with Pistachios

PREP TIME: 10 MIN	COOK TIME: 1 HR 30 MIN	YIELD: 6 SERVINGS

INGREDIENTS

1¼ cups (225g) soft wheat berries

3 cups (720mL) milk or almond milk

½ cup (87g) pomegranate arils

2 tablespoons (30mL) agave nectar

½ cup (62g) plain shelled pistachios, finely chopped

DIRECTIONS

1 Bring a large saucepan ¾ full of water to boil over high heat. Add the wheat berries and cook for 20 to 30 minutes, or until tender.

2 Combine the cooked wheat berries with the milk in a medium saucepan and stir. Cover and cook the mixture over low heat for 1 hour, until most of the milk has evaporated and the wheat berries are creamy, stirring every 15 minutes or so. Allow to cool to almost room temperature.

3 Stir in the pomegranate arils, agave nectar, and most of the pistachios. Place the pudding in small dessert bowls and garnish with the remaining pistachios.

NOTE: Wheat berries, which are traditional in Mediterranean breakfasts and desserts, are a whole grain rich in fiber, B vitamins, and minerals like iron and magnesium. The fiber content supports digestive health, while the nutrients contribute to overall energy metabolism and red blood cell formation.

VARY IT! Use rice or barley instead of wheat berries. Swap the pomegranate for your favorite fruit.

NOTE: Figure 12-1 shows how to seed a pomegranate.

PER SERVING: Calories 306 (From Fat 87); Fat 10g (Saturated 3g); Cholesterol 12mg; Sodium 53mg; Carbohydrate 48g (Dietary Fiber 9g); Protein 12g; Sugars 15g.

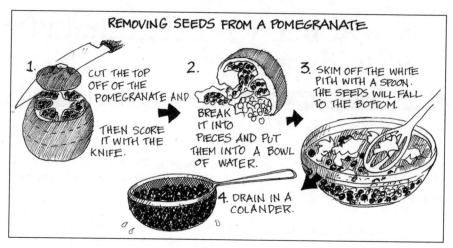

Illustration by Liz Kurtzman

Creating Comfort Desserts: Crisps and Cobblers

In the United States, crisps and cobblers are among the first baked treats that many people learn how to make. Especially popular in summer and fall when fresh fruit is plentiful, these dishes bring a touch of comfort to dessert.

Many people get the two items confused. Here's a quick comparison:

>> **Crisps** get their name primarily from their crisp, streusel crumb topping.

>> **Cobblers,** on the other hand, are soft-centered and often include a biscuit dough crust on the bottom.

Here are a few crisp and a couple cobbler recipes in the following section:

>> **Blueberry Cream Cobbler:** Perfect for summertime, or whenever fresh blueberries are plentiful

>> **Sweet Peach Cobbler:** A warm weather dessert when peaches are at their peak

>> **Apple Cinnamon Crisp:** A touch of spicy sweetness to fall and winter meals with this easy crisp

>> **Strawberry Basil Crisp:** A perfect crowd-pleaser to serve at summer gatherings

🍅 Blueberry Cream Cobbler

PREP TIME: 5 MIN	COOK TIME: 40 MIN	YIELD: 8 SERVINGS

INGREDIENTS

4 cups (592g) fresh (or frozen) blueberries

1 cup (320g) maple syrup

Zest of 1 lemon

Juice of 1 lemon

2 teaspoons (8.4g) pure vanilla, divided

1 tablespoon (8g) cornstarch dissolved in 2 tablespoons (27g) water

1 cup (156g) old fashioned oats, gluten-free if desired

1 cup (141g) finely chopped almonds

1 tablespoon (10g) whole flaxseeds

1 cup (112g) almond flour

⅓ cup (71g) Amy Riolo Selections or other EVOO

2 cups (200g) vanilla Greek yogurt, for garnish

DIRECTIONS

1 Preheat the oven to 350 degrees F (175 degrees C). In a large bowl, mix the blueberries, ½ cup (160g) maple syrup, lemon zest and juice, and vanilla. Then add the cornstarch and toss in the blueberries. Spoon the berries into an 8-x-8-inch pan.

2 In another bowl, mix the oats, almonds, flaxseeds, and almond flour. Stir in the remaining maple syrup, EVOO, and vanilla until well combined. Spread the cobbler topping on top of the blueberries mixture until most of the blueberries are covered.

3 Bake for 40 to 45 minutes or until golden brown. Cool for 15 minutes before eating. Store the leftovers in the fridge. Garnish with ¼ cup of yogurt to serve.

VARY IT! Swap blueberries for raspberries, blackberries, or strawberries, or your favorite combination.

PER SERVING: *Calories 548 (From Fat 242); Fat 27g (Saturated 3g); Cholesterol 0mg; Sodium 29mg; Carbohydrate 65g (Dietary Fiber 8g); Protein 16g; Sugars 40g.*

🍅 Sweet Peach Cobbler

PREP TIME: 15 MIN | COOK TIME: 45 MIN | YIELD: 8 SERVINGS

INGREDIENTS

4 cups (616g) sliced fresh peaches

¼ cup (80.5g) plus 1 tablespoon (20g) maple syrup

Zest of 1 lemon

Juice of 1 lemon

1 teaspoon (4.2g) pure vanilla

1 teaspoon (2.6g) plus 1 tablespoon (8g) cinnamon, divided

1 tablespoon (8g) cornstarch dissolved in 2 tablespoons (30mL) water

1 cup (156g) old fashioned oats, gluten-free if desired

1 cup (141g) finely chopped almonds

1 tablespoon (10g) whole flaxseeds

1 cup (112g) almond flour

⅓ cup (71g) Amy Riolo Selections or other EVOO

DIRECTIONS

1 Preheat the oven to 350 degrees F (175 degrees C). In a large bowl, mix the peaches, ¼ cup (80.5g) maple syrup, lemon zest and juice, vanilla, and cinnamon. Then add the cornstarch and toss in the peaches. Spoon the peach mixture into an 8-×-8-inch pan.

2 In another bowl, mix the oats, almonds, flaxseeds, and almond flour. Stir in the 1 tablespoon (20g) maple syrup, EVOO, and cinnamon until well combined. Spread the cobbler topping on top of peaches until most of the peaches are covered.

3 Bake in the oven for 40 to 45 minutes or until the topping is golden brown. Cool for 15 minutes before eating. Store leftovers in the fridge.

TIP: Use fresh peaches when they're in season for this recipe.

PER SERVING: *Calories 417 (From Fat 241); Fat 27g (Saturated 3g); Cholesterol 0mg; Sodium 3mg; Carbohydrate 38g (Dietary Fiber 8g); Protein 11g; Sugars 15g.*

Apple Cinnamon Crisp

PREP TIME: 15 MIN	COOK TIME: 55 MIN	YIELD: 8 SERVINGS

INGREDIENTS

1 teaspoon (4.5g) plus ¼ cup (54g) Amy Riolo Selections or other EVOO

⅓ cup (53g) oat flour

½ cup (78g) old fashioned rolled oats, gluten-free if desired

⅓ cup (60g) date sugar

1 teaspoon (2.6g) cinnamon

¼ teaspoon (2.4g) sea salt

½ cup (56g) raw chopped pecans

5 to 6 medium apples, peeled, cored, and very thinly sliced

⅓ cup (104g) maple syrup

1 teaspoon (2.6g) cinnamon

¼ teaspoon (.5g) ground cloves

1 tablespoon (13g) pure vanilla extract

DIRECTIONS

1 Preheat the oven to 350 degrees F (175 degrees C). Generously grease an 8×8-inch baking pan with 1 teaspoon EVOO and set aside.

2 To make the topping, combine the flour, oats, date sugar, cinnamon, sea salt, and pecans in a large bowl until well combined. Add the ¼ cup EVOO, mix until the mixture resembles wet sand, and then place in the fridge. To make the filling, place the apples, maple syrup, cinnamon, cloves, and vanilla in a large bowl and toss to combine. Allow to sit for 5 to 10 minutes.

3 Take ⅓ cup of the topping mixture and toss with the apple mixture. Place the apple mixture in the pan and sprinkle evenly with topping. Bake the crisp on a baking sheet (just in case the filling bubbles over) for 45 to 55 minutes, or until the topping is golden brown and the filling is bubbling. Remove and cool 10 minutes on a wire rack. Serve warm.

NOTE: Top with Vanilla Frozen Yogurt or Vanilla Gelato from Chapter 14.

PER SERVING: *Calories 308 (From Fat 124); Fat 14g (Saturated 2g); Cholesterol 0mg; Sodium 121mg; Carbohydrate 43g (Dietary Fiber 6g); Protein 4g; Sugars 27g.*

Strawberry Basil Crisp

INGREDIENTS

1 teaspoon (4.5g) plus ¼ cup (54g) Amy Riolo Selections or other EVOO

⅓ cup (53.5g) oat flour

½ cup (78g) old fashioned rolled oats, gluten-free if desired

2 tablespoons (14g) ground flaxseeds

⅓ cup (60g) date sugar

½ cup (56g) raw chopped macadamia nuts

1 teaspoon (2.6g) cinnamon

¼ teaspoon (1.2g) sea salt

5 cups (830g) hulled fresh strawberries, very thinly sliced

⅓ cup (104g) honey

2 teaspoons (1.5g) finely chopped fresh basil, divided

1 tablespoon (13g) pure vanilla extract

DIRECTIONS

1 Heat the oven to 350 degrees F (175 degrees C). Grease an 8×8-inch baking pan with 1 teaspoon EVOO and set aside.

2 To make the topping, combine the flour, oats, flaxseeds, date sugar, macadamia nuts, cinnamon, and sea salt in a large bowl until well combined. Add the ¼ cup EVOO, mix until the mixture resembles wet sand, and then place in the fridge. To make the filling, place the strawberries, honey, 1 teaspoon (.75g) basil, and vanilla in a large bowl and toss to combine. Allow to sit for 5 to 10 minutes.

3 Take ⅓ cup of the topping mixture and toss with the strawberry mixture. Place the strawberry mixture in the pan and sprinkle evenly with topping. Bake the crisp on a baking sheet (just in case the filling bubbles over) for 45 to 55 minutes, or until the topping is golden brown and the filling is bubbling. Remove and cool 10 minutes on wire rack. Garnish with remaining 1 teaspoon (.75g) basil and serve warm.

PER SERVING: *Calories 299 (From Fat 132); Fat 15g (Saturated 2g); Cholesterol 0mg; Sodium 63mg; Carbohydrate 38g (Dietary Fiber 6g); Protein 4g; Sugars 23g.*

Adding Fruit to Traditional Dessert Recipes

Chapter 9 focuses on transforming fruit into dessert, but this section takes those recipes a step further, incorporating them into traditional recipes in unique ways. Passionfruit, berries, cherries, and pumpkin are just a few of the scores of fresh fruits that make dessert recipes sing.

This section contains the following recipes:

» **Passionfruit Tiramisu:** Rich, indulgent flavors of traditional tiramisu are reserved for special occasions in Italy. This version combines yogurt and passionfruit for a light, uplifting version that's perfect for a healthy indulgence any time of year.

» **Strawberry Shortcake:** This summer classic is enriched with almonds to make it healthier and more satisfying.

» **Pumpkin Gingerbread Trifle:** This is a perfect fall and winter holiday dessert.

» **Mixed Berry and Mascarpone Parfaits:** This delicious parfait does double duty at breakfast and brunch.

» **Ricotta and Berry Cheesecake Torte:** This torte is a lovely way to end a special meal.

» **Almond and Cherry Clafoutis:** A *clafoutis* is a typical home-style French dessert resembling a thick cakey baked custard, sometimes called a French flan.

Passionfruit Tiramisu

PREP TIME: 10 MIN	COOK TIME: OVERNIGHT CHILLING	YIELD: 8 SERVINGS

INGREDIENTS

One 7-ounce (198g) package lady fingers (24 total)

1 cup (237mL) passion fruit juice

20 ounces (591mL) fresh or frozen passion fruit pulp

2 cups (200g) full-fat vanilla yogurt

1 teaspoon (2.6g) cinnamon

1 teaspoon (1.8g) natural unsweetened cocoa powder

8 fresh mint sprigs

DIRECTIONS

1 Line the bottom of an 8-inch-wide bowl with 12 lady fingers (you may need to break a few to get them to fit into holes) making an even layer. Pour ½ cup of the passion fruit juice evenly over the lady fingers.

2 Combine the yogurt with the cinnamon in a medium bowl. Spoon the yogurt mixture over the lady fingers evenly. Scatter the passion fruit pulp over the yogurt, reserving 1 tablespoon for garnish. Line the top of the passion fruit with the remaining 12 lady fingers. Pour the remaining ½ cup passionfruit juice over the lady fingers.

3 Place the cocoa powder in a small sieve and sift over the top of the lady fingers. Place the remaining tablespoon of passionfruit pulp in the center of the tiramisu.

4 Refrigerate overnight. Serve 8 equal portions in small dessert cups and garnish each with a mint sprig.

VARY IT! You can use pineapple and pineapple juice instead of passion fruit.

PER SERVING: *Calories 223 (From Fat 25); Fat 3g (Saturated 1g); Cholesterol 55mg; Sodium 81mg; Carbohydrate 42g (Dietary Fiber 8g); Protein 9g; Sugars 26g.*

🍓 Strawberry Shortcake

PREP TIME: 15 MIN	COOK TIME: 10 MIN	YIELD: 5 SERVINGS

INGREDIENTS

¾ cup (84g) almond flour

½ cup (60g) tapioca flour

1 teaspoon (4.6g) baking powder

½ teaspoon (2.3g) baking soda

¼ cup (48g) date sugar

2½ tablespoons (35.5g) cold unsalted butter, cut into small pieces

¼ cup (59mL) whole milk

1 teaspoon (4.9g) lemon juice

1 large egg

1 pound fresh (454g) strawberries, hulled and sliced

¼ cup (85g) plus 1 tablespoon (21g) honey

½ cup (118mL) heavy whipping cream or cream from raw milk

½ teaspoon (2.1g) vanilla

DIRECTIONS

1 Preheat the oven to 400 degrees F (205 degrees C). Add all the dry ingredients to a large mixing bowl and mix well and then add the butter. Using two forks or a pastry cutter, mix in the butter until it's well incorporated, but some chunks remain intact. Add all the wet ingredients to a small bowl and whisk them together. Pour the wet ingredients into the dry ingredients and mix until well combined.

2 Use a large spoon or a ¼ cup measuring cup to form about ¼ cup of the dough and drop it onto a parchment paper–lined baking sheet. Bake for 10 minutes or until a toothpick comes out clean. While the shortcake is baking, drizzle honey over the strawberries in a bowl and stir.

3 To make the whipped topping, add the whipping cream, 1 tablespoon honey, and vanilla to a large bowl. Mix with a hand mixer on high until stiff peaks form. Slice the biscuit in half and scoop the strawberries in the middle and top with whipped topping. Replace the biscuit top and add more strawberries and whipped topping.

PER SERVING: *Calories 390 (From Fat 182); Fat 20g (Saturated 8g); Cholesterol 75mg; Sodium 250mg; Carbohydrate 48g (Dietary Fiber 6g); Protein 6g; Sugars 31g.*

Pumpkin Gingerbread Trifle

PREP TIME: 15 MIN	COOK TIME: 2 HRS CHILLING	YIELD: 8 SERVINGS

INGREDIENTS

1 Chocolate and Pumpkin Snack Cake (see Chapter 17), cut into 1-inch cubes

3 tablespoons (1 ounce) (42g) mascarpone

2 cups (200g) vanilla yogurt

2 cups (490g) pureed pumpkin

1 tablespoon (12g) date sugar

1 teaspoon (1.8g) ginger

1 teaspoon (1.7g) pumpkin pie spice

¾ cup (83g) no-sugar-added granola

½ teaspoon (.9g) ground ginger

¼ cup (26g) sliced almonds

DIRECTIONS

1 Place ½ of the Chocolate and Pumpkin Snack Cake cubes on the bottom of an 8-inch clear trifle bowl.

2 Stir the mascarpone and the yogurt together. Spoon ½ of the mixture on top of the cake. Mix the pumpkin, date sugar, ginger, and pumpkin pie spice together in a medium bowl. Spread ½ on top of the yogurt mixture.

3 Scatter the remaining Chocolate and Pumpkin Snack Cake over the pumpkin puree. Spoon the remaining yogurt mixture over the top and then the rest of the pumpkin puree. Place the granola in a small bowl, stir in the ginger and scatter over the top, followed by the almonds.

4 Cover with plastic wrap and refrigerate a minimum of 2 hours or a maximum of overnight before serving.

TIP: If you don't have pumpkin pie spice, you can substitute ½ teaspoon cinnamon, ¼ teaspoon ground cloves, and ¼ teaspoon allspice instead.

VARY IT! Substitute regular gingerbread or pumpkin bread for the Chocolate and Pumpkin Snack Cake.

PER SERVING: *Calories 555 (From Fat 190); Fat 21g (Saturated 6g); Cholesterol 60mg; Sodium 558mg; Carbohydrate 77g (Dietary Fiber 11g); Protein 22g; Sugars 26g.*

⌚ Mixed Berry and Mascarpone Parfaits

PREP TIME: 15 MIN	COOK TIME: 2 HRS CHILLING	YIELD: 6 SERVINGS

INGREDIENTS

½ cup (72g) trimmed strawberries, thinly sliced, divided

½ cup (74g) blueberries, divided

½ cup (62g) raspberries, divided

3 tablespoons (1 ounce) (42g) mascarpone

1 tablespoon (12g) date sugar

1 teaspoon (2.6g) cinnamon

1 cup (227g) full-fat Greek yogurt with 1 teaspoon (4.2g) pure vanilla extract stirred in

¾ cup (83g) lowfat almond granola

DIRECTIONS

1 Place ¼ cup strawberries, ¼ cup blueberries, ¼ cup raspberries, mascarpone, date sugar, and cinnamon in a blender and whip until light. Stir in the yogurt and set aside.

2 Pour ⅓ cup of the yogurt mixture into 6 clear parfait glasses.

3 Top with 1 layer of remaining strawberry slices (reserving 6 for garnish), blueberries, and raspberries. Scatter 1 tablespoon granola on top of the berries in each glass. Top each glass with another layer of remaining strawberry mixture. Garnish with 1 remaining strawberry. Cover with plastic wrap and refrigerate a minimum of 2 hours or a maximum of overnight before serving.

PER SERVING: *Calories 156 (From Fat 72); Fat 8g (Saturated 4g); Cholesterol 10mg; Sodium 21mg; Carbohydrate 17g (Dietary Fiber 2g); Protein 6g; Sugars 7g.*

Ricotta and Berry Cheesecake Torte

PREP TIME: 15 MIN	COOK TIME: 30 MIN PLUS 2 HRS CHILLING	YIELD: 10 SERVINGS

INGREDIENTS

1 cup (125g) all-purpose flour, plus extra for rolling out dough

¼ cup (28g) almond flour

2 tablespoons (14g) ground flaxseeds

2 tablespoons (18g) date sugar

½ teaspoon (2.4g) sea salt

½ teaspoon (2.3g) baking powder

4 tablespoons (57g) cold, unsalted butter, cut into pieces

⅓ cup (79mL) whole milk

1 egg yolk mixed with 1 tablespoon (14mL) water

1 recipe Mixed Berry Compote (see Chapter 9)

2¼ cups (554g) whole milk ricotta

½ teaspoon (1.3g) cinnamon

3 tablespoons (63g) honey

2 cups (296g) mixed fresh berries (blackberries, raspberries, blueberries, strawberries)

DIRECTIONS

1 In a food processor, pulse together the flour, almond flour, flaxseeds, date sugar, sea salt, and baking powder. Add the butter and process until the largest pieces are the size of small peas. With the machine running, add the milk until the dough holds together. If the mixture is too dry, add additional milk, a teaspoon at a time. Pat the dough into a disk and wrap it in plastic wrap. Refrigerate the dough for 1 hour or up to overnight.

2 On a lightly floured surface with a floured rolling pin, roll out the dough to ¼ inches thick. If the dough starts to break and crack around the edges, simply push it together. Sprinkle the surface of the dough and the rolling pin with flour. Continue rolling out the dough until it's 10 inches in diameter.

3 Preheat the oven to 375 degrees F (190 degrees C). Fit the dough into a 9-inch tart pan with a removable bottom. Gently press down to cover the bottom and sides. Patch any broken holes or cracks with your fingers. Use a fork to prick holes in the dough. Freeze for 15 minutes. Line with parchment paper and fill with pie weights. Bake the shell for 15 minutes.

4 Remove the parchment and weights and brush with the egg yolk mixture. Bake until golden brown, another 15 minutes, and let cool. Spread with the Mixed Berry Compote. Puree the ricotta with the cinnamon and honey in a food processor or blender. Pour the mixture over the top of the compote and use a table knife or spatula to spread it out. Top with the berries. Chill for 2 hours and serve cold.

NOTE: This tart crust gets its characteristic flavor from the combination of almond meal and flaxseeds. However, you may substitute this crust for one of the ones in Chapter 8.

TIP: For quicker prep time, make and bake the tart shell a day in advance.

NOTE: If you leave the dough in the refrigerator overnight, it will need to stand at room temperature for up to an hour prior to rolling out.

NOTE: The combination of healthful fats and protein found in the almonds, flaxseeds, and ricotta, along with carbohydrates from the berries and honey help to balance the sugar.

VARY IT! You can use 2 cups unsweetened berry preserves instead of the Mixed Berry Compote.

PER SERVING: *Calories 393 (From Fat 224); Fat 25g (Saturated 10g); Cholesterol 62mg; Sodium 172mg; Carbohydrate 36g (Dietary Fiber 3g); Protein 10g; Sugars 20g.*

☙ Almond and Cherry Clafoutis

PREP TIME: 10 MIN	COOK TIME: 30 MIN	YIELD: 4 SERVINGS

INGREDIENTS

1 teaspoon (4.5g) Amy Riolo Selections or other EVOO

5 tablespoons (65g) organic coconut sugar, divided

2 extra-large eggs

½ cup (56g) finely ground almond flour

1 cup (237mL) heavy cream

1 teaspoon (4.2g) pure vanilla extract

1 teaspoon (2g) orange zest

1 teaspoon (4.2g) almond extract

Pinch of sea salt

1 cup (154g) pitted cherries, fresh or frozen

1 teaspoon (2.5g) confectioners' sugar, for dusting

DIRECTIONS

1 Preheat the oven to 375 degrees F (190 degrees C). Oil an 8-inch (20 cm) baking dish. Sprinkle 2 tablespoons coconut sugar over the bottom.

2 Beat the eggs and the remaining 3 tablespoons sugar in the bowl of an electric mixer fitted with the paddle attachment on medium-high speed, until light and fluffy, about 3 minutes. With the mixer running on low speed, add in the flour, cream, vanilla extract, orange zest, almond extract, and sea salt. Increase the speed to high and beat for 2 to 3 minutes until very frothy.

3 Add the cherries to the bottom of the baking dish, turn to coat in coconut sugar, and pour the batter over the top. Bake for 20 to 30minutes, until the top is golden, and the custard is set. Serve warm, sprinkled with confectioners' sugar.

NOTE: Remember the general formula of your favorite baking recipes — as well as how they look and smell while baking so that you can recreate them anytime, anywhere.

VARY IT! Swap out the almond flour for other types of flour and the cherries for raspberries or blackberries.

PER SERVING: *Calories 430 (From Fat 297); Fat 33g (Saturated 15g); Cholesterol 200mg; Sodium 121mg; Carbohydrate 28g (Dietary Fiber 3g); Protein 8g; Sugars 22g.*

Chapter **13**

Creating Truffles and Fruit-Based Sweet Treats

RECIPES IN THIS CHAPTER

- **Date, Almond, and Cocoa Balls**
- **Chocolate Peanut Clusters**
- **Peanut Butter and Coconut Bombs**
- **Yogurt Kisses**
- **Coconut Chocolate "Fudge"**
- **Quinoa and Macadamia Clusters**
- **Chocolate Swirl Bark**
- **Chocolate-Covered Stuffed Dates**
- **Stuffed Figs Dipped in Chocolate**
- **Dark Chocolate–Covered Cherries**

Many confections such as truffles, chocolate bark, and chocolate-covered fruit are often made with high sugar ingredients and are therefore normally off-limits for individuals with diabetes.

This chapter explains how you can make decadent interpretations of classic desserts like fudge and chocolate peanut clusters that will satisfy your cravings while also providing unexpected health benefits.

Satisfying Your Sweet Tooth with Bite-Sized Treats

Dark chocolate (80 percent or higher), fresh and dried fruit, nutritious nuts, Greek yogurt, and even extra-virgin olive oil (EVOO) are high quality ingredients that are especially beneficial for people with diabetes.

Here are some of the health benefits of the ingredients in the following recipes:

➤ **EVOO:** Enjoying a few or even several tablespoons of EVOO each day is ideal in order to gain its benefits in cooking, flavoring, drizzling, and even replacing butter or margarine. You can safely cook at all normal temperatures with EEVO, exactly as they do in the Mediterranean; the antioxidant compounds protect the oil from burning or degrading and combine healthily with other nutrients in the foods you're cooking. Having a large container of EVOO in the kitchen is economical. Just store it away from light and heat and seal it after you use it. You may want a smaller bottle of fine EVOO for finishing dishes with delicious flavors and healthful polyphenols. The more delightfully peppery and subtly bitter, the more likely it is that the oil is high in polyphenols.

➤ **Greek yogurt:** is a great prebiotic and acts as food for the microbiome. Probiotics, such as fermented foods including yogurt, add specific beneficial species to your microbiome. Try to include them in every meal.

➤ **Fruit:** Fruit has much less kilocalories (half the amount) than even the simplest of cakes and can be the base of many confections.

➤ **Nuts:** The following selections are about the same kilocalories as that piece of fruit:

  - 6 almonds

  - 1 tablespoon cashews

  - 2 whole pecans

  - 10 large peanuts

  - 2 whole walnuts

➤ **Dark chocolate:** The polyphenols in dark chocolate (80 percent or higher) may improve *insulin sensitivity,* or how well insulin works in the body, which may delay or prevent the onset of diabetes and may help control blood sugar.

Here are the recipes in this section:

➤ **Date, Almond, and Cocoa Balls:** Healthful no-bake desserts make wonderful beginner recipes for young children and can also be enjoyed as snacks in between meals.

➤ **Chocolate Peanut Clusters:** These healthful sweet treats make great gifts at holiday time.

➤ **Peanut Butter and Coconut Bombs:** This is a delicious and nutritious snack for palates of all ages.

➤ **Yogurt Kisses:** These make great after-school snacks as well as dessert.

Date, Almond, and Cocoa Balls

INGREDIENTS

1 pound (454g) soft Medjool dates, pitted

2 tablespoons (27g) Amy Riolo Selections or other EVOO

¼ cup (59mL) water

½ pound (227g) blanched almonds

1 teaspoon (4.2g) vanilla extract

1 teaspoon (2g) ground cardamom

½ teaspoon (1.3g) ground cinnamon

½ cup (43g) unsweetened dark cocoa

DIRECTIONS

1 Place the dates, EVOO, water, almonds, vanilla, cardamom, and cinnamon in a food processor. Pulse to form a smooth paste. Shape the dough into date-size balls.

2 Spread cocoa onto a plate. Roll the date balls into the cocoa to coat and then arrange on a serving platter. Store in an airtight container in the refrigerator for up to a week.

TIP: If you can only find dates that are hard and dry, soak them in water overnight before using the recipe. Even if you buy pitted dates, always double-check; occasionally you may still find a pit or two.

VARY IT! You can use dried figs instead of dates if preferred.

PER SERVING: *Calories 367 (From Fat 167); Fat 19g (Saturated 2g); Cholesterol 0mg; Sodium 10mg; Carbohydrate 52g (Dietary Fiber 9g); Protein 8g; Sugars 39g.*

Chocolate Peanut Clusters

PREP TIME: 15 MIN PLUS 30 MIN COOLING TIME	COOK TIME: 6 TO 8 MIN	YIELD: 24 SERVINGS

INGREDIENTS

1½ cup (384g) natural, fresh peanut butter

6 ounces (170g) dark chocolate (80 percent or higher)

10 ounces (283g) peanuts

Fleur de sel, for sprinkling (optional)

DIRECTIONS

1 Set a heatproof bowl over a pan of water over high heat. Bring to a simmer and reduce the heat to low. Add the peanut butter and the chocolate to the bowl and stir until melted and smooth.

2 Add the peanuts and stir to coat in the chocolate. Drop 24 rounded spoonfuls onto a waxed paper–lined baking sheet.

3 Sprinkle with the fleur de sel, if desired. Place the clusters in the refrigerator and chill until firm, about 30 minutes.

TIP: Store the clusters in a covered container in the fridge for up to a week or freeze them for several months.

NOTE: Both dark chocolate and peanuts are diabetes-friendly foods. Peanuts and peanut butter have a low glycemic index, which means they don't cause blood sugar to rise sharply.

VARY IT! Swap raw blanched almonds and natural, fresh almond butter for peanuts and peanut butter.

PER SERVING: *Calories 203 (From Fat 152); Fat 17g (Saturated 4g); Cholesterol 0mg; Sodium 77mg; Carbohydrate 8g (Dietary Fiber 3g); Protein 8g; Sugars 4g.*

Peanut Butter and Coconut Bombs

PREP TIME: 15 MIN | YIELD: 12 SERVINGS

INGREDIENTS

2 tablespoons (18g)
maple syrup

1½ cup (384g) fresh, natural
creamy peanut butter

½ cup (78g) rolled oats

¼ cup (28g) ground flaxseeds

1 teaspoon (2.6g) cinnamon

1 teaspoon (4.2g) vanilla extract

⅓ cup (28g) natural
desiccated coconut

DIRECTIONS

1 In a large mixing bowl add the maple syrup, peanut butter, oats, flaxseeds, cinnamon, and vanilla. Mix well to combine with a wooden spoon.

2 Using a spoon or a small melon baller, scoop out the dough to form 24 equal-sized balls. Roll in your hands to make the balls smooth and uniform.

3 Place the coconut on a plate. Roll the balls in coconut and place them on a serving platter. Serve immediately or store in the refrigerator for up to a week.

TIP: You can find desiccated coconut in organic and health stores and online. It's a great option because it doesn't usually contain sugar or unwanted ingredients and has a dry texture compared to the shredded coconut normally purchased in stores.

NOTE: Desiccated coconut is made by grating the flesh of mature coconuts and then drying it out in hot air. The result is a dry, finely grated coconut that works well when coating and topping dessert recipes.

VARY IT! Substitute the coconut for a mixture of ground cinnamon and cocoa.

PER SERVING: *Calories 248 (From Fat 172); Fat 19g (Saturated 5g); Cholesterol 0mg; Sodium 149mg; Carbohydrate 13g (Dietary Fiber 4g); Protein 10g; Sugars 4g.*

🍅 Yogurt Kisses

PREP TIME: 15 MIN PLUS 2 HRS FREEZING TIME	YIELD: 8 SERVINGS

INGREDIENTS

1½ cups (340g) plain Greek yogurt

3 tablespoons (60g) maple syrup

2 teaspoons (8.4g) vanilla extract

1 teaspoon (2.6g) ground cinnamon

½ teaspoon (1g) ground cardamom

DIRECTIONS

1 Mix all the ingredients together in a medium bowl. Spoon the mixture into a plastic, sealable bag and snip off one corner or put into a pastry bag. Line a baking sheet with parchment paper.

2 Pipe the "kisses" (to look like the chocolate candy) onto lined tray. Freeze for 2 hours and serve or store in the refrigerator for up to a week.

VARY IT! Add ¼ cup (37.9g) dark cocoa to make chocolate kisses.

PER SERVING: *Calories 64 (From Fat 18); Fat 2g (Saturated 1g); Cholesterol 0mg; Sodium 16mg; Carbohydrate 8g (Dietary Fiber 0g); Protein 4g; Sugars 6g.*

Pleasing Your Palate with Fudge, Clusters, and Bark

Rich, sweet fudge, clusters, and bark are seemingly the most off-limits of all confections for people with diabetes. Thanks to the use of nuts, dark chocolate, and dried fruit, however, these recipes are energy boosters and palate pleasers that won't spike your blood sugar levels.

TIP

Make them ahead of time and keep them in the freezer for when needed. They're a wonderful alternative to purchased chocolates for people looking to balance their blood sugar.

Try the following recipes:

>> **Coconut Chocolate "Fudge":** Cocoa powder, dark chocolate, and coconut oil replace the butter and large amounts of sugar in the original recipe.

>> **Quinoa and Macadamia Clusters:** Macadamia nuts are a tasty, low-glycemic index snack packed with healthy monounsaturated fats. They also help lower the GI of carbohydrates in meals and snacks.

>> **Chocolate Swirl Bark:** Dark chocolate gets a flavor and a nutrient boost with the addition of healthful sesame seeds, pumpkin seeds, walnuts, and cranberries.

🥥 Coconut Chocolate "Fudge"

PREP TIME: 15 MIN PLUS 4 HRS COOLING TIME

YIELD: 16 SERVINGS

INGREDIENTS

1 cup (218g) semi-solid unrefined coconut oil

½ cup (43g) cocoa powder

3 tablespoons (63g) honey

2 teaspoons (8.4g) vanilla extract

Pinch sea salt

4 ounces (113g) dark chocolate (80 percent or higher), cut into small pieces.

¼ cup (23g) desiccated coconut

DIRECTIONS

1 Place the coconut oil in a bowl. Using a standing mixer fitted with a paddle attachment or a hand mixer, beat the oil until smooth and fluffy, about two minutes.

2 Add the cocoa powder, honey, vanilla, and salt and beat to combine.

3 Pour the mixture into an 8-inch glass baking dish and use a spatula to spread evenly and smooth out the top. Sprinkle the chocolate and coconut on top. Refrigerate 4 hours or overnight to set. To serve, dip a sharp knife into warm water and cut the fudge into 16 equal-sized squares.

TIP: Look for unrefined, cold-pressed, organic coconut oil for the healthiest option.

NOTE: The fudge will be quite hard when you remove it from the refrigerator. Let it sit out for a few minutes before serving.

NOTE: In addition to adding great flavor and texture in baking, coconut oil is also great for your hair and skin.

PER SERVING: *Calories 189 (From Fat 161); Fat 18g (Saturated 15g); Cholesterol 0mg; Sodium 17mg; Carbohydrate 8g (Dietary Fiber 2g); Protein 1g; Sugars 5g.*

Quinoa and Macadamia Clusters

PREP TIME: 15 MIN PLUS 30 MINS COOLING TIME | YIELD: 8 SERVINGS

INGREDIENTS

1 tablespoon (13.5g) unrefined coconut oil

½ cup (85g) quinoa, rinsed

½ cup (67g) raw macadamia nuts, chopped

1 teaspoon (5g) sea salt

1 teaspoon (2.6g) cinnamon

3½ ounces (99g) dark chocolate (80 percent or higher), cut into pieces

Grated zest of 1 orange

DIRECTIONS

1 Line a baking sheet with parchment paper and set aside. Heat a large skillet over medium heat and add the coconut oil to melt. Add the quinoa, stirring often, for about 5 minutes, until it becomes golden brown. Transfer to a medium bowl and add the macadamia nuts, sea salt, and cinnamon.

2 Place the chocolate in the top of a double boiler over medium heat. Heat until melted, stirring often to prevent burning. Stir in the orange zest and carefully remove from the double boiler.

3 Add the melted chocolate to the quinoa and macadamia mixture and stir well until combined. Drop 8 even spoonfuls (you can use a small melon baller if you want to make additional, smaller clusters) onto the baking sheet. Refrigerate 30 minutes, or until hardened. Store clusters in an airtight container in the refrigerator for up to a week.

NOTE: Instead of a double boiler, you can use a metal or glass bowl over a pot of boiling water.

VARY IT: Swap out almonds or walnuts for the macadamia nuts.

PER SERVING: *Calories 189 (From Fat 126); Fat 14g (Saturated 6g); Cholesterol 0mg; Sodium 259mg; Carbohydrate 14g (Dietary Fiber 3g); Protein 3g; Sugars 3g.*

Chocolate Swirl Bark

INGREDIENTS

12 ounces (340g) dark chocolate (80 percent or higher)

¾ cup (113g) sesame seeds

¼ cup (11g) unsweetened dried cranberries

2 tablespoons (17g) pumpkin seeds

2 tablespoons (16g) roughly chopped walnuts

DIRECTIONS

1 Place the chocolate in the top of a double boiler over medium heat (you can also use a metal or glass bowl over a pot of boiling water). Heat until melted, stirring often to prevent burning.

2 Place a piece of parchment paper on a large rimmed baking sheet.

3 After the chocolate melts, use a rubber spatula to spread the melted chocolate into an even layer about ¼-inch (.64-cm) thick.

4 Sprinkle and swirl in the sesame seeds, cranberries, pumpkin seeds, and walnuts on top of the chocolate. Gently press the ingredients into the chocolate. Place the baking sheet on a flat surface in the refrigerator for 30 minutes. When the chocolate is completely hardened, use your hands to break it apart into the desired amount of pieces.

TIP: Be sure to use the best quality chocolate that you like the most in this recipe.

NOTE: In Step 3, when spreading the melted chocolate, don't worry if the chocolate doesn't reach the edges of the baking sheet or if it's not a perfect rectangle.

NOTE: You can store the pieces of bark in between sheets of waxed or parchment paper in an airtight container in the refrigerator for up to a week.

VARY IT! Swap out the sesame seeds for hemp or flaxseeds and the unsweetened dried cranberries for cherries or figs.

PER SERVING: *Calories 242 (From Fat 163); Fat 18g (Saturated 8g); Cholesterol 1mg; Sodium 10mg; Carbohydrate 16g (Dietary Fiber 5g); Protein 4g; Sugars 7g.*

Dipping Fruit in Chocolate

Sometimes the simplest desserts are the most impressive. Fruit dipped in chocolate is always a popular choice, especially for gift giving. Birthdays, Valentine's Day, and Christmas time are times when chocolate-dipped fruit is always welcomed. They make wonderful gifts for those hosting parties and dinners too.

This section includes the following recipes:

>> **Chocolate-Covered Stuffed Dates:** A decadent classic from the Middle East

>> **Stuffed Figs Dipped in Chocolate:** A traditional Christmas recipe in Southern Italy

>> **Dark Chocolate–Covered Cherries:** The quintessential American romantic edible gift

Chocolate-Covered Stuffed Dates

PREP TIME: 5 MIN PLUS COOLING TIME | **YIELD: 12 SERVINGS**

INGREDIENTS

24 soft Medjool dates, pitted

24 whole almonds

8 ounces (227g) dark chocolate (80 percent or higher)

DIRECTIONS

1 Place the pitted dates on a parchment paper–lined 11-x-17-inch baking sheet.

2 Place an almond where the pit would have been.

3 Heat the chocolate in a glass bowl over a pot of simmering water or in a double boiler over medium heat until melted.

4 Carefully remove the bowl and set onto a surface. Use tongs to pick up the dates and dip them into the chocolate to cover. Repeat with all the dates. Set on a baking sheet to dry. Refrigerate for an hour or until serving. Store in the fridge for a week.

TIP: If your dates aren't soft when you purchase them, soak them in water overnight to soften. If you get called away while dipping the dates in chocolate, the chocolate may harden again and will need to be remelted.

NOTE: I first experienced this recipe in Saudi Arabia, where a wide variety of delicious dates are sold in confectioner's boxes like elegant chocolate candies and enjoyed with coffee.

VARY IT! Use dried figs instead of dates.

PER SERVING: *Calories 260 (From Fat 84); Fat 9g (Saturated 5g); Cholesterol 1mg; Sodium 4mg; Carbohydrate 45g (Dietary Fiber 6g); Protein 3g; Sugars 37g.*

☺ Stuffed Figs Dipped in Chocolate

PREP TIME: 20 MIN	COOK TIME: 5 MIN	YIELD: 10 SERVINGS

INGREDIENTS

20 dried figs

¼ cup (20g) slivered almonds

Zest of 1 orange

1 teaspoon (2.6g) ground cinnamon

½ teaspoon (1.3g) ground cloves

4 ounces dark chocolate (80 percent or higher)

DIRECTIONS

1 Preheat the oven to 350 degrees F (180 degrees C). Line two baking sheets with parchment paper.

2 With the fig upright, make an incision halfway down to the bottom and open with your fingers. In a small bowl, combine the almonds, orange zest, cinnamon, and cloves. Stuff each of the figs with the filling. Press the figs closed and place them an inch (2.5 cm) apart on one baking sheet. Bake until slightly softened and darkened, 5 to 8 minutes.

3 Place the chocolate in the top of a double boiler over low heat. Heat, stirring constantly, just until chocolate is melted, 2 to 3 minutes.

4 Remove the figs from the oven and using tongs or holding figs by the stem, dip them quickly into the warm chocolate. Place on the second baking sheet and allow to cool. Store in an air-tight container in the refrigerator. Allow to stand at room temperature for at least 20 minutes before serving.

NOTE: This recipe is usually reserved for Christmas and New Year's Day, but I like to make them as edible gifts for my loved ones throughout the year. Dried figs contain a very concentrated amount of vitamins and minerals and just one of these chocolate-covered figs is satisfying.

VARY IT! Swap out dates or unsulphured apricots in this recipe.

PER SERVING: *Calories 179 (From Fat 59); Fat 7g (Saturated 3g); Cholesterol 0mg; Sodium 6mg; Carbohydrate 30g (Dietary Fiber 5g); Protein 3g; Sugars 21g.*

Dark Chocolate–Covered Cherries

PREP TIME: 10 MIN PLUS 2 HRS COOLING TIME	COOK TIME: 2 MIN	YIELD: 8 SERVINGS

INGREDIENTS

24 fresh cherries with stems

1 cup (168g) dark chocolate (80 percent or higher) pieces

2 tablespoons (27g) Amy Riolo Selections, or other EVOO

DIRECTIONS

1 Carefully remove the pit from each cherry while keeping the stem intact.

2 Place the chocolate in a microwave-safe bowl. Add the olive oil and stir. Heat the mixture in the microwave for about 20 seconds. Remove and stir and repeat until the chocolate is mostly melted. Stir well to combine.

3 Line a baking sheet with parchment paper. Dip each cherry in the dark chocolate and place it on the baking sheet. Repeat with the remaining cherries. Place in the refrigerator and allow to set for a few hours before serving.

TIP: Cherries have a low glycemic index, making them a good choice for diabetes-friendly desserts.

NOTE: Adding EVOO to the chocolate helps to lessen the glycemic load.

VARY IT! You can use this method with any dried fruit.

PER SERVING *(3 cherries): Calories 171 (From Fat 111); Fat 12g (Saturated 6g); Cholesterol 1mg; Sodium 4mg; Carbohydrate 14g (Dietary Fiber 3g); Protein 2g; Sugars 8g.*

Chapter **14**

Whipping Up Frozen Desserts

RECIPES IN THIS CHAPTER

☺ **Vanilla Frozen Yogurt**

☺ **Vanilla Gelato**

☺ **Pineapple Frozen Yogurt Pops**

☺ **Strawberry, Yogurt, and White Balsamic Semifreddo**

☺ **Orange and Greek Yogurt Creamsicles**

☺ **Strawberry Swirl Ice Cream**

☺ **Coffee Ice Cream**

☺ **Chocolate "Ice Cream"**

☺ **Pistachio Honey Ice Cream**

☺ **Banana and Peanut Butter "Ice Cream"**

Frozen desserts have roots in ancient Persia and are now enjoyed all over the world. Nowadays, many frozen desserts are so readily available that people don't think about making them at home.

Because modern commercially prepared frozen desserts are often laden with sodium, sugar, and unhealthful fats as well as artificial ingredients, they're considered off-limits for people with diabetes. By making your own desserts and using quality ingredients such as natural fruit and frozen yogurt, you don't need to miss out on frozen desserts in order to keep your blood sugar balanced.

This chapter explains how to make delicious frozen treats like frozen yogurt, ice cream, gelato, sorbet, granita, and more that fit into a diabetes-friendly meal plan.

⏱ **Lemon Granita**

⏱ **Espresso Granita**

⏱ **Raspberry Sorbet**

⏱ **Frozen Peanut Butter and Vanilla Cups**

⏱ **Blackberry Banana Soft Serve**

⏱ **Red, White, and Blue Creamsicles**

Having Fun with Frozen Yogurt

Most people appreciate frozen desserts in warmer months. The best thing about serving frozen yogurt recipes to guests is that you can make them in advance and have them ready when needed. These desserts have a sweet spot in everyone's heart, whether they have diabetes or not.

I chose Greek yogurt for these recipes because it has a high amount of protein and is a healthy source of fat and carbohydrate. Not only will eating it not cause your blood sugar to spike, but it can also help to stabilize glucose levels.

One of the challenges for people who are trying to eat healthfully is the desire for a large, sweet dessert. By keeping healthier versions such as these recipes on hand in the freezer, you don't have to deprive yourself of anything, and you're more likely to steer clear of the high fat and high sugar desserts that cause a spike in blood sugar:

>> **Vanilla Frozen Yogurt:** This is a classic, base recipe for frozen desserts and a great one to have on hand in the summertime.

>> **Vanilla Gelato:** This healthier version on the traditional Italian frozen treat is a delight for the taste buds that doesn't derail your diet.

>> **Pineapple Frozen Yogurt Pops:** Greek yogurt, pineapple, and cardamom make a bright and vibrant flavor profile to enjoy anytime.

>> **Strawberry, Yogurt, and White Balsamic Semifreddo:** *Semifreddo* is a genre of Italian semi-frozen desserts that are made with a mousse-like base. Popular in restaurants because they can be made in advance, they're also easy to reproduce at home.

>> **Orange and Greek Yogurt Creamsicles:** This recipe is a great way to cool off during the summer.

TIP

Many different popsicle molds are available on the market and depending on the size you use determines how many servings you make for these recipes that require molds. Look for molds that hold about four-tenths fluid ounces to make a standard American popsicle size.

Vanilla Frozen Yogurt

PREP TIME: 10 MIN PLUS 6 HRS CHILL TIME	YIELD: 4 SERVINGS

INGREDIENTS

2 cups (238g) plain Greek yogurt

⅓ cup (112g) honey

1 teaspoon (5g) vanilla paste

DIRECTIONS

1 Whisk the yogurt, honey, and vanilla paste together.

2 If you have an ice cream maker, spoon the mixture into the machine and process according to your machine's directions. If you don't have an ice cream maker, freeze the yogurt mixture in an ice cube tray, and then blend in a blender on high speed until smooth and creamy.

3 Store in an airtight container in the freezer for up to a month but is best served just after chilling. Thaw any leftovers 15 to 20 minutes before serving.

TIP: If you don't have a blender or prefer to make frozen yogurt the old fashioned way, skip Step 2 and freeze the mixture in a shallow container. Stir the slush once every 30 minutes for three hours and serve when solid and creamy. This was how I originally learned to make it.

NOTE: Because of the Greek yogurt content, this recipe is balanced and doesn't need to be eaten with a meal. You can enjoy it as a snack or between meals.

VARY IT! Top with chopped almonds, dark chocolate, sliced bananas, or berries.

PER SERVING: *Calories 141 (From Fat 25); Fat 3g (Saturated 2g); Cholesterol 0mg; Sodium 22mg; Carbohydrate 26g (Dietary Fiber 0g); Protein 5g; Sugars 25g.*

Vanilla Gelato

INGREDIENTS

3½ cups (826mL) whole milk

1 cup (237mL) heavy cream

1 cup (176g) allulose, divided

7 egg yolks

Pinch sea salt

1½ teaspoons (7.5g) vanilla bean paste or vanilla extract

2 tablespoons (27g) Amy Riolo Selections or other EVOO

DIRECTIONS

1 Combine the milk and cream in a large heavy-bottomed saucepan and bring to a simmer over medium heat. Remove from the heat. Add ¾ cup (132g) of the allulose to the milk and bring to a simmer over medium heat, stirring to dissolve the allulose.

2 Whisk the egg yolks, the remaining ¼ cup (44g) allulose, and the sea salt together in a medium heatproof bowl. Gradually whisk in about 1 cup (236.5mL) of the hot milk mixture, then return the mixture to the saucepan and cook, stirring constantly with a heatproof spatula or a wooden spoon, until the custard registers 185 degrees F (85 degrees C) on an instant-read thermometer.

3 Immediately strain the custard through a fine-mesh strainer into a heatproof bowl. Add the vanilla, and chill over an ice bath, stirring occasionally, until cold. Cover and refrigerate for at least 6 hours, or, preferably, overnight.

4 Freeze the gelato in an ice cream maker according to the manufacturer's instructions, stopping to add the EVOO about halfway through the freezing process. Pack into a freezer container and freeze for at least 1 hour before serving. Sprinkle a few flakes of sea salt and drizzle with EVOO.

NOTE: The gelato is best served the day it's made.

PER SERVING: *Calories 489 (From Fat 392); Fat 44g (Saturated 21g); Cholesterol 470mg; Sodium 187mg; Carbohydrate 13g (Dietary Fiber 0g); Protein 13g; Sugars 11g.*

Pineapple Frozen Yogurt Pops

INGREDIENTS

2 cups (330g) fresh pineapple chunks, chopped into small pieces divided

3 cups (680g) plain Greek yogurt

½ cup (88g) allulose

1 teaspoon (4.2g) pure vanilla extract

1 teaspoon (2g) ground cardamom

DIRECTIONS

1 Combine 1 cup of the pineapple chunks with the Greek yogurt, allulose, vanilla, and cardamom and mix well in a bowl.

2 Fill popsicle molds ¼ full with the yogurt mixture and add a little more than a tablespoon of the remaining pineapple chunks. Continue to fill with the yogurt mixture until the popsicle molds are full. Place the popsicle stick down the middle. Freeze approximately 6 hours, or until solid.

TIP: Choose classic popsicle molds with 4-ounce capacity per hole.

VARY IT! If you don't have allulose on hand, use organic vanilla and coconut sugar.

PER SERVING: *Calories 66 (From Fat 13); Fat 1g (Saturated 1g); Cholesterol 8mg; Sodium 22mg; Carbohydrate 7g (Dietary Fiber 1g); Protein 7g; Sugars 3g.*

Strawberry, Yogurt, and White Balsamic Semifreddo

PREP TIME: 15 MIN PLUS 6 HRS FREEZING TIME	YIELD: 8 SERVINGS

INGREDIENTS

1 cup (144g) plus 8 strawberries, hulled

1 cup (176g) plus 1 tablespoon (13g) allulose powder, divided

2 tablespoons (32g) Amy Riolo Selections White Balsamic or your favorite no-sugar-added balsamic

6 egg yolks

1 cup (238g) whipping cream

1 teaspoon (4.2g) pure vanilla extract

DIRECTIONS

1 Combine the strawberry pieces (reserving 8 small pieces for garnish) and 1 tablespoon allulose with the white balsamic and allow to stand for 20 minutes at room temperature.

2 In a medium bowl combine the egg yolks and 1 cup allulose. Beat with an electric mixer on medium speed for 5 minutes or until the mixture is creamy and lemon colored. Add the whipping cream and continue mixing until it becomes thick and mousse-like but not too stiff. Add the vanilla extract and mix well to combine. Fold in the strawberry-balsamic mixture.

3 Transfer the mixture into 8 ramekins or serving cups that are about 3-inches wide and 1 ⅓-inches (approximately 7.5cm by 3.5cm) tall. Chill in the refrigerator for a minimum of 6 or up to 24 hours if that works better with your schedule. Garnish with a strawberry each and serve chilled.

VARY IT! Substitute other berries, dried fruit, nuts, or dark chocolate for the strawberries and use your favorite natural sugar instead of the allulose.

PER SERVING: *Calories 158 (From Fat 130); Fat 14g (Saturated 8g); Cholesterol 198mg; Sodium 19mg; Carbohydrate 4g (Dietary Fiber 1g); Protein 3g; Sugars 2g.*

Orange and Greek Yogurt Creamsicles

PREP TIME: 15 MIN PLUS 6 HRS FREEZING | YIELD: 8 SERVINGS

INGREDIENTS

Juice and zest of 1 orange

3 cups (680g) plain
Greek yogurt

¼ cup (48g) coconut sugar

1 teaspoon (4.2g) pure
vanilla extract

DIRECTIONS

1 Combine the orange juice and zest with the Greek yogurt, sugar, and vanilla and mix well in a bowl.

2 Add the yogurt mixture to the popsicle molds until they're full. Place the popsicle stick in the middle. Freeze approximately 6 hours, or until solid.

NOTE: Be sure to use freshly squeezed orange juice for the best results.

VARY IT! Swap out coconut sugar with organic vanilla and coconut sugar.

PER SERVING: *Calories 88 (From Fat 16); Fat 2g (Saturated 1g); Cholesterol 10mg; Sodium 28mg; Carbohydrate 4g (Dietary Fiber 0g); Protein 9g; Sugars 1g.*

Transforming Ice Cream into a Healthful Finale

Like with all other culinary recipes, not all ice creams are created equal. In theory, when made with wholesome ingredients and eaten in appropriate portions, ice cream can be a part of a diabetes meal plan. Some studies show that consuming certain ice creams before bed can help keep blood sugar levels even throughout the night when eaten as a late-night snack. Make sure you quantify which type of ice cream as well as how it's made that are the determining factor.

The easiest way to ensure that you can enjoy ice cream without spiking your blood sugar or eating unhealthful ingredients is to make it yourself. Making ice cream is easy and fun; it just takes a bit of advance prep work, but the results are worth the effort.

The use of Greek yogurt in these recipes is intentional because it contains each of the three macronutrients. That means that you can enjoy the ice cream after or in-between meals without worrying about eating something else to balance the effects of the sugar. If you don't tell people how healthful they are when serving them, these recipes will pass for being tasty homemade treats. You can then surprise people with the health benefits after they've enjoyed them.

TIP

If you substitute nondairy yogurts for the Greek yogurt, be sure to add a scoop or two of unsweetened vanilla protein powder to the mix.

The following recipes appear in this section:

>> **Strawberry Swirl Ice Cream:** A beautiful and tasty summer treat for kids and adults alike.

>> **Coffee Ice Cream:** A sophisticated twist on a classic satisfies your sweet tooth and coffee cravings.

>> **Chocolate "Ice Cream":** This nutrient-dense recipe is a delicious indulgent that you can feel good about.

>> **Pistachio Honey Ice Cream:** Try serving this Middle Eastern-inspired favorite following a Mediterranean-style meal.

>> **Banana and Peanut Butter "Ice Cream":** This recipe appeals to all ages!

🍓 Strawberry Swirl Ice Cream

PREP TIME: 15 MIN PLUS OVERNIGHT FREEZING	YIELD: 8 SERVINGS

INGREDIENTS

2 cups (288g) fresh strawberries, cleaned, hulled and divided in half

¼ cup (85g) honey, divided

2 tablespoons (30mL) water

1¼ cups (296mL) whole milk

1 cup plain (227g) Greek yogurt, drained

2 teaspoons (8.4g) vanilla extract

1 pinch sea salt

DIRECTIONS

1 Puree 1 cup (144g) strawberries, 2 tablespoons (42.5g) honey, and 2 tablespoons (30mL) water in a blender or food processor until smooth. Cover and place in refrigerator. Finely chop the remaining cup of strawberries.

2 In a medium bowl, whisk the milk, Greek yogurt, remaining 2 tablespoons (42.5g) of honey, vanilla, and sea salt. Stir in the chopped strawberries and refrigerate 1 to 2 hours or overnight.

3 Turn on the ice cream maker, pour the mixture into the frozen freezer bowl, and let the maker run until a soft, creamy consistency is achieved, about 20 minutes. Slowly pour in the strawberry puree from the refrigerator. Turn off as soon as the puree is swirled in but not blended, a few seconds.

4 Transfer the ice cream to an airtight container and freeze for at least 3 hours, or until it achieves the desired consistency. Serve in dessert bowls.

PER SERVING: *Calories 90 (From Fat 17); Fat 2g (Saturated 1g); Cholesterol 7mg; Sodium 56mg; Carbohydrate 14g (Dietary Fiber 1g); Protein 4g; Sugars 13g.*

Coffee Ice Cream

INGREDIENTS

1 tablespoon (6g) finely ground espresso

1 cup (236.5mL) whole milk

1 cup (176g) allulose

1 cup (284g) coconut cream

DIRECTIONS

1 Place the coffee grounds in a small saucepan with the milk and bring to a boil over medium heat. Let the pan cool and strain it into another bowl. Add the allulose. Gently fold the coconut cream in the cooled coffee mixture. Pour into a large, wide container (plastic 9-x-13 with lid is fine). Place it in the freezer for at least 2 hours. Remove from the freezer and stir with a fork to break up any crystals that have formed.

2 Smooth out the surface and return to the freezer for at least another hour. Remove from the freezer and mix again to ensure crystals are broken. Pack the ice cream into another (smaller) container and freeze until serving.

NOTE: If not serving the ice cream immediately, allow leftovers to thaw for 15 minutes before serving.

PER SERVING: *Calories 301 (From Fat 126); Fat 14g (Saturated 13g); Cholesterol 6mg; Sodium 53mg; Carbohydrate 42g (Dietary Fiber 0g); Protein 3g; Sugars 3g.*

BUYING STORE-BOUGHT ICE CREAM

Choosing healthful ice creams at the supermarket can be challenging because there's so much variation. Many conventional brands are full of not only sugar, but sodium, chemicals, and fake dyes. Others contain lower sugar and fewer ingredients so read the label and the nutritional profile. Here are a few ways to make sure that you're choosing the best store-bought ice cream:

- Look for ice cream low in sugar, sodium, and free of artificial sweeteners and flavors and lower in carbohydrates and saturated fat.

- Select ice creams that are higher in protein.

- Stick to a serving size, which is usually ½ cup.

Chocolate "Ice Cream"

PREP TIME: 10 MIN PLUS OVERNIGHT FREEZING

YIELD: 4 SERVINGS

INGREDIENTS

2 ripe medium-size bananas

2 ripe medium-size avocados

⅓ cup (78.6mL) full-fat coconut milk

⅓ cup (28g) dark cocoa powder

1 tablespoon (15g) cold coffee or espresso

1 teaspoon (4.2g) pure vanilla extract

½ teaspoon (.25g) pure stevia extract powder

DIRECTIONS

1 Add the bananas, avocados, coconut milk, cocoa powder, coffee, vanilla, and stevia extract to a food processor or blender and blend until completely smooth, stopping occasionally to scrape the sides with a spatula.

2 If using a homemade ice cream maker, blend the mixture in the ice cream maker according to package instructions, and then pack into a container and freeze. If making without an ice cream maker, place the mixture in a shallow metal baking pan lined with plastic wrap and freeze 6 hours or overnight.

TIP: Remove the ice cream from the freezer about 20 minutes before serving to slightly thaw so it's easier to scoop.

TIP: Because this ice cream doesn't contain a significant amount of protein, be sure to pair it with a handful of almonds or another quality protein source.

VARY IT! Swap out coconut milk for Greek yogurt.

PER SERVING: Calories 266 (From Fat 179); Fat 20g (Saturated 6g); Cholesterol 0mg; Sodium 12mg; Carbohydrate 27g (Dietary Fiber 11g); Protein 4g; Sugars 8g.

🍅 Pistachio Honey Ice Cream

PREP TIME: 15 MIN PLUS 3 HRS FREEZING | **YIELD: 6 SERVINGS**

INGREDIENTS

1 cup (236mL) whole milk

2 cups (454g) plain
Greek yogurt

½ cup (170g) honey

¼ cup (44g) allulose

1 tablespoon (15g) vanilla
paste, or pure vanilla extract

¼ teaspoon (1.2g) sea salt

1 cup (123g) unsalted roasted
pistachios

DIRECTIONS

1   In a large bowl, whisk together the milk, Greek yogurt, honey, allulose, vanilla, and sea salt. Add the pistachios to a food processor and pulse a few times until the nuts are broken down but not yet a powder consistency. Add the pistachios to the bowl.

2   If using an ice cream maker, pour the mixture into your ice cream maker and follow the manufacturer's instructions for proper use. If making without an ice cream maker, pour into a large, wide container (plastic 9-x-13 with lid is fine). Place it in the freezer for at least 2 hours. Remove from the freezer and stir with a fork to break up any crystals that have formed. Smooth out the surface and return to the freezer for at least another hour. Remove from the freezer and mix again to ensure crystals are broken.

3   Transfer to a smaller freezer-safe container and freeze for at least 4 hours before serving.

NOTE: The combination of milk, yogurt, and pistachios provide healthful fats, protein, and carbohydrates, making it balanced in terms of macronutrients.

VARY IT! Swap out milk and yogurt with nondairy options.

PER SERVING: *Calories 281 (From Fat 111); Fat 12g (Saturated 3g); Cholesterol 13mg; Sodium 123mg; Carbohydrate 33g (Dietary Fiber 2g); Protein 13g; Sugars 27g.*

Banana and Peanut Butter "Ice Cream"

PREP TIME: 5 MIN	COOK TIME: 2-4 HOURS FREEZING TIME	YIELD: 4 SERVINGS

INGREDIENTS

3 large very ripe bananas, sliced

¼ cup (64g) unsweetened natural peanut butter

1 teaspoon (4.2g) pure vanilla

¼ cup (60mL) whole milk

DIRECTIONS

1 Arrange the banana slices in a single layer on a large plate or baking sheet. Freeze for 1 to 2 hours.

2 Place the frozen banana in a food processor or blender. Puree the banana, scraping down the bowl as needed. Puree until the mixture is creamy and smooth. Add the peanut butter, vanilla, and milk and puree to combine.

TIP: For soft-serve ice cream consistency, serve immediately. If you prefer harder ice cream, place it in an airtight container and freeze for a few hours and then serve.

TIP: Whenever you have leftover bananas that are ripening too quickly, peel and freeze them to make this recipe at a later date.

VARY IT: Swap out regular milk for unsweetened almond or oat milk if desired.

PER SERVING: Calories 191 (From Fat 86); Fat 10g (Saturated 2g); Cholesterol 2mg; Sodium 79mg; Carbohydrate 23g (Dietary Fiber 4g); Protein 5g; Sugars 12g.

Trying Granita and Sorbet Recipes

Nothing beats a refreshing granita or sorbet in the hot weather. These recipes are better made at home because they're simple and they allow you to control costs and the use of unwanted ingredients.

Although both granita and sorbet are ice-based desserts, the way that they're made differs in technique. Granita and sorbet are made from fruit, sugar, and water, but they differ in texture and preparation method. Here's a quick rundown:

>> **Granita:** It's an originally Sicilian dessert, which is now popular all over Italy. It consists of a granular, icy texture that's made by pouring the mixture into a pan or freezing it on a sheet, then scraping it repeatedly while it freezes. In the summer, granita is often enjoyed for breakfast with warm brioche and whipped cream in place of a hot coffee. Granita is usually made with a 2-part water to 1 part sugar mix.

>> **Sorbet:** Also known as *sorbetto* as it's called in Italian, sorbet is a smooth, soft frozen dessert made by churning the mixture in a similar way to ice cream. Sorbet is lighter than ice cream because it doesn't contain cream or milk, but it's still sweet because of the sugar, and the healthful alternatives in this book will prevent your blood sugar from spiking. Lemon, orange, and raspberry are among the most popular sorbet flavors.

The following section contains a few recipes you can try on a hot day when you're attempting to cool off:

>> **Lemon Granita:** This Italian summertime classic is a popular way to end a seafood-based meal.

>> **Espresso Granita:** When it's too hot to enjoy traditional espresso at breakfast or at the end of the meal, most people opt for granita, often served with a dollop of fresh whipped cream.

>> **Raspberry Sorbet:** Sorbets are an elegant way to finish a meal, especially in the summer. If you have an ice cream maker and want a smoother consistency, you can use it to make this sorbet.

🍅 Lemon Granita

PREP TIME: 30 MIN PLUS FREEZING   **YIELD: 4 SERVINGS**

INGREDIENTS

1¼ cups (300mL) freshly squeezed lemon juice

½ cup (100g) organic vanilla and coconut sugar

1¾ cup (415mL) water

½ cup (118mL) heavy cream

1 teaspoon (4.2g) vanilla

DIRECTIONS

1   Place the lemon juice in a medium bowl and set aside. In a medium saucepan, combine the sugar and water. Make a syrup by heating the mixture until it starts to boil. Remove from the heat and let cool for about 30 minutes. Pour the mixture into a freezer-proof container. Place flat in the freezer.

2   Remove from the freezer every hour and whisk to break up the larger ice crystals until all the liquid is frozen, about 2 to 3 hours, depending on your freezer temperature. If you continue to stir every hour, until frozen, it shouldn't freeze solid. If you run into that problem, however, you can pulse the lemon ice in the food processor.

3   Make the whipped cream by placing the heavy cream in a blender with the vanilla and whipping until fluffy. Otherwise place in a bowl and whisk by hand until you reach the desired consistency.

4   To serve, scoop a small amount of the frozen granita into old-fashioned glasses or champagne flutes. Top with a teaspoon of whipped cream and another scoop of granita. Top with another teaspoon of whipped cream. Allow to melt slightly for a few minutes and serve. Store remaining granita covered in the freezer.

NOTE: In addition to having a refreshing taste on the palate, which is always appreciated after a meal, lemon juice has an alkalizing effect on the body.

NOTE: The most popular granita flavors are lemon and coffee, but nowadays many chefs and pastry chefs are using local produce and specialties to make their own versions. I even had a chili pepper granita while working in Calabria, Italy once!

PER SERVING: *Calories 201 (From Fat 101); Fat 11g (Saturated 7g); Cholesterol 41mg; Sodium 24mg; Carbohydrate 26g (Dietary Fiber 0g); Protein 1g; Sugars 25g.*

Espresso Granita

INGREDIENTS

1¼ cups (300mL) cold espresso

½ cup (100g) organic coconut sugar

1¾ cup (415mL) water

½ cup (118mL) heavy cream

1 teaspoon (4.2g) vanilla

4 roasted coffee beans, for garnish

DIRECTIONS

1 Place the cold espresso in a medium bowl and set aside. In a medium saucepan, combine the sugar and water. Make a syrup by heating the mixture until it starts to boil. Remove from the heat and add the sugar-water mixture to the espresso. Stir and let cool for about 30 min. Pour the mixture into a freezer-proof container. Place flat in the freezer.

2 Remove the mixture from the freezer every hour and whisk to break up the larger ice crystals until all the liquid is frozen, about 2 to 3 hours, depending on your freezer temperature. If you continue to stir every hour, until frozen, it shouldn't freeze solid. If you run into that problem, however, you can pulse the coffee ice in the food processor.

3 Make the whipped cream by placing the heavy cream in a blender with the vanilla and whipping until fluffy. Otherwise place in a bowl and whisk by hand until you reach the desired consistency.

4 To serve, scoop the frozen granita, topped, or layered with whipped cream into old-fashioned glasses. Top with an espresso bean. Store covered in the freezer.

NOTE: Coffee contains antioxidants, such as chlorogenic acid, and caffeine, which may have cognitive and mood-enhancing effects. Moderate coffee consumption has been associated with a reduced risk of certain diseases, including Parkinson's and Alzheimer's.

PER SERVING: *Calories 201 (From Fat 101); Fat 11g (Saturated 7g); Cholesterol 41mg; Sodium 24mg; Carbohydrate 26g (Dietary Fiber 0g); Protein 1g; Sugars 25g.*

🍓 Raspberry Sorbet

PREP TIME: 10 MIN PLUS 3 HRS FREEZING | YIELD: 4 SERVINGS

INGREDIENTS

12 ounces (340g) fresh raspberries

Juice and zest of 1 lemon

¼ cup (60mL) no-sugar-added white grape juice

1 tablespoon (21g) honey

¼ cup organic coconut sugar

DIRECTIONS

1 Wash the raspberries and place them in a blender or food processor. Puree until smooth. Add the lemon juice, grape juice, honey, and vanilla and coconut sugar. Puree for another minute.

2 Pass the mixture through a fine-mesh sieve, stirring and pushing the raspberry pulp into the sieve to separate the seeds. Place the strained mixture in a large plastic container and put in the freezer for 1 hour.

3 Remove the sorbet from the freezer and spoon it back into the blender. Puree to break down the ice crystals that have formed. Freeze for another 2 to 3 hours or until the mixture is frozen.

4 To serve, distribute the sorbet in fruit glasses and top with lemon zest.

NOTE: Raspberries are rich in antioxidants, including quercetin and ellagic acid, which may have anti-inflammatory and anticancer properties. They also provide vitamin C, fiber, and manganese. Blackberries are high in vitamins C and K, fiber, and antioxidants like anthocyanins. They contribute to immune health, support bone health, and may have anti-inflammatory effects.

VARY IT! Use blackberries instead of raspberries. You can also swap out the grape juice with prosecco.

PER SERVING: *Calories 91 (From Fat 7); Fat 1g (Saturated 0g); Cholesterol 0mg; Sodium 2mg; Carbohydrate 22g (Dietary Fiber 7g); Protein 2g; Sugars 13g.*

Freezing Delightful Frozen Classics

Unexpected guests, busy days, and cravings call for making some frozen classics in advance. The desserts in this section are great to have on hand for when you crave something sweet or want to impress guests.

These recipes are fun at all ages, but children especially enjoy making and eating them. Dark chocolate, nuts, fruit, and Greek yogurt are nutritious ingredients, especially for people with diabetes to eat, and they also add flavor and depth. Be sure to stock up on them in order to make preparing these desserts easier.

Even if you've never made frozen desserts before, these recipes can enable you to expand your repertoire and satisfy your sweet tooth in a healthful manner:

» **Frozen Peanut Butter and Vanilla Cups:** A fan favorite and a hit with guests of all ages

» **Blackberry Banana Soft Serve:** A smooth, creamy, and fruity treat to enjoy in the warmer months

» **Red, White, and Blue Creamsicles:** Perfect to celebrate summer holidays with these festive sweet treats

Frozen Peanut Butter and Vanilla Cups

PREP TIME: 10 MIN PLUS 1 HR FREEZING	YIELD: 5 SERVINGS

INGREDIENTS

12 ounces (340g) dark chocolate (80 percent or more), chopped

1 tablespoon (13g) coconut oil

½ cup (112g) Greek yogurt

½ cup (128g) organic creamy peanut butter

1 tablespoon (15g) pure vanilla extract

¼ cup (85g) honey

DIRECTIONS

1 Line a cupcake pan with 10 paper liners. In a medium saucepan, melt the chocolate and coconut oil over low heat, stirring with a wooden spoon.

2 Spoon 1 tablespoon of melted chocolate into each liner and freeze for 10 minutes.

3 Mix the yogurt, peanut butter, vanilla, and honey in a medium bowl.

4 When the chocolate is frozen, spoon the yogurt-peanut butter mixture evenly over the top of each chocolate base. If you have leftover chocolate, you can drizzle that over top. Freeze until firm, about 1 hour. Keep covered in the freezer or refrigerator until serving. Allow to rest at room temperature 5 minutes before serving. Serve 2 cups per person.

NOTE: Peanut butter is a good source of protein, healthy fats, and essential nutrients like vitamin E, magnesium, and potassium. The monounsaturated fats contribute to heart health, and the protein supports muscle development.

VARY IT! Swap almond butter or pistachio cream for the peanut butter.

PER SERVING: *Calories 654 (From Fat 411); Fat 46g (Saturated 22g); Cholesterol 2mg; Sodium 140mg; Carbohydrate 51g (Dietary Fiber 9g); Protein 14g; Sugars 33g.*

Blackberry Banana Soft Serve

PREP TIME: 10 MIN PLUS OVERNIGHT FREEZING

YIELD: 6 SERVINGS

INGREDIENTS

3 cups (680g) plain Greek yogurt

1 cup (151g) frozen blackberries

1 cup (225g) mashed ripe frozen banana

2 teaspoons (8.4g) pure vanilla extract

¼ cup (81g) maple syrup

Pinch of sea salt

½ cup (118mL) unsweetened full-fat coconut milk

DIRECTIONS

1 Spoon the yogurt into an ice cube tray and freeze, covered with plastic wrap, overnight.

2 Place the yogurt ice cubes with the frozen blackberries, banana, vanilla, maple syrup, sea salt, and coconut milk in the blender. Blend until creamy, stopping and carefully opening the lid to scrape down the sides and redistribute the mixture a few times, if necessary.

3 Serve immediately as is or transfer to a piping bag and pipe swirls into a cup. Store any remaining ice cream in an airtight container in the freezer.

TIP: Blending time varies depending upon the type of blender that you have.

NOTE: The coconut milk helps the mixture to be extra creamy and have a "soft-serve" like consistency. You can leave it out for a firmer texture.

VARY IT! Use blueberries instead of blackberries and fresh berries instead of frozen when in season. You can also swap out the Greek yogurt for a nondairy yogurt.

PER SERVING: *Calories 206 (From Fat 59); Fat 7g (Saturated 5g); Cholesterol 13mg; Sodium 80mg; Carbohydrate 26g (Dietary Fiber 2g); Protein 12g; Sugars 15g.*

☺ Red, White, and Blue Creamsicles

PREP TIME: 15 MIN PLUS 6 HRS FREEZING | **YIELD: 10 SERVINGS**

INGREDIENTS

1½ cups (249g) sliced fresh strawberries

1 cup (148g) fresh blueberries

3 cups (680g) plain Greek yogurt

¼ cup (81g) maple syrup

1 teaspoon (4.2g) pure vanilla extract

DIRECTIONS

1 Rinse the strawberries and blueberries and pat dry. Combine the Greek yogurt with the maple syrup and vanilla and mix well in a bowl.

2 Add the yogurt about ¼ of the way up the popsicle mold. Place the berries in the mold so that they're visible on the outside. Place the popsicle stick in the middle. Add more yogurt and berries until the popsicle mold is full.

3 Freeze approximately 6 hours, or until solid.

NOTE: Fresh, in-season berries are perfect for serving during spring and summertime holidays. Because these popsicles use yogurt as a base, they're balanced in macronutrients and can also be enjoyed as a snack without having to pair them with protein.

VARY IT! If you aren't concerned about a red, white, and blue theme, then use fresh pineapple, mango, and kiwi as delicious and nutritious additions to the popsicles.

PER SERVING: *Calories 87 (From Fat 14); Fat 2g (Saturated 1g); Cholesterol 8mg; Sodium 23mg; Carbohydrate 12g (Dietary Fiber 1g); Protein 7g; Sugars 8g.*

Chapter **15**

Mastering Pies and Tarts

RECIPES IN THIS CHAPTER

Ⓢ **Mixed Berry Crostata**

Ⓢ **Creamy Lemon Crostata**

Ⓢ **Apple, Raisin, and Nut Strudel**

Ⓢ **Strawberry, Citrus, and Ricotta Tart**

Ⓢ **Almond and Apricot Tart**

Ⓢ **Cinnamon-Scented Apple Pie**

Ⓢ **Key Lime Pie Jars**

Ⓢ **Blackberry Lemon Pie Pots**

Pies and tarts have a special place in many people's hearts. Most countries around the globe have their own traditional sweet treats made with doughs. Often times, however, these recipes are laden with so much sugar and fat that for someone watching their weight or with diabetes, they're strictly off-limits except for the holidays.

That doesn't mean you have to go without. You just need to make some modifications. This chapter explores how you can make classic Italian crostata, an innovative strudel recipe made with phyllo dough, master the art of tarts and pies, and create sweet jars and pots that are as nutritious as they are delicious.

Creating Crostata and Strudel

Italian *crostate* (plural word for crostata) are open-faced pies made in a tart shell. Sometimes they include lattice-dough on the top, but many times they only contain crust on the bottom. Usually made with fresh, seasonal fruit and relatively low sugar, they're a great addition to the repertoire of someone looking to balance their blood sugar.

Strudel is the national dessert of the country of Austria as well as an international classic. Years ago I created a lighter version for my father by swapping out the traditional dough for phyllo dough brushed with olive oil. The result was a lovely, flaky pastry that compliments the soft, sweet fruit filling perfectly. It's a great solution for someone who loves the flavor of strudel but doesn't want to derail their diet.

REMEMBER

Be sure to read through these recipes in this section to ensure that you have the proper equipment and choose the best recipe for your occasion and schedule:

>> **Mixed Berry Crostata:** A go-to summer fruit favorite to enjoy indoors or out

>> **Creamy Lemon Crostata:** An elegant Italian finale to any meal

>> **Apple, Raisin, and Nut Strudel:** A classic, delicious, and nutritious dessert

Mixed Berry Crostata

PREP TIME: 10 MIN	COOK TIME: 35 MIN	YIELD: 10 SERVINGS

INGREDIENTS

1 cup (148g) fresh berries (¼ cup (37g) each of trimmed sliced strawberries, blackberries, raspberries, and blueberries)

3 teaspoons (8g) cornstarch divided in ¼ cup (59mL) water

1 cinnamon stick

2 teaspoons (5g) pure monk fruit

1 recipe Homemade Pie Crust (see Chapter 8)

1 teaspoon (4.5g) Amy Riolo Selections or other EVOO

2 tablespoons (16g) unbleached, all-purpose flour for dusting surface

1 egg white, lightly beaten

5 fresh mint leaves

DIRECTIONS

1 Combine the berries in a medium saucepan. Add the cornstarch mixture, cinnamon stick, and monk fruit. Bring to a boil over high heat, reduce the heat to medium, stirring slowly, and continue to cook 3 to 5 minutes until the mixture becomes thick like a pie filling. Remove from the heat and allow to cool. Discard the cinnamon stick.

2 Preheat the oven to 400 degrees F (205 degrees C). Grease a 10-inch tart pan with the EVOO. Lightly flour a clean work surface and a rolling pin. Roll the dough out into a 12-inch circle. Use the tart pan as a cookie cutter to cut out a circle from the dough to fit the pan. Press the dough down into the tart shells and prick with a fork. Line with parchment paper and fill with pie weights or a bag of rice or dried beans. Bake for 20 minutes.

3 Remove from the oven, remove the pie weights or rice or beans, and brush with egg white. Return to oven and bake another 10 minutes. Allow to cool slightly and carefully remove from the pans. Fill with berry filling and top with mint sprig in the middle. Serve at room temperature.

TIP: Keep the prepared Homemade Pie Crust from Chapter 8 covered in plastic in the freezer. Thaw in the fridge overnight or at room temperature for a few hours before using.

PER SERVING: *Calories 145 (From Fat 97); Fat 11g (Saturated 1g); Cholesterol 21mg; Sodium 60mg; Carbohydrate 9g (Dietary Fiber 3g); Protein 5g; Sugars 4g.*

🍅 Creamy Lemon Crostata

PREP TIME: 10 MIN	COOK TIME: 45 MIN	YIELD: 10 SERVINGS

INGREDIENTS

2 cups (473mL) whole milk

1 teaspoon (4.2g) pure vanilla

4 egg yolks, plus 1 egg white, whisked

½ teaspoon (.5g) pure powdered stevia extract

4 tablespoons (31g) all-purpose flour

Juice and zest of 2 lemons

1 recipe Homemade Pie Crust (see Chapter 8)

1 teaspoon (4.5g) Amy Riolo Selections or other EVOO

DIRECTIONS

1 To make the pudding, pour the milk into a saucepan. Add the vanilla and bring to a boil. In a medium bowl, beat the egg yolks with the stevia. Then whisk in the flour. Stir in the lemon juice and zest. After the milk begins to boil, remove it from the heat and slowly add the egg white, stevia, and flour mixture, whisking as you go. The resulting mixture should be soft and creamy.

2 Transfer the mixture to the stove over medium heat. Stir continuously until the cream becomes dense and coats the back of a spoon, about 10 to 15 minutes and can be done a day ahead of time. After it's ready, transfer the cream to a bowl and cover with plastic wrap and let cool in refrigerator. Be sure to cover the bowl well so that a film doesn't form on the surface of the cream.

3 To make the shell, preheat the oven to 400 degrees F (205 degrees C). Grease a 10-inch tart pan with 1 teaspoon (4.5g) EVOO. Lightly flour a clean work surface and a rolling pin. Roll the dough out into a 12-inch circle. Use the tart pan as cookie cutter to use as a guide to cut the dough into the same size as the tart shell. Press the dough into the tart shells and prick with a fork. Line with parchment paper and fill with pie weights or a bag of rice or dried beans. Bake for 20 minutes.

4 Remove from the oven, remove the pie weights or rice or beans, and brush with the egg white. Return to the oven and bake another 10 minutes. Allow to cool slightly, and then carefully remove from the pans. Fill with lemon pudding and allow to cool to room temperature before serving.

PER SERVING: *Calories 194 (From Fat 127); Fat 14g (Saturated 3g); Cholesterol 110mg; Sodium 84mg; Carbohydrate 11g (Dietary Fiber 2g); Protein 8g; Sugars 5g.*

Apple, Raisin, and Nut Strudel

PREP TIME: 15 MIN	COOK TIME: 1 HR 10 MIN	YIELD: 12 SERVINGS

INGREDIENTS

¾ cup honey (254g) and 1 tablespoon (21g) for garnish

1 cup (237mL) water

One 2-x-3-inch (5-7.6cm) strip lemon peel

¼ cup (59mL) lemon juice

1 cup (120g) chopped walnuts

4 Golden Delicious apples, peeled, cored, and cut into 1-inch pieces

½ cup (73g) golden raisins

4 tablespoons (54g) Amy Riolo Selections, or other good quality EVOO

7 sheets phyllo dough, at room temperature

¾ cup (81g) dried plain breadcrumbs

DIRECTIONS

1 Combine the honey with the water and lemon peel in a large saucepan over medium heat. Cook, stirring occasionally, until the honey has dissolved completely. Add the walnuts, stir to combine, and cover the saucepan. Reduce the heat to low and simmer for 20 minutes.

2 Add in the apples, stir, and simmer, covered, for another 20 minutes. Remove the pan from the heat and stir in the raisins. Allow the mixture to cool completely. When mixture is cooled to room temperature, remove the lemon peel, and preheat the oven to 375 degrees F (190 degrees C).

3 Line a baking sheet with parchment paper or a silicone liner. Carefully unfold the phyllo dough and lay 1 sheet down on a clean work surface. Place the EVOO in a small bowl and using a pastry brush, lightly oil the phyllo, working from the outside in. Sprinkle with 2 tablespoons (13g) of breadcrumbs.

4 Continue layering the phyllo dough, brushing each with EVOO and sprinkling with breadcrumbs. Spoon the filling evenly down the long side of the phyllo sheet, about 2 inches (5cm) from the bottom edge and 1 inch (2.5cm) from both sides, creating a 12-x-13-inch log. Carefully fold the bottom edge and the side flaps over the filling. Slowly roll up the phyllo sheets like a jelly roll and place on a baking sheet.

5 Lightly brush the top of the strudel with additional EVOO and drizzle remaining tablespoon of honey across the top. Make 12 (1-inch; 2.5-cm) evenly spaced diagonal slits across the top of the strudel to reveal the filling. Bake for 25 minutes and then rotate pan. Bake another 10 to 15 minutes, or until golden. Remove from the oven and let rest for at least 10 minutes. Serve warm or at room temperature.

TIP: Keep phyllo dough on hand in the freezer to make nutritious, flaky, pastries when needed.

NOTE: Phyllo dough is free of trans fat, saturated fat, and cholesterol, making it an excellent alternative to butter-laden dough and crusts. Many people actually prefer its light, crunchy, and flaky texture for soft, moist fillings. Experiment by replacing some of the traditional dough and crust in your favorite recipes with phyllo dough. The combination of fruit and nuts make for a balanced sweet treat that can be enjoyed after a meal or as an occasional snack.

VARY IT! Swap out dates for raisins and pears for apples.

PER SERVING: Calories 280 (From Fat 109); Fat 12g (Saturated 1g); Cholesterol 0mg; Sodium 105mg; Carbohydrate 43g (Dietary Fiber 2g); Protein 4g; Sugars 29g.

SOME INTERESTING TIDBITS ON STRUDEL

Years ago I had the opportunity to watch Austrian-born Certified Global Master Chef Wilhelm Jonach serve classic strudel at the Austrian Embassy in Washington, D.C. My father mentioned how much he loved strudel. At the time, I was working on another diabetes-friendly cookbook and wanted to create a version that would fit into my mom's diabetes-friendly diet requirements and also satisfy my dad's cravings, so I came up with the phyllo version.

I was surprised to learn the history of strudel. Even though it's associated with Austrian cuisine, it gained popularity in the 18th century and spread throughout the Habsburg Empire (which lasted from the 13th until the 19th century) — many cuisines nowadays also enjoy strudel. *Strudel* comes from the German word for "whirlpool" because when you cut into the cooked, rolled strudel, the layers of pastry resembles the inside of a whirlpool. The dessert is also believed to have evolved after Turkish baklava arrived in Austria in the 15th century (making my healthier version even more appropriate)!

Apple strudel (said to be a Viennese creation) is the national dessert of Austria and the official state pastry of Texas. You can create variations on the classic by using pears or cherries in the Apple, Raisin, and Nut Strudel recipe or by swapping out vanilla cream for a filling as well. You can even make savory versions by adding mushrooms and cheese, spinach and cheese, or your favorite fillings.

Making Tarts and Pies

If you're looking to up your dessert game, impress guests, or just enjoy tarts and pies that might otherwise be off-limits, this section is for you. The following recipes use the base tart and pie dough recipes from Chapter 8 along with wholesome and mouthwatering ingredients that will enchant your taste buds while ensuring that your blood sugar doesn't spike.

The recipes here include the following:

>> **Raspberry, Citrus, and Ricotta Tart:** Great for after a light dinner or for breakfast

>> **Almond and Apricot Tart:** A wonderful way to end a nutritious meal in springtime or whenever apricots are in season

>> **Cinnamon-Scented Apple Pie:** A perennial favorite to serve in autumn or whenever the mood strikes

REMEMBER

Be sure to read the variations in the recipes to create even more delicious variations.

TART VERSUS PIE: WHAT'S THE DIFFERENCE?

A *pie* is a baked dish featuring a fruit filling encased in dough, which is called a pie crust after it's baked. Raw pie doughs can be made into a double-crust, single-crust on the bottom, or a bottom crust with an intricate lattice crust on top. Pie recipes can be sweet or savory.

A *tart* is a freestanding shallow open-faced pastry, often baked in a fluted tart pan with a removable bottom. Smaller tarts are served as individual portions and referred to as *tartlets*. Normally tarts and tartlets are served with unbaked fillings, such as custard, pastry cream, or fruit fillings.

Strawberry, Citrus, and Ricotta Tart

INGREDIENTS

1 teaspoon (4.5g) Amy Riolo Selections or other EVOO

2 teaspoons (7.5g) all-purpose flour

1 recipe Basic Tart Crust (see Chapter 8)

4 cups (984g) fresh ricotta cheese (whole milk)

Juice and zest of 1 orange

3 tablespoons (43g) plain Greek yogurt

¼ cup (85g) raw honey

1 teaspoon (4.2g) vanilla paste or vanilla extract

2½ cups (415g) sliced fresh or frozen strawberries

1 teaspoon (2.5g) confectioners' sugar

DIRECTIONS

1 Preheat the oven to 350 degrees F (175 degrees C). Lightly grease a (9-inch) tart pan with 1 teaspoon (4.5g) EVOO.

2 Place parchment paper on a worksurface. Using a rolling pin lightly dusted with flour, roll the dough out into a 10-inch circle. Press the dough down into tart shells and prick with a fork. Line with parchment paper and fill with pie weights or a bag of rice or dried beans. Bake for 10 minutes. Remove the weights and return to the oven for another 5 to 6 minutes, or until lightly golden. Carefully remove from the pan and cool on a wire rack.

3 In a medium glass bowl or the bowl of a standing mixer using the whisk attachment, whip together the ricotta, orange juice and zest, yogurt, honey, and vanilla until smooth and fluffy. When ready to serve, fill the pastry shell with the ricotta and top with the strawberries, placing each in a circular pattern to cover the surface of the tart. Place confectioners' sugar in a small fine-mesh sieve and dust the top of the tart. Drizzle with Chocolate Ganache if desired.

VARY IT: You can use one recipe of Dark Chocolate Ganache (see Chapter 8) for garnish.

PER SERVING: *Calories 350 (From Fat 183); Fat 20g (Saturated 11g); Cholesterol 59mg; Sodium 86mg; Carbohydrate 29g (Dietary Fiber 2g); Protein 14g; Sugars 16g.*

Almond and Apricot Tart

PREP TIME: 15 MIN | COOK TIME: 30 MIN | YIELD: 10 SERVINGS

INGREDIENTS

2 cups (224g) almond flour

¼ cup (55g) coconut oil

2 tablespoons (42g) honey

1 pinch unrefined sea salt

6 fresh fresh apricots, halved, pitted, and sliced into quarters

¼ cup (27g) sliced almonds, toasted

1 teaspoon (4.2g) vanilla extract

1 teaspoon (2.6g) ground cardamom or cinnamon

¼ cup (72g) sugar-free apricot preserves melted in 2 tablespoons hot water

2 tablespoons (15g) finely chopped unsalted pistachios

DIRECTIONS

1 Preheat the oven to 350 degrees F (175 degrees C). In a large bowl combine the almond flour, coconut oil, honey, and sea salt. Mix by hand or with a food processor until a dough forms.

2 Press the dough into a 9-inch tart pan, spreading it evenly across the bottom and up the sides. Arrange the apricot slices on the dough.

3 In a small bowl, mix the sliced almonds, vanilla extract, and cardamom and spoon this mixture over the apricots. Brush the apricot preserves over the tart.

4 Bake for 25 to 30 minutes or until the crust is golden and the apricots are tender. Sprinkle the chopped pistachios over the top. Allow to cool before serving.

TIP: Make the dough a day in advance and store in the refrigerator.

VARY IT!: Substitute the almond flour for coconut flour.

VARY IT! Fresh apricots are usually available and at their best in the springtime. Use fresh peaches, nectarines, or plums when they're in season.

PER SERVING: *Calories 235 (From Fat 169); Fat 19g (Saturated 6g); Cholesterol 0mg; Sodium 24mg; Carbohydrate 14g (Dietary Fiber 4g); Protein 6g; Sugars 9g.*

🍅 Cinnamon-Scented Apple Pie

PREP TIME: 15 MIN	COOK TIME: 40 MIN	YIELD: 10 SERVINGS

INGREDIENTS

6 cups sliced green, or other tart apples

1 cup (145g) blanched almonds, roughly chopped

½ cup (72g) pure maple sugar

1 tablespoon (8g) cornstarch dissolved in 2 tablespoons (15mL) water

1 teaspoon (4.2g) pure vanilla

Zest and juice of 1 lemon

2 teaspoons (5g) pure cinnamon

1 tablespoon (13.5g) plus 1 teaspoon (4.5g) Amy Riolo Selections, or other EVOO

2 recipes Homemade Pie Crust (see Chapter 8)

DIRECTIONS

1 Preheat the oven to 425 degrees F (220 degrees C). In a large bowl combine the apple, almonds, maple sugar, cornstarch mixture, vanilla, lemon zest and juice, and cinnamon.

2 Lightly flour a clean work surface and a rolling pin. Roll each piece of dough out into a 10-inch circle. Press the dough down into a pie dish greased with 1 teaspoon EVOO and prick with a fork. Pour the apple mixture into the unbaked pie crust.

3 Cover with the remaining crust and seal the edges. Using a knife or a cookie cutter, make a few slits or designs on the top of the crust to prevent it from bursting while baking. Brush 1 tablespoon EVOO over the top and sides of pie. Sprinkle with the additional cinnamon.

4 Bake for 15 minutes. Lower the temperature to 350 degrees F (175 degrees C) and continue baking for an additional 30 to 40 minutes.

TIP: If you're allergic to almonds, swap out nuts with flaxseeds or raisins.

NOTE: The addition of almonds not only provides crunch and flavor, but it also ensures that there are enough protein and healthful fats to balance out the carbohydrates and natural sugars.

PER SERVING: *Calories 311 (From Fat 175); Fat 19g (Saturated 2g); Cholesterol 21mg; Sodium 56mg; Carbohydrate 32g (Dietary Fiber 7g); Protein 8g; Sugars 21g.*

Serving Jars and Pots

Jars and pots are fun and popular ways to serve deconstructed individual pies that can be eaten with a spoon. These no-bake desserts aren't only trendy to serve at parties, but they also can be made quickly and ahead of time, making them a host's favorite. Keep in mind that these recipes — Key Lime Pie Jars and the Blackberry and Lemon Pie Pots — are just two examples in a world full of inspiration. After you become used to the technique in making these desserts, follow the variations and create your own versions.

REMEMBER

When making jars and pots, make sure you have the right equipment on hand. Of course, you can always make one larger version of these desserts in a pretty glass bowl in the same way that British puddings and trifles are served. If you like the idea of serving them individually, stock up on miniature Mason jars from container or art supply stores, or save the ones that you buy other products in. Nowadays a lot of yogurt and pudding companies sell their products in glass jars in the refrigerator section of supermarkets. You could use those, or even any small, clear drinking glass that you have at home. For the pots, I like to use small ramekins as in French Pots de Crème recipes.

This section includes these recipes:

>> **Key Lime Pie Jars:** A fruity and fun summer dessert to enjoy outside

>> **Blackberry Lemon Pie Pots**: Creamy and citrusy individual desserts to add an elegant touch to any meal

Key Lime Pie Jars

INGREDIENTS

1 cup (112g) almond flour

¼ cup (54g) Amy Riolo Selections or other EVOO

3 tablespoons (30g) all natural monk fruit sweetener, divided

One 16-ounce (454g) package silken tofu, drained

2 teaspoons (8.4g) vanilla extract, divided

2 ounces (57g) cream cheese

Zest and juice of 3 key limes, divided

1 cup (237mL) heavy cream

DIRECTIONS

1 To make the crust in a skillet over medium-high heat, add the almond flour, EVOO, and 2 tablespoons (20g) monk fruit. Stirring often, toast until golden brown, about 3 to 5 minutes. Remove from the heat and set aside to cool.

2 For the filling, using a hand mixer with the whisk attachment and a bowl or a stand mixer fitted with a bowl and the whip attachment, combine the silken tofu, 1 teaspoon (4.2g) vanilla, cream cheese, and remaining 1 tablespoon (10g) monk fruit until smooth and creamy. Add the key lime juice and two-thirds of lime zest and continue mixing. Increase the mixer to high and pour in ½ cup of the heavy cream. Whip until light and fluffy.

3 To make the whipped cream, whip the remaining ½ cup heavy cream, and remaining 1 teaspoon (4.2g) vanilla until it's creamy and thick. Be careful not to overbeat. If you overwhip the cream, it will become dense and clumpy like butter.

4 Divide the crust ingredients evenly into 8 small dessert jars or 6 (8-ounce) ramekins. Spoon equal portions of the key lime filling over each. Top each with a dollop of whip cream and a sprinkling of the remaining third of the lime zest. Store in the refrigerator until serving.

NOTE: The heavy cream and cream cheese give this recipe a higher fat content than many of the desserts in this book. While the tofu and the almonds provide protein, don't consume too much fat. Enjoy this dessert after a light meal consisting of low-carb vegetables, fresh greens, and lean protein.

PER SERVING: *Calories 408 (From Fat 345); Fat 38g (Saturated 12g); Cholesterol 65mg; Sodium 50mg; Carbohydrate 10g (Dietary Fiber 2g); Protein 9 g; Sugars 3g.*

Blackberry Lemon Pie Pots

PREP TIME: 20 MIN	COOK TIME: 5 MIN	YIELD: 6 SERVINGS

INGREDIENTS

1 cup (112g) coconut flour

¼ cup (59mL) pure organic coconut oil

3 tablespoons (30g) all-natural monk fruit sweetener, divided

One 16-ounce (454g) package silken tofu, drained

2 teaspoons (8.2g) pure vanilla extract

2 ounces (57g) cream cheese, at room temperature

Zest and juice of 3 lemons, divided

¼ cup (60mL) whole milk

1 cup (144g) blackberries

DIRECTIONS

1 For the crust, in a skillet over medium-high heat, add the coconut flour, coconut oil, and 2 tablespoons (20g) monk fruit. Stirring often, toast until golden brown, about 3 to 5 minutes. Remove from the heat and set aside to cool.

2 For the filling, using a hand mixer with the whisk attachment and a bowl or a stand mixer fitted with a bowl and the whip attachment, combine the silken tofu, vanilla, cream cheese, and remaining 1 tablespoon (10g) monk fruit until smooth and creamy. Add the lemon juice and two-thirds of the lemon zest and continue mixing. Increase the mixer to high and pour in the heavy cream. Whip until light and fluffy.

3 Divide crust ingredients evenly into 6 (8-ounce) ramekins. Spoon equal portions of the lemon filling over each. Top each with a sixth of blackberries and a sprinkling of the remaining third of the lemon zest. Store in the refrigerator until serving.

TIP: Make a day in advance and top with blackberries just before serving.

NOTE: Tofu is low in fat and high in protein, making it an excellent choice to balance carbs and natural sugars in recipes.

VARY IT! Substitute any berries that you like.

PER SERVING: *Calories 259 (From Fat 157); Fat 17g (Saturated 13g); Cholesterol 11mg; Sodium 52mg; Carbohydrate 18g (Dietary Fiber 9g); Protein 8g; Sugars 6g.*

Chapter **16**

Sipping on Sweet Drinks

RECIPES IN THIS CHAPTER

☙ Moroccan Avocado Smoothie

☙ Pineapple Cardamom Crush

☙ Zero-Proof Sgroppino

☙ Apricot and Ginger Cooler

☙ Papaya, Banana, and Orange Smoothie

☙ Almond and Banana Smoothie

☙ Hot Spiced Chocolate

☙ Creamy Chai

☙ Spiced Hot Cider

S weet drinks can be the perfect finale to a delicious meal. They can quench your thirst, satisfy your sweet tooth, aid in digestion, and help you wind down at the end of the day. For people with diabetes and other health concerns as well as individuals trying to lose weight, however, drinks (other than water, plain coffee, tea, and herbal teas) can be problematic. Often times, sweet drinks are laden with sugar, lack nutrients, and add very little to your diet.

This chapter introduces several dessert drink recipes that you can enjoy in a wide variety of settings without derailing your diet.

Crafting Some Sweet Fruit Sips

Fruity drinks can be good to taste and good for you when made properly. The right amounts of fresh, seasonal fruit combined with healthful ingredients like flaxseeds, yogurt, and spices can be heavenly. Use these drink recipes as after dinner desserts or as pre-or post-workout fuel.

This section includes these recipes:

>> **Moroccan Avocado Smoothie:** A great way to use leftover ripe avocados

>> **Pineapple Cardamom Crush:** A cooling and refreshing drink to enjoy during the warmer months

Moroccan Avocado Smoothie

PREP TIME: 5 MIN	YIELD: 4 SERVINGS

INGREDIENTS

1 ripe avocado (pitted and peeled)

1 overripe banana

1 cup (237mL) unsweetened almond milk

1 cup (236g) ice

DIRECTIONS

1 Place the avocado, banana, milk, and ice into a blender. Blend until there are no pieces of avocado remaining and the mixture is smooth and frothy.

2 Divide into chilled glasses and enjoy.

NOTE: Avocados may not be your first thought when it comes to sweets and desserts, but remember that they're actually a fruit, not a vegetable, and that their texture adds creaminess to smoothies. Research shows that avocados can help people manage their diabetes and improve their health because they're a good source of healthful fats, contain antioxidants, and help stabilize blood sugar.

VARY IT! You can use any other nondairy milk in place of almond milk for a lower carb, vegan beverage. Or, for something sweeter and fruitier, you can use orange or pineapple juice.

PER SERVING: *Calories 114 (From Fat 73); Fat 8g (Saturated 1g); Cholesterol 0mg; Sodium 4mg; Carbohydrate 12g (Dietary Fiber 4g); Protein 2g; Sugars 4g.*

🍍 Pineapple Cardamom Crush

PREP TIME: 5 MIN | YIELD: 4 SERVINGS

INGREDIENTS

2 cups (330g) fresh pineapple chunks

1 cup (227g) plain Greek yogurt

¼ cup (28g) ground flaxseeds

1 teaspoon (2g) ground cardamom

1 teaspoon (4.2g) vanilla

1 cup (236g) ice

1 tablespoon (21g) honey, if desired

DIRECTIONS

1 Combine all the ingredients in blender. Whip on high speed until smooth and frothy. Divide into 4 glasses and enjoy!

NOTE: The flaxseeds and Greek yogurt in this recipe transform a simple drink into a balanced snack that you can enjoy for dessert or before or after workouts.

TIP: If your drink is too thick, you can add some cold water or a few more ice cubes of ice until you achieve the consistency that you like.

NOTE: Use fresh pineapple and not canned or sweetened versions. Pineapple has a great deal of vitamin C, manganese, and enzymes that may improve digestion. It's also immune boosting. People with diabetes should consume less than 100 grams of pineapple per day so that it doesn't cause a rise in blood sugar.

VARY IT! You can substitute fresh strawberries for pineapple.

PER SERVING: *Calories 139 (From Fat 38); Fat 4g (Saturated 1g); Cholesterol 7mg; Sodium 22mg; Carbohydrate 19g (Dietary Fiber 3g); Protein 7g; Sugars 13g.*

Cooling Down with Drinks

Nothing's better and more refreshing than sipping on a cooling drink during a hot day. Whether the drink is cool because it's made from cold ingredients or from flavors that are naturally refreshing, cool drinks are the stuff everyone craves when temperatures soar.

A common misconception is that people with diabetes need to drink more than others, but that's not necessarily the case. To stay hydrated, men should drink about 15.5 cups (3.7 liters) of fluids a day and women should drink about 11.5 cups (2.7 liters) of fluids a day.

TIP

Keep in mind that these fluid recommendations also include foods and other beverages that contain water. For example, foods like yogurt and soups contain water.

Although drinking the majority of your fluids from water is important, you can enjoy other types of drinks from time to time. This section contains the following recipes:

» **Zero-Proof Sgroppino:** An alcohol-free version of an elegant Italian drink that's sometimes served between courses to cleanse your palate

» **Apricot and Ginger Cooler:** A thirst-quenching sweet drink with Middle Eastern roots

» **Papaya, Banana, and Orange Smoothie:** A delicious and satisfying drink that will transport your tastebuds to the tropics

» **Almond and Banana Smoothie:** A filling drink for a sweet snack or post-workout for recovery

Zero-Proof Sgroppino

PREP TIME: 5 MIN | YIELD: 4 SERVINGS

INGREDIENTS

1 recipe Lemon Granita (see Chapter 14), or 2 cups purchased Lemon Sorbet

1 cup (237mL) sparkling water

Grated zest of 1 lemon

DIRECTIONS

1 Place all the ingredients in a blender and blend on high until frothy.

2 Taste and serve.

NOTE: A *sgroppino* is a Venetian cocktail usually made from lemon sorbet, vodka, and prosecco.

NOTE: This recipe uses sparkling water and lemon zest instead of the alcohol. This drink is often served after heavy meals and is known for cleansing the palate and aiding in digestion.

TIP: Add a teaspoon of honey in Step 2 if you want it to be sweeter.

PER SERVING: *Calories 215 (From Fat 99); Fat 11g (Saturated 7g); Cholesterol 41mg; Sodium 24mg; Carbohydrate 7g (Dietary Fiber 0g); Protein 1g; Sugars 2g.*

🍅 Apricot and Ginger Cooler

PREP TIME: 5 MIN	YIELD: 4 SERVINGS

INGREDIENTS

3 ripe apricots, peeled and pitted

1 cup (237mL) sparkling water

1 cup (236g) ice

¼ inch (.6cm) fresh ginger, peeled and grated

DIRECTIONS

1 Chill cocktail glasses in the refrigerator until serving. Combine the ingredients in a blender over high speed and blend until frothy.

TIP: Fresh ginger root is sold in the produce aisle of the grocery store and is a great ingredient to have on hand for flavor and anti-inflammatory benefits.

NOTE: Apricots provide a good amount of dietary fiber and plant compounds. They're believed to help protect your eyesight, digestive tract, and gut health. The ginger in this recipe contains anti-inflammatory benefits.

VARY IT! In a pinch, or when apricots are out of season, you can substitute no-sugar added apricot juice, but whole apricots are preferable for their nutrients.

PER SERVING: *Calories 13 (From Fat 1); Fat 0g (Saturated 0g); Cholesterol 0mg; Sodium 13mg; Carbohydrate 3g (Dietary Fiber 1g); Protein 0g; Sugars 2g.*

Papaya, Banana, and Orange Smoothie

PREP TIME: 5 MIN	YIELD: 4 SERVINGS

INGREDIENTS

1 cup (140g) fresh papaya chunks

1 ripe banana

1 cup (227g) plain Greek yogurt

1 orange, zested and juiced

1 teaspoon (4.2g) pure vanilla extract

1 cup (236g) ice

DIRECTIONS

1 Combine the ingredients in a blender over high speed. Blend until frothy and enjoy!

TIP: Papaya has a medium glycemic index (see Chapter 2), but studies suggest that eating it may help to lower blood sugar.

NOTE: A single serving of papaya is rich in vitamin C, folate, vitamin A, magnesium, fiber, and antioxidants.

VARY IT! If you can't find fresh papaya, swap out fresh kiwi or pineapple.

PER SERVING: *Calories 90 (From Fat 12); Fat 1g (Saturated 1g); Cholesterol 7mg; Sodium 20mg; Carbohydrate 14g (Dietary Fiber 1g); Protein 6g; Sugars 7g.*

◌ Almond and Banana Smoothie

PREP TIME: 5 MIN	YIELD: 4 SERVINGS

INGREDIENTS

2 ripe bananas

⅓ cup (85g) almond butter

¼ cup (28g) ground flaxseeds

1 cup (227g) plain Greek yogurt

1 cup (236g) ice

DIRECTIONS

1 Combine the ingredients in a blender over high speed. Blend until frothy. Enjoy!

TIP: As bananas begin to brown, keep them in the fridge to use in smoothie recipes.

NOTE: The combination of almond butter and Greek yogurt in this recipe balances out the carbs and sugars in the banana with protein.

VARY IT! Swap out whole raw almonds for almond butter or silken tofu, if desired.

VARY IT! Add ½ cup dark cacao powder to make a chocolate version of this recipe.

PER SERVING: *Calories 265 (From Fat 152); Fat 17g (Saturated 2g); Cholesterol 7mg; Sodium 117mg; Carbohydrate 22g (Dietary Fiber 4g); Protein 11g; Sugars 8g.*

Warming Up with Hot Drinks

Set the scene: You're nuzzled under a thick blanket sipping on a hot drink on a cold day or night, and you begin to warm up immediately. Curling up with even a cup of hot tea or hot chocolate can be comforting to take the bite out of the outside chill. Here, I include some of the world's most popular hot drinks. Laden with lavish spices that hold anti-inflammatory and antioxidant benefits and steeped in age-old traditions, these drinks will warm your heart and your body with every sip.

One of the things I love the most about these drinks is that they satisfy your sweet tooth enough to curb the craving for heavier desserts. You can also enjoy them on occasion with a balanced breakfast on chilly mornings.

This section has the following recipes:

>> **Hot Spiced Chocolate:** A cold-weather family favorite

>> **Creamy Chai:** Rich in antioxidants and flavor, perfect to sip during the winter

>> **Spiced Hot Cider:** A tasty and warming drink

Hot Spiced Chocolate

PREP TIME: 3 MIN	COOK TIME: 5 MIN	YIELD: 4 SERVINGS

INGREDIENTS

2 tablespoons (11g) unsweetened cocoa powder

1 teaspoon (2.6g) cinnamon

¼ teaspoon (.5g) ground cloves

¼ teaspoon (.5g) ground ginger

¼ teaspoon (.5g) ground cardamom

Pinch of black pepper

Pinch of sea salt

Pinch of cayenne or ground crushed red pepper

3 cups (710mL) whole milk

4 tablespoons (80g) maple syrup

DIRECTIONS

1 Combine the cocoa, spices, milk, and maple syrup in a medium saucepan over medium–high heat.

2 Bring to a boil, whisking, and then reduce the heat to low. Continue to whisk until all the ingredients are incorporated. Strain mixture through a fine mesh strainer into 4 mugs and serve.

TIP: I like to keep large batches of the cocoa and spice blend in a glass jar in the cupboard so that I can make hot chocolate on a regular basis in the colder months.

NOTE: The combination of cocoa and spices stirred into hot milk provide powerful antioxidant and anti-inflammatory benefits as well as an explosion of flavors.

VARY IT! You can swap out honey or sugar for the maple syrup if desired. Use your own favorite combination of spices.

PER SERVING: *Calories 172 (From Fat 58); Fat 6g (Saturated 4g); Cholesterol 18mg; Sodium 140mg; Carbohydrate 24g (Dietary Fiber 1g); Protein 6g; Sugars 22g.*

☕ Creamy Chai

PREP TIME: 5 MIN	COOK TIME: 5 MIN, PLUS 10 MINS STEEPING	YIELD: 4 SERVINGS

INGREDIENTS

2½ (591mL) cups water

3 cups (710mL) whole milk

¼ cup (85g) honey

1 teaspoon (2.6g) ground cinnamon

1 teaspoon (2.6g) ground cardamom

½ teaspoon (1g) ground nutmeg

½ teaspoon (1g) ground cloves

½ teaspoon (1g) ground ginger

4 tea bags (black tea) regular or decaf

DIRECTIONS

1 In a medium saucepan, bring water, milk, honey, and spices to a gentle boil. Whisk well to ensure that all the ingredients dissolve.

2 Remove from the heat, add the tea bags, and cover the pan. Let steep for 10 minutes.

3 Place each tea bag between two spoons and squeeze gently to extract the tea from each bag and remove them.

4 Pour the chai through a fine mesh strainer to remove the spice solids. Serve hot or cold.

TIP: Chai is the Hindi word for tea, and this sumptuous drink is a daily staple for several countries. It's sweet enough to end a meal but tastes great at breakfast as well.

NOTE: Tea can stay fresh in a covered container in the refrigerator for up to 4 days.

VARY IT! You may omit the tea and enjoy just the warm spices in milk.

VARY IT: You can substitute almond or rice milk for the whole milk.

PER SERVING: *Calories 180 (From Fat 55); Fat 6g (Saturated 4g); Cholesterol 18mg; Sodium 80mg; Carbohydrate 27g (Dietary Fiber 1g); Protein 6g; Sugars 27g.*

Spiced Hot Cider

PREP TIME: 5 MIN	COOK TIME: 15 MIN	YIELD: 5 SERVINGS

INGREDIENTS

1 quart (946mL) unsweetened apple cider

3 cinnamon sticks

4 whole cloves

1 star anise

3 green cardamom pods

1 strip orange zest

DIRECTIONS

1 Add all the ingredients to a large saucepan or pot at medium-high heat. After the mixture begins to simmer, cover, reduce the heat to low, and cook for 15 minutes to allow the flavors to develop. Serve hot.

TIP: When entertaining in the cooler months, keep the cider cooking in a slow cooker so that guests can help themselves.

NOTE: One 6-ounce serving of this cider is an appropriate portion for maintaining blood sugar levels. Be sure to consume this drink just after a complete meal or with a handful of nuts or other healthful protein to help with the digestion of the natural sugar in the recipe.

PER SERVING: *Calories 93 (From Fat 2); Fat 0g (Saturated 0g); Cholesterol 0mg; Sodium 6mg; Carbohydrate 23g (Dietary Fiber 0g); Protein 0g; Sugars 22g.*

NOTING THE BENEFITS OF HOT BEVERAGES

In addition to their comforting effect, hot beverages, even plain water, can offer great health benefits. They can help with aiding digestion, maintaining your body temperature, alleviating sore throats, and more.

A glass of hot water can do the following:

- Aid digestion
- Improve circulation
- Promote weight loss
- Act as a detoxifier
- Reduce stress and nasal congestion
- Improve hydration
- Combat constipation
- Improve brain and dental health
- Alleviate asthma and menstrual cramps
- Boost metabolism
- Help prevent colds

Chapter **17**

Baking Cakes

RECIPES IN THIS CHAPTER

🍥 **Italian Sponge Cake**

🍥 **Angel Food Cake**

🍥 **Carrot Pecan Spice Cake**

🍥 **Apple, Cinnamon, and Olive Oil Cake**

🍥 **Orange, Almond, and Olive Oil Cake**

🍥 **Upside-Down Kiwi Cake**

🍥 **Chocolate and Pumpkin Snack Cake**

🍥 **Banana Chocolate Chip Cake**

🍥 **Mini Flourless Olive Oil and Chocolate Cakes**

🍥 **Gluten-Free Chocolate Cupcakes**

So many of life's celebrations call for cake. You may have heard the saying "A party without a cake is just a meeting." And I believe that sums it up best. Celebrating with cake can be especially tricky for people with diabetes because many types of modern cakes are filled with artificial ingredients, copious amounts of sugar, and unhealthful fats.

You can still have your cake and eat it even if you have diabetes. You just need to make choices that don't spike your blood sugar. This chapter explores how you can incorporate nutritious ingredients in unique ways to produce flavorful and healthful classic cakes, fruit cakes, and chocolate cakes.

Experimenting with Classic Cake Recipes

Cakes are among the most popular of all desserts. Because they require some chemistry and skill, many people are insecure about baking for the first time. The thought of making diabetes-friendly cakes can be even more intimidating. But there's no need to worry, with the easy tips and techniques here you can create favorites that please your friends and family while helping you achieve your health goals.

This section includes these recipes:

» **Italian Sponge Cake:** A true classic in the Italian kitchen that's used as a base for more intricate desserts and also eaten plain at breakfast

» **Angel Food Cake:** No introduction needed for this light, airy cake that fits into a diabetes-friendly lifestyle when made properly

» **Carrot Pecan Spice Cake:** Classic cake with autumnal flavors and health benefits

LOOKING AT THE HISTORY OF CAKES

What people commonly refer to cakes dates back to ancient Egypt. Old Kingdom (2700–2600 BC) tomb scenes depict bread being shaped and produced in mass quantities. Ramses II's tomb revealed pictures of elegant pastries, cakes, and pies being made in bakeries that catered specifically to royalty. Sweets were also prepared in communal ovens and sweetened with honey and molasses, instead of sugar, which was extremely expensive at the time because the Persians had just introduced it.

Roman philosopher Cato wrote about cakes after Romans took control of Egypt and gained access to wheat and sugar. Ancient Greek cakes were made of honey and fruits. Typically, the Roman and Greek cakes were used as offerings to the gods.

In Medieval England the terms bread and cake were synonymous, and cake usually referred to small bread. During the renaissance in Italy, baking really took off and caused both English and French to import Italian pastry chefs to work for them. By the 17th century, baking pans consisted of round rings that were placed on flat surfaces. The round symbol has been used since antiquity as a symbol of the life cycle itself. As a result, people still use cakes as a way of marking life's most monumental events.

In the mid 18th century, eggs replaced yeast as the most common leavening agent in Europe — many cakes from the rest of the world still use yeast.

By the 19th century the Industrial Revolution changed the world of cake making. Baking powder was invented, and the modern cake was born. In the 20th century industrialization created a market for the boxed cake, and a generation of cooks, especially in the United States, stopped making cakes from scratch. Baking cakes, however, is fun and rewarding. With the recipes in this chapter, you can whip up mouthwatering creations in minutes.

🍅 Italian Sponge Cake

PREP TIME: 10 MIN	COOK TIME: 40 MIN	YIELD: 8 SERVINGS

INGREDIENTS

Butter or oil spray for greasing pan

6 large eggs, separated

1 cup (176g) allulose

2 teaspoons (8.4g) vanilla

1⅛ cup (141g) unbleached all-purpose flour

DIRECTIONS

1 Preheat the oven to 350 degrees F (175 degrees C). Grease a 1.5-quart loaf pan (8.25-x-9-x-2.75 inches) with the spray oil. Beat the egg whites in a large bowl until they're stiff and set aside. Cream the allulose and egg yolks together and continue beating until they're very light yellow in color.

2 Stir in the vanilla. Gently fold the egg whites into the batter. Sprinkle the flour on top of the mixture and carefully incorporate it into the batter until just combined.

3 Pour into prepared baking pan and bake for 40 minutes or until the cake is golden and the sides begin to pull away from the pan or until a toothpick inserted comes out clean.

4 Remove from the oven and allow to cool completely.

TIP: This recipe is normally made with table sugar and is a popular breakfast treat enjoyed in Italy with cappuccino or caffe latte in the morning. Be sure to eat a serving of raw almonds or other protein along with this cake when enjoying it to prevent blood sugar from spiking.

TIP: You can double the recipe and freeze one cake wrapped in plastic wrap for another time.

NOTE: In Italy, *Pan di Spagna*, or Bread from Spain, is the Italian name for what Americans call Sponge Cake and the French spell Genoise.

VARY IT! You can make a chocolate sponge cake by adding ¼ cup dark cocoa to the mix. You can also swap out the allulose for organic vanilla and coconut sugar or organic coconut sugar.

PER SERVING: *Calories 121 (From Fat 35); Fat 4g (Saturated 1g); Cholesterol 159mg; Sodium 53mg; Carbohydrate 14g (Dietary Fiber 0g); Protein 7g; Sugars 0g.*

Angel Food Cake

INGREDIENTS

1 teaspoon (4.5g) Amy Riolo Selections or other EVOO

12 egg whites

1½ teaspoons (4.5g) cream of tarter

1 teaspoon (4.2g) pure vanilla extract

1 cup (176g) allulose

½ teaspoon (2.4g) sea salt

1 cup (137g) cake flour

DIRECTIONS

1   Heat the oven to 325 degrees F (160 degrees C). Grease the insides and center of an angel food cake pan with the EVOO.

2   In a mixing bowl with the beater attachment or in a bowl of a standing mixer with the whisk attachment whip together the egg whites until stiff peaks begin to form. Then add the cream of tartar, water, and vanilla extract and whip until whites are completely stiff.

3   While your ingredients are mixing, sift together the cake flour, allulose, and sea salt in another large bowl.

4   Carefully fold the egg whites into the flour mixture. Pour the batter into your prepped pan and bake for 50 to 60 minutes or until golden.

5   To cool, invert the cake by placing the fluted hole over a bottle and allow it to sit for about an hour until cool. Run a butter knife around the edges to loosen the cake and invert on a plate to serve.

TIP: If you don't have cake flour and don't want to buy it for this recipe, remove two tablespoons from one cup of all-purpose flour, add two tablespoons of cornstarch or arrowroot powder, and sift together.

VARY IT! You can make Angel Food Cupcakes by placing the same batter in lined muffin tins and baking at 325 degrees F (160 degrees C) for 20 to 25 minutes or until golden and cooked through.

PER SERVING: *Calories 83 (From Fat 6); Fat 1g (Saturated 0g); Cholesterol 0mg; Sodium 178mg; Carbohydrate 13g (Dietary Fiber 0g); Protein 6g; Sugars 0g.*

Carrot Pecan Spice Cake

PREP TIME: 15 MIN	COOK TIME: 40 MIN	YIELD: 9 SERVINGS

INGREDIENTS

2 cups (274g) whole-wheat pastry flour

¼ cup (28g) ground flaxseeds

2 teaspoons (9g) baking powder

1 tablespoon (5.6g) pumpkin pie spice

½ teaspoon (2.4g) sea salt

2 large eggs

½ cup (122g) unsweetened applesauce

½ cup (161g) maple syrup

½ cup (118mL) milk

½ cup (108g) Amy Riolo Selections or other good quality EVOO

2 teaspoons (8.4g) pure vanilla extract

2 cups (220g) finely grated carrots

1 cup (109g) pecans, chopped

1 tablespoon (8g) confectioners' sugar, for garnish

DIRECTIONS

1 Preheat the oven to 350 degrees F (175 degrees C) and grease a 9-inch round baking pan or an 8-x-8 square pan. In a large bowl, whisk together the flour, flaxseeds, baking powder, pumpkin pie spice, and sea salt.

2 In a medium bowl, whisk the eggs and then whisk in the applesauce, maple syrup, milk, EVOO, and vanilla. Stir in the carrots and pecans.

3 Pour the wet ingredients into the bowl of dry ingredients and stir until just combined. Pour the batter into the baking dish and bake for 35 to 38 minutes, or until a toothpick inserted comes out clean. Let the cake cool completely. Sift powdered sugar over the top and serve.

NOTE: The combination of wholesome wheat flour, flaxseeds, nuts, olive oil, carrots, and anti-inflammatory spices make this a healthier dessert that you can enjoy on its own or after a balanced meal.

PER SERVING: *Calories 411 (From Fat 215); Fat 24g (Saturated 3g); Cholesterol 48mg; Sodium 257mg; Carbohydrate 45g (Dietary Fiber 3g); Protein 6g; Sugars 15g.*

Baking Fruit Cakes

Fruit cakes have been popular for centuries in the Mediterranean region. A favorite of homemakers, they usually incorporate seasonal fruit and were eaten on Sundays and special occasions. I like to make one of these types of cake each week to have on hand for guests or to bring as hosts' gifts when invited to dinner or a party.

You can find the following recipes in this section:

>> **Apple, Cinnamon, and Olive Oil Cake:** The perfect fall cake to enjoy at breakfast, brunch, or teatime

>> **Orange, Almond, and Olive Oil Cake:** A wholesome finale to an elegant meal

>> **Upside-Down Kiwi Cake:** A fun twist on the classic

>> **Chocolate and Pumpkin Snack Cake:** Cake with balanced macronutrients that you can also eat between meals

>> **Banana Chocolate Chip Cake:** A sweet, moist, and dense cake that travels well and is a crowd-pleaser

Apple, Cinnamon, and Olive Oil Cake

PREP TIME: 15 MIN	COOK TIME: 45 MIN	YIELD: 10 SERVINGS

INGREDIENTS

⅓ cup (71g) EVOO, plus 1 teaspoon (4.5g) for coating pan

¾ cup (252g) raw agave nectar

3 large eggs

3 cups (336g) almond flour

1 teaspoon (4.6g) baking powder

2 teaspoons (5g) cinnamon

1 teaspoon (4.2g) vanilla

4 large Golden Delicious apples, cored, peeled, and diced

1 tablespoon (8g) confectioners' sugar, for dusting

DIRECTIONS

1 Preheat the oven to 350 degrees F (175 degrees C). Grease a 10-inch springform cake pan with 1 teaspoon (4.5g) olive oil. Place the EVOO, agave nectar, and eggs in a medium bowl, and mix to combine. Stir in the almond flour and baking powder, mixing well to combine. Add the cinnamon and vanilla and mix well to combine. Stir in the apples.

2 Spoon the batter into the greased cake pan, spread the mixture evenly, and smooth the top. Shake the pan to ensure that there are no gaps in the batter. Bake on the center rack of the oven for 40 to 45 minutes, or until a knife or toothpick inserted in the center of the cake comes out clean.

3 Remove cake from the oven and allow to cool to room temperature. Sprinkle with confectioners' sugar and serve.

NOTE: The almond flour helps to balance the sweetness.

VARY IT! Use pears instead of apples.

PER SERVING: *Calories 407 (From Fat 234); Fat 26g (Saturated 3g); Cholesterol 63mg; Sodium 71mg; Carbohydrate 40g (Dietary Fiber 7g); Protein 9g; Sugars 31g.*

🍊 Orange, Almond, and Olive Oil Cake

PREP TIME: 10 MIN	COOK TIME: 45 MIN	YIELD: 9 SERVINGS

INGREDIENTS

½ cup (108g) plus 1 teaspoon (4.5g) Amy Riolo Selections or other EVOO

½ cup (47.5g) sliced almonds

2 eggs, separated

⅓ cup (79mL) orange juice

2 teaspoons (4g) grated orange zest

1 cup (176g) allulose

2 teaspoons (8.4g) pure vanilla extract

1 teaspoon (4.2g) almond extract

2⅓ cups (261g) almond flour

1 teaspoon (4.6g) baking powder

½ teaspoon (2.4g) sea salt

½ cup (123g) whole milk ricotta

2 tablespoons (16g) confectioners' sugar, to serve

DIRECTIONS

1 Preheat the oven to 350 degrees F (175 degrees C). Line with parchment paper and brush both sides with EVOO and sprinkle one side with sliced almonds.

2 In the bowl of a standing mixer with the whisk attachment or in a large metal bowl using a hand mixer, beat the egg whites until stiff peaks form. Set aside. In a separate bowl, combine the orange juice and zest, allulose, remaining olive oil, egg yolks, vanilla, and almond extract.

3 In a large bowl, sift together the flour, baking powder and sea salt. Stir in the orange mixture and fold in the ricotta. Fold in the egg whites. Pour the batter into the prepared pan and smooth out with a spatula. Bake until a toothpick inserted into the middle comes out clean and the cake begins to pull away from the sides of the pan, 40 to 45 minutes. Cool completely and then invert the cake onto a platter and release the sides of the pan. Remove the parchment paper, sprinkle with confectioners' sugar, and serve.

TIP: Make an extra cake in advance and wrap it in the freezer to enjoy at a later date.

NOTE: The eggs, ricotta cheese, and almond flour add protein and healthful fats to this recipe so that a portion could be enjoyed on its own or after a meal.

VARY IT! Swap out the orange for lemon and the almonds for walnuts, if desired. You can also add blueberries to this cake.

PER SERVING: *Calories 364 (From Fat 292); Fat 32g (Saturated 5g); Cholesterol 54mg; Sodium 186mg; Carbohydrate 11g (Dietary Fiber 4g); Protein 10g; Sugars 4g.*

Upside-Down Kiwi Cake

PREP TIME: 10 MIN	COOK TIME: 30 MIN	YIELD: 8 SERVINGS

INGREDIENTS

½ cup (108g) plus 1 teaspoon (4.5g) Amy Riolo Selections or other EVOO, divided

1¾ cups (219g) unbleached, all-purpose flour

2 teaspoons (9g) baking powder

1 pinch (.6g) sea salt

1 cup (176g) allulose

1 cup (237mL) whole milk

1 teaspoon (4.2g) vanilla extract

3 kiwis peeled and sliced into thin rounds

DIRECTIONS

1 Heat the oven to 350 degrees F (175 degrees C). Grease an 8-inch round cake pan with 1 teaspoon EVOO. Line with parchment paper. Turn the parchment over to coat the other side with EVOO as well.

2 Combine the flour, baking powder, sea salt, allulose, milk, ½ cup (108g) EVOO, and vanilla in a large mixing bowl. Mix well until incorporated.

3 Arrange the kiwi slices on the bottom of the pan. Pour the batter on top of the kiwi slices and smooth the top with a spatula.

4 Bake for 30 minutes or until a toothpick inserted in the middle comes out clean. Allow to cool completely. Use a butter knife to loosen the edge of the pan and invert on to a plate and tap on the bottom to release the cake.

TIP: Enjoy this cake after a meal that consists of lean protein, leafy greens, and cruciferous vegetables. To increase the protein content, use a nut flour instead of the all-purpose flour.

NOTE: Kiwis have a moderate glycemic index (GI) of 50, which means they're digested at a moderate pace and cause a modest increase in blood sugar levels yet their fiber content helps to lessen the glycemic load (GL) as does the use of healthful olive oil in this recipe.

VARY IT! Substitute almond flour for the all-purpose flour and plant-based milk for the whole milk.

PER SERVING: *Calories 262 (From Fat 139); Fat 15g (Saturated 3g); Cholesterol 3mg; Sodium 166mg; Carbohydrate 27g (Dietary Fiber 2g); Protein 4g; Sugars 4g.*

✪ Chocolate and Pumpkin Snack Cake

PREP TIME: 15 MIN	COOK TIME: 30 MIN	YIELD: 20 SERVINGS

INGREDIENTS

2 eggs

½ cup (118mL) egg whites

1 large yellow squash, trimmed, cut into pieces

One 15-ounce (444mL) can pumpkin puree

⅓ cup (83g) almond butter

1 teaspoon (4.2g) pure vanilla extract

2½ cups (405g) oat flour

1 tablespoon (5.6g) pumpkin pie spice

½ cup (43g) dark cocoa powder

2 teaspoon (9g) baking powder

¼ teaspoon (1.2g) sea salt

¼ cup (81g) maple syrup

⅓ cup (55g) dark chocolate chips, divided

1 teaspoon (4.5g) Amy Riolo Selections or other EVOO

DIRECTIONS

1 Preheat the oven to 350 degrees F (175 degrees C). Grease a 9-x-13-inch baking pan with the EVOO and line with parchment paper. Turn the parchment paper and coat the other side with EVOO.

2 Whisk your eggs and whites in a large mixing bowl. Place the squash, pumpkin puree, and almond butter into a food processor and puree until smooth. Add the pureed mixture and vanilla to the egg white bowl. Mix well. Add the oat flour, pumpkin pie spice, cocoa powder, baking powder, and sea salt and mix until combined. Add the maple syrup and stir in half of the chocolate chips.

3 Pour the batter in the pan, top with the remaining chocolate chips, and bake for 30 minutes, or until golden and a toothpick inserted in the middle comes out clean.

PER SERVING: *Calories 159 (From Fat 56); Fat 6g (Saturated 1g); Cholesterol 21mg; Sodium 146mg; Carbohydrate 22g (Dietary Fiber 3g); Protein 6g; Sugars 5g.*

Banana Chocolate Chip Cake

PREP TIME: 10 MIN	COOK TIME: 50 MIN	YIELD: 9 SERVINGS

INGREDIENTS

⅓ cup (71g) plus 1 teaspoon (4.5g) Amy Riolo Selections or other EVOO

½ cup (96g) coconut sugar

3 ripe bananas, mashed

2 eggs

¼ teaspoon (1.2g) sea salt

1 teaspoon (4.2g) vanilla

1 teaspoon (4.6g) baking powder

1¾ cups (284g) oat flour

¼ cup (28g) ground flaxseeds

½ cup (84g) dark chocolate chips

DIRECTIONS

1 Preheat oven to 350 degrees F (175 degrees C). Coat a 9-inch round or square cake pan with 1 teaspoon (4.5g) EVOO and coat pan.

2 Combine ⅓ cup (71g) EVOO and coconut sugar in a large bowl. Stir with a wooden spoon until combined. Add the bananas, eggs, sea salt, vanilla, baking powder, oat flour, and flaxseeds. Mix well to combine and then add the chocolate chips.

3 Bake for 50 minutes or until the cake is golden and cooked through (until a toothpick inserted in the middle comes out clean). Allow to cool and serve.

TIP: You can pour this batter into muffin tins lined with paper to make Banana Chocolate Chip Muffins.

VARY IT! Make it into a chocolate cake by adding ⅓ cup (30g) dark cocoa powder to the batter.

PER SERVING: *Calories 351 (From Fat 150); Fat 17g (Saturated 4g); Cholesterol 47mg; Sodium 130mg; Carbohydrate 36g (Dietary Fiber 4g); Protein 7g; Sugars 10g.*

Relishing Chocolate Cakes

Chocolate cakes became popular in the United States in the early 20th century, and they continue to be a favorite of many. Some keys to making chocolate cakes diabetes-friendly include

>> Use dark cocoa and chocolate pieces that are high in antioxidants and low in sugar.

>> Use nutritious flours, such as almond, oat, whole wheat, and so on.

>> Incorporate healthful sweeteners, such as allulose and coconut sugar.

>> Use EVOO instead of other oils.

>> Add in high protein ingredients, such as nuts, Greek yogurt, and so on.

You can find these recipes in this section:

>> **Mini Flourless Olive Oil and Chocolate Cakes:** These desserts are quite decadent and should be only enjoyed on occasion, after a meal consisting of lean protein and green leafy vegetables.

>> **Gluten-Free Chocolate Cupcakes:** Chocolate cupcakes are welcome additions to dessert buffets, elegant affairs, and children's parties.

Mini Flourless Olive Oil and Chocolate Cakes

PREP TIME: 15 MIN	COOK TIME: 15 MIN	YIELD: 6 SERVINGS

INGREDIENTS

½ cup (108g) plus 1 teaspoon (4.5g) Amy Riolo Selections or other EVOO

5 ounces (142g) bittersweet (not unsweetened) or semisweet chocolate, chopped

3 large eggs

3 large egg yolks

1 cup (175g) allulose

½ cup (56g) almond flour

1 cup (123g) raspberries, for decoration

DIRECTIONS

1 Preheat the oven to 450 degrees F (230 degrees C). Grease six ¾-cup soufflé dishes or custard cups with 1 teaspoon (4.5g) EVOO. Stir the chocolate and remaining EVOO in a heavy medium saucepan over low heat until melted. Cool slightly.

2 Whisk the eggs and egg yolks in a large bowl to blend. Whisk in the allulose, and then the chocolate mixture and the flour. Pour the batter into the dishes, dividing equally. The batter can be refrigerated at this point and baked the next day, if desired.

3 Bake the cakes until the sides are set but the center remains soft and runny, about 11 minutes or up to 14 minutes for batter that was refrigerated. Run a small knife around the cakes to loosen. Immediately turn the cakes out onto plates. Garnish with raspberries and serve.

TIP: These desserts are quite decadent and should be only enjoyed on occasion, after a meal consisting of lean protein and green leafy vegetables.

PER SERVING: *Calories 406 (From Fat 318); Fat 35g (Saturated 9g); Cholesterol 211mg; Sodium 42mg; Carbohydrate 20g (Dietary Fiber 4g); Protein 8g; Sugars 14g.*

⊘ Gluten-Free Chocolate Cupcakes

PREP TIME: 15 MIN	COOK TIME: 20 MIN	YIELD: 12 SERVINGS

INGREDIENTS

6 tablespoons (81g) plus
2 teaspoons (9g) Amy Riolo
Selections or other EVOO,
divided

One 15-ounce (425g) can black
beans, rinsed and drained

5 eggs

1 tablespoon (13g) pure vanilla
extract

½ teaspoon (2.4g) sea salt

1 teaspoon (2.3g) baking
powder

½ teaspoon (23g) baking soda

1 cup (192g) coconut sugar

⅓ cup (31g) cocoa powder

1 tablespoon (8g) confectioners'
sugar, for dusting

1 cup (144g) strawberries,
sliced

DIRECTIONS

1 Preheat the oven to 325 degrees F (165 degrees C). Grease a 12-hole muffin tin with 2 teaspoons (9g) EVOO. Place all the ingredients into a blender and blend until well mixed.

2 Fill the muffin holes about halfway full of batter. Bake for 15 to 20 minutes, or until a toothpick inserted comes out clean. Allow to cool, dust with confectioners' sugar, and top with strawberries.

TIP: This recipe can also be made into a single 8-inch layer cake. Increase bake time to 30 minutes.

NOTE: Beans are a great way to add fiber and protein to cake and brownie recipes.

PER SERVING: *Calories 201 (From Fat 89); Fat 10g (Saturated 2g); Cholesterol 88mg; Sodium 224mg; Carbohydrate 8g (Dietary Fiber 3g); Protein 6g; Sugars 2g.*

4
The Part of Tens

IN THIS PART . . .

Find out how you can enjoy dessert even when you have diabetes.

Debunk common myths about diabetes and desserts.

Discover ingredients you can use in your desserts to make them diabetes-friendly.

Chapter **18**

Ten Ways to Enjoy Desserts When You Have Diabetes

D esserts are a taboo topic in the world of diabetes because many people erroneously believe that indulging in a sweet treat every now and then is what causes diabetes. The truth is that if you discover how to create wholesome desserts as well as when and how to eat them, you can enjoy sweet treats without fear of derailing your diet. This chapter gives you strategies to make it easy to "have your cake and eat it too"!

Relishing Desserts

If you eat a balanced diet and get plenty of exercise, wholesome and nutritious desserts can be a part of your lifestyle plan. Be sure to always eat small portions of desserts. Choose sweets made from whole grains, small amounts of natural sweeteners, eggs, nuts, seeds, and good quality fat such as EVOO. Enhance their flavor with nutrient rich dark cocoa, fresh fruit, and sweet-tasting spices.

Consuming All Three Macronutrients during Each Meal

This simple trick often gets overlooked. Desserts affect blood sugar differently, depending upon whether or not they're eaten alone (strictly carbs and sugar) or whether or not they contain healthful fats and lean protein. By balancing small amounts of sugar (preferably natural sources) with good fats and quality proteins, you can avoid spikes in your sugar.

REMEMBER

This means that if you have a piece of cake, for example, enjoying it with a handful of almonds can help to balance your blood sugar. The same thing is true if you eat a pie made from wholesome grains and a low-fat protein. Both the quality of the individual ingredients and the way in which you combine them play a role in balancing blood glucose.

Monitoring Your Blood Glucose Levels

Before eating dessert, always test your blood glucose levels. If your glucose is high, then now isn't the time to indulge. Walk around, drink water, listen to peaceful music, meditate, and be sure that you're taking your medicine and/or insulin properly. Only indulge in desserts and foods with a higher glycemic index (GI) or glycemic load (GL) when your glucose levels are within a normal range. (Chapter 2 discusses GI and GL in greater detail and identifies foods that have higher levels.)

TIP

Alternately, if you test your blood glucose after eating dessert and it spikes, figure out why. Perhaps the spike is because you ate a serving too big, a dessert that was too sugary, or a carb-heavy meal. Perhaps you ate the dessert as a snack and you didn't eat something to balance out the sugar. Try to figure out the reason so that you can avoid the same types of spikes.

Eating More Fruit-Based Desserts

Fruit is nature's dessert. When fresh and in season, fruit is the best option. A large amount of the recipes in Part 3 focus on fruit-based recipes because they're the healthiest. The high amount of fiber and other nutrients in fruit make it the perfect food for people on the go.

The National Center for Chronic Disease Prevention and Health Promotion states that a diet high in fruits and vegetables may help people manage their weight, in addition to lowering the risk for chronic diseases and improving overall health. According to researchers, the water and fiber in fruits increase volume and therefore reduce *energy density* (calories per weight) of the food. That's important because foods with high energy density have a high number of calories per weight of food and cause weight gain. Fruits make you feel fuller faster with fewer calories. Consuming dietary fiber also plays a significant role in weight regulation. Whole fruit not only contains more fiber because of the peel, but it's also considered lower in energy density and more fulfilling than fruit juices, making it the top choice, when available.

TIP

A diet high in soluble fiber can slow the absorption of sugar and control blood sugar levels. Be sure to choose fresh, seasonal, organic fruit whenever possible. Always vary the types of fruit that you eat so that you enjoy a wide range of nutrients.

REMEMBER

The key to eating fresh fruit is moderation. Even though you need it for its fiber and antioxidant content, too much of a good thing can be harmful to people with diabetes. Avoid consuming large quantities of fruit that contain carbs and sugars. Instead, opt for a single serving of fresh fruit at a time, preferably balanced with a serving of protein.

Paying Attention to Portion Sizes

Being cognizant of portion sizes may sound like a no-brainer, but many people have some difficulty understanding portion sizes thanks to the amount of prepared foods and restaurant portion sizes available. Restaurants, for example, make much more profit on dessert if they serve large portions (you can't charge $15 for a small slice of cake), so people get used to the particular size as being appropriate. Those serving sizes, however, have nothing to do with physical portions when applied to nutrition and your health. Most modern restaurant dessert servings could easily feed four. So, if you do order a decadent dessert at a restaurant, share it with everyone at the table where everyone gets one or two bites.

Each recipe in Part 3 gives nutritional information for the specific portion size. The old adage that "too much of a good thing . . ." is definitely true with desserts. The key is to allow yourself a little indulgence of nutritious desserts so that you don't go overboard with unhealthful options after refraining from eating any dessert for a long time.

Substituting Butter with EVOO Whenever Possible

I've been baking with EVOO ever since I was a child. I can't tell you how many times people told me that it wasn't possible because it would "change the flavor of the food." They were right; it often did change the flavor, for the better, that is. Olives, after all, are a natural fruit. The different varieties come in a multitude of flavor profiles that can enhance many baking recipes while helping to improve your health.

Using EVOO in place of butter or margarines more often is an obvious choice. As an unprocessed healthy monounsaturated fat from fruit, EVOO isn't solid at room temperature, and it's a much healthier option when baking cakes, sweet breads, crusts, tortes, and more.

REMEMBER

Experiment with adding it to desserts like those made with dark chocolate, and drizzling it over vanilla ice cream or gelato, or even plain, full-fat Greek yogurt makes for a tasty treat with added health benefits. Adding EVOO to desserts even helps lessen its GL and extracts more nutrients already present in the dessert. That means that it slows the digestion of carbohydrates in the dessert due to its healthy fats, thus delaying the absorption of sugar into the bloodstream. In this sense, the EVOO acts as a buffer to prevent a rapid rise in glucose that's caused when eating desserts.

Making It a Team Effort

Labeling desserts diabetes-friendly is a turnoff for many people, because the term denotes sacrifice and a lack of sugar. If, however, you let your friends and family know that you're now focusing on nourishing desserts that are as good tasting as they are good for you, you set yourself up for success.

TIP

Invite your loved ones into the kitchen to whip up some desserts with you. The quality time is therapeutic, and you may just find some new favorites in the meantime. When serving the desserts in this book, or other diabetes-friendly desserts, just call them by their name, such as "Strawberry-Studded Blondies" or "Banana Chocolate Chip Cake" and refrain from using the words "healthy" or "diabetes-friendly," which unfortunately turn people off. Let them enjoy the desserts first before telling them how they were made!

Exploring New Tastes and Dessert Styles

Human beings begin craving sweet flavors at their first taste of their mother's milk. The sweet notes that humans first experienced when being held as babies is then associated with comfort, safety, and nourishment. For that reason, sweet flavors are an easy sell for the rest of their lives and ones that they continue to crave.

In many parts of the world overly sweet desserts that were once prepared only for festivals and enjoyed sporadically are being served daily, and they're hard to resist. The key to success is to find healthful sweeteners to use sparingly along with other healthful ingredients which enhance sweet flavors. By gradually cutting down on added sugars in recipes, you can train yourself to enjoy healthier sweeteners.

Triple chocolate cake or fried glazed stuffed donuts may be your favorite sweet treats (up until know, that is). But those desserts have no place in a wholesome diabetes-friendly meal plan. By exploring new flavors — fruits, nuts, and lowfat cheeses that are new to you — you can jump-start your taste buds to form new flavor memories. As you enjoy new healthful ingredients, the old favorites won't cause such strong cravings.

If cake and donuts are the only way you've been enjoying desserts, I have good news for you: A whole world of treats is just waiting for you. Fruit-based desserts, pies, tarts, custards, dozens of styles of cookies, bars, brownies, blondies, and even sweet sips can broaden your repertoire.

Planning Ahead

If you want to enjoy desserts, you need to accept that if you have diabetes, choosing which type of desserts to eat and when you eat them is an important part of your daily life. That means if you want to eat a dessert after a meal, including those in Part 3, you have to plan for it.

If, for example, you plan on eating a dessert that's high in sugar and carbs and has a high GL, eat a meal of predominately lean protein and green leafy vegetables. If you eat a high-sugar/high-carb dessert after a meal that contains a significant amount of sugar and carbs, your blood sugar will spike.

Exercising on a Regular Basis

Regular physical activity is important for everyone, but it's extremely important for individuals with diabetes who wish to maintain healthy blood glucose levels. Activities such as walking, bike riding, playing sports, gardening, running, jogging, working out at the gym, yoga, Pilates, and dancing before or after consuming desserts can help your body to metabolize them better. If you exercise in fresh air, your body gets even more benefit from it. According to the Centers for Disease Control and Protection (CDC), you want at least 150 minutes of moderate-intensity physical activity every week or 30 minutes on most days.

Chapter **19**

Ten Myths Debunked about Diabetes and Desserts

I n the most recent editions of *Diabetes For Dummies* and *Diabetes Meal Planning & Nutrition For Dummies*, my coauthor Dr. Simon Poole and I describe the management of diabetes in detail as well as how to plan daily meal plans to keep you on track with blood glucose levels.

REMEMBER

Doctors consider your blood glucose *normal* when it's less than 100 mg/dl (5.5 mmol/L) if you've eaten nothing for 8 to 12 hours. If you've eaten, your blood glucose is normal if it's less than 140 mg/dl (7.8 mmol/L) 2 hours after eating. If you never see a blood glucose level higher than 140, you're doing very well, indeed.

You can use many tricks to achieve this level of control. In this chapter, I dispel the many myths around diabetes and desserts.

Knowing Your Current Blood Glucose Levels Doesn't Matter

You should always know your blood glucose levels. The number of glucose meters you can choose is vast, and they're all good. Your insurance company may prefer one type of meter, or your doctor may have computer hardware and software for only one type. Other than those limitations, the choice is yours.

REMEMBER

Testing in the morning before breakfast, in the evening before dinner, and preferably before dessert can tell you which types of foods you can afford to eat. If your blood sugar is very high before a meal, then that's not the time to enjoy dessert. Rather you need to eat a very balanced, diabetes-friendly meal, take your medications as prescribed, and get physical exercise to help lower the blood glucose levels. Testing at bedtime is also necessary in order to select your snack and insulin dose, if you're using insulin.

If pre-meal testing reveals that your blood sugar is already in a good place, then you can enjoy a serving of the desserts in Part 3. I include instructions on how you can pair the desserts with the meal that you eat prior to it. For example, I mention whether the dessert is balanced in terms of macronutrients or not. If it is, then you can enjoy the dessert anytime. If the dessert is slightly carb-heavy, however, it should only follow a meal that's based on lean protein and nonstarchy vegetables and not one that's carb-heavy.

Exercising to Control Your Glucose Doesn't Help

Exercise is imperative, not just for controlling your blood glucose but also for improving your physical and mental state in general. Research suggests that even individuals with a genetic predisposition to develop diabetes because both parents had it were able to avoid developing diabetes thanks to regular exercise.

TIP

If you've been diagnosed with diabetes, are looking to avoid it, or just want to be healthy, take a brisk walk, lasting no more than 60 minutes, every day, and not necessarily all at once.

Exercise can provide several benefits to your overall health, and it also helps you metabolize the carbohydrates, sugar, and fat in recipes more properly. Exercise does the following:

>> Lowers the blood glucose by using it for energy

>> Helps with weight loss

>> Lowers bad cholesterol and triglyceride fats and raises good cholesterol

>> Lowers blood pressure

>> Reduces stress levels

>> Improves mood

>> Reduces the need for drugs and insulin shots

Increasing Medications Enables You to Eat Anything

If your doctor has prescribed medications for your diabetes, taking them according to instructions is an essential part of your diabetes plan. Many people, however, are under the assumption that they can simply eat what they like and self-medicate with extra pills or insulin shots to make up for it.

That's one of the worst ways to manage your blood glucose levels. Taking the right dosages at the right time is important to maintain level amounts as much as possible.

TIP

If you want to be able to enjoy desserts and occasional unhealthy foods, here's what you can do to stay on track while taking your medications as prescribed:

>> **Maintain a positive attitude.** The mind-body connection is important. Choose your thoughts wisely. Decide that you're worthy and deserving of good health and seek to search for things and thoughts that make you feel good daily. Use positive affirmations about your health.

>> **Be grateful.** Give thanks for your food, your body, and your health as often as possible.

>> **Get help.** If needed, seek a therapist and/or health coach to help you maintain a healthy mindset and keep you on track with your health goals.

>> **Exercise daily.** Refer to the preceding section for more information.

>> **Get enough sleep and take short afternoon naps when possible.** Research has shown that sleep affects your hormones, endocrine system, and metabolism. If you can't get a solid night's sleep, seek medical and/or mental help.

>> **Eat as healthfully as possible the majority of the time.** Check out my books *Diabetes Meal Planning & Nutrition For Dummies* and the *Diabetes Cookbook For Dummies* written with co-author Dr. Simon Poole (John Wiley & Sons, Inc.) to help make sure that most of your meals are as nutritious as possible. That way when you're forced to be in a situation where you need to eat less than desirable foods, it won't have as negative of an impact.

>> **Eat communally and socialize as much as possible.** Eating with friends and family has an impact on your mental and physical health.

>> **Eat as many green leafy vegetables as possible throughout the day.** Choose lean proteins, legumes, whole grains, and beans daily. Use herbs, spices, and extra-virgin olive oil (EVOO) as flavor enhancers.

>> **Spend as much time doing what you love.** Hobbies and pleasurable activities help you to keep blood glucose in check.

>> **Manage stress.** Yoga, deep breathing, meditation, mindfulness techniques, and so on can help lower stress, which has a negative effect on blood sugar levels and health in general.

>> **Get fresh air as much as possible.** Even 10 minutes a day can offer health benefits, but at least 30 minutes a day is ideal because it offers mental and psychological benefits.

>> **Choose small amounts of the best quality desserts.** The recipes in Part 3 are a great place to start.

>> **Harness the power of happiness hormones.** Refer to Chapter 2.

Using Alternative or Artificial Sweeteners Is Okay

Recent studies have proven that artificial sweeteners can be even more harmful than sugar in recipes. Although artificial sweeteners don't contain table sugar and may be zero-calorie, they often include more sodium, fat, and chemical substances than the traditional counterpart. In fact, the sodas, desserts, drinks, and snacks that use them shouldn't be considered any safer than the regular variety. If you have diabetes or want to avoid developing it, avoid these items.

In a recent Harvard study of 103,388 people in which 80 percent were women at an average age of 42, each participant recorded their food intakes daily along with their medical history and health habits. More than one-third (37 percent) used artificial sweeteners, and they consumed about 42 milligrams per day, on average — an amount roughly equal to the contents of one tabletop packet or just under a quarter-cup of diet soda. The follow-up lasted for approximately 9 years, and participants were asked to fill out questionnaires and report changes in health biannually. Scientists' findings concluded that "artificial sweeteners were linked to a 9 percent higher risk of any type of cardiovascular problem (including heart attacks) and an 18 percent greater risk of stroke."

Refer to Chapter 6 for more information about what alternative, artificial, and regular sugar mean.

Regardless of whether a sugar or sweetening agent is natural or not, enjoy it at a minimum and in combination with foods that contain healthful fats and lean protein in order to balance blood sugar in individuals with diabetes.

Preparing Desserts in Advance or Thinking about Them Is Taboo

How many times have you heard someone say "I'm watching what I eat (or I'm on a diet), and I can't even think about food."? Nothing, though, is further from the truth. In modern societies, the more that you're watching what you eat, the more that you have to think about what you put into your mouth and when you eat.

By planning ahead of time (see Chapter 7), you can make better choices. When following any diet plan, having the best versions of desserts available is important in order to avoid buying the kinds that aren't good for you. Fantastic desserts and pastries are available everywhere nowadays, and people are biologically designed to crave sweet flavors.

By stocking up on nutritious ingredients (refer to Chapter 6), taking control of cravings — I discuss more in Chapter 3), and allowing yourself to enjoy sweets on occasion, you can avoid binging and completely derailing your meal plan. The key is to discovering how to make these desserts for yourself and others to enjoy.

Making "Healthful Desserts" Taste Good Is Impossible

Enjoying good-tasting desserts that are also good for you is possible. Just like healthful food can taste good when prepared properly, so can healthful desserts. The recipes in Part 3 rely on the delicious flavors of fresh fruit, sweet spices like cinnamon and cloves, citrus, as well as proteins and healthful fats from almonds and other nuts, Greek yogurt, and EVOO, to balance the nutrition and enhance the depth of flavor.

After you have a few preparation techniques under your belt, you can start to create desserts that both look and taste great while satisfying your sweet tooth. Whether you're craving cookies, brownies, fruit-based desserts, pies and tortes, cakes, or sweet drinks, you can enjoy them and good health too.

Planning for the Unexpected Isn't Necessary

One of the key factors that often derails the best intentions when it comes to eating well is the unexpected. Sometimes major life events happen that cause you to shift your attention elsewhere. Other times and most often, however, the small daily choices add up over a long period of time and get in the way of meeting your health goals.

In a perfect world you'd have time to make all your food from the best ingredients possible daily. However, busy schedules, harried days, after-school activities, caregiving, traffic, and mishaps are the reality. Finding pockets of time — once a week or once or twice a month — to prepare and freeze nutritious desserts in advance can really help you to achieve your long-term goals.

Chapter 7 explores ways to set aside some time to bake and prepare desserts in advance so that they're ready when you need them. Setting aside time to bake and make desserts may sound counterintuitive for someone with diabetes, or someone who's trying to avoid it to spend time on homemade desserts. If the recipes in Part 3 were the only types of desserts and sweets available, fewer people would be living with diabetes. By prepping wholesome versions in advance and enjoying them on occasion, you won't feel deprived and you may gain a new hobby or passion in the meantime.

Thinking That Desserts Can't Be Good for You

When eaten in small amounts, at times when your blood sugar levels are within a healthy range and combined with other nutritious foods, healthful desserts can be good for you. Here are some things to keep in mind:

» **Plan ahead for eating dessert by ensuring that what you eat prior is balanced and not carb- or fat-heavy.** Refer to Chapter 7.

» **Enjoy desserts made from nutritious ingredients.** The recipes in Part 3 rely on fresh and dried fruit, dark chocolate, almonds and nuts, seeds, Greek yogurt, EVOO, and sweet spices in their preparation. These ingredients contain antioxidants that positively impact your health and are known to help balance blood sugar while adding flavor and essential nutrients.

» **Eat desserts that are good sources of the three macronutrients — carbohydrate, fat, and protein.** Examples of complex carbohydrates include whole grains, examples of healthful fat include EVOO, nuts, seeds, and Greek yogurt, and examples of protein include ricotta cheese, yogurt, and seeds. See Chapter 4 for more about macronutrients.

Prepping Tasty Diabetes-Friendly Desserts Is Hard

Nothing could be further from the truth! Just like with preparing all desserts, planning and preparation is your key to success. Here are some steps to make it easier:

» **Build a pantry of healthful baking ingredients.** See Chapter 6.

» **Figure out what works best for you when preparing your desserts.** Use Chapter 7 to help you plan ahead.

» **Read recipes thoroughly and prep all ingredients before making them.** Doing so sets you up for success, keeps you organized, and saves time as well.

» **Try recipes and experiment before you entertain.** Even professional cooks and bakers rely on tried-and-true recipes when serving food to others for the first time.

>> **Start slow.** If you're new to the kitchen, start with making sweet drinks (Chapter 16) and fruit-based desserts (Chapter 9), then move on to brownies and bars in Chapter 10. Eventually you can work your way up to cakes and pies.

>> **Seek help.** If you're intimidated by baking or cooking, ask a kitchen-savvy relative or friend for help or enroll in cooking classes. Watch cooking and baking videos so that you become familiar with the process. Cooking and baking are learned skills, so just like other new activities, having a coach along with this book can really help.

Avoiding What Is Problematic Is Difficult

Some desserts aren't fit for human consumption. For example, commercially prepared, overly sweet birthday cakes should be limited to once a year — if that, by anyone, regardless of a diabetes diagnosis. Can you imagine that just a few hundred years ago teaspoons of sugar were sold in apothecaries in France and used "to pick people up" a teaspoon at a time when they were sick? Today's processed foods contain tablespoons and cups full of sugar in single serving portions and people are living the results of the opposite extreme. Unhealthful amounts of sugar are consumed daily in many places around the world. Be aware of anything that has large amounts of sugar and unhealthful fats. Vowing to make your own desserts at home is the best way to avoid the temptation of what is truly harmful.

TIP

If you need help deciding which recipes and foods are best for you in your own life and health journey, bring your concerns and this book to your nutrition professional to help create the best plan for your individual needs.

Chapter **20**

Ten Best Ingredients for Diabetes Desserts

K eeping ingredients that offer powerful nutrition benefits on hand is the best way to create delicious and healthful desserts. This chapter explores how kitchen staples like dairy, dark chocolate, nuts, seeds, and Greek yogurt can transform your decadent desserts into diabetes-friendly indulgences. I also explain how you can swap out some standard ingredients for better, more nutritious, options. Making small dietary changes daily can offer the rewards of good flavor and good health.

REMEMBER

The *superfoods* such as extra-virgin olive oil (EVOO), berries, leafy green vegetables, and so forth that I mention in this chapter are only a small sample of what you can (and should) enjoy for desserts in a diabetes-friendly diet. Furthermore, all spices are *free foods,* meaning that you can incorporate them into any dessert without worrying about counting their calories and tracking carbs or sugar. In addition, wholesome whole grains such as oats, barley, and whole wheat are good additions/swap outs for other grains.

REMEMBER

To date, raw honey is the most healthful sweetening option for people with diabetes or those trying to avoid a diagnosis. Small amounts of raw honey consumed by individuals with diabetes actually has benefits for them because of its antioxidant properties.

Cinnamon

Pure cinnamon, often labelled *Ceylon cinnamon* in the United States, has been shown to help regulate blood sugar levels. It's also an anti-inflammatory ingredient, which is important for anyone dealing with any type of illness. Studies have shown that taking 1, 3, or 6 grams of cinnamon per day reduces fasting serum glucose levels in people with type 2 diabetes. Another study found that cinnamon can significantly reduce fasting blood sugar levels and insulin resistance. Cinnamon is also known to reduce triglyceride, LDL cholesterol, and total cholesterol levels in people with type 2 diabetes and to help insulin connect with cells which, in turn, assists them in taking in glucose.

From a dessert and pastry standpoint, this research is exciting because cinnamon is a common baking ingredient. In addition, the taste of cinnamon has been shown to trick a person's taste buds into thinking that they're eating something sweet.

Add cinnamon (make sure it's pure and use a teaspoon more than normal) to recipes to add sweet notes to a recipe without sweeteners.

TIP

In addition to cinnamon, dried cardamom, cloves, ginger, are all wonderful additions to baked goods.

REMEMBER

Dark Chocolate

A square or two of dark chocolate is a great addition to your day and can help you keep cravings for less beneficial sweet treats at bay. If you prefer milk chocolate to dark, you can train yourself to appreciate the higher quality, higher cocoa content chocolate by gradually increasing the percentage of cocoa in the chocolate that you consume. After you get used to the dark chocolate's decadent flavor, you won't want to go back to milk chocolate, and even better, you'll have a better sweet treat to enjoy. Chapter 2 discusses dark chocolate in greater detail.

Some of the recipes in Part 3 also feature dark processed cocoa powder. Purchasing dark, black, or unsweetened (different brands use different names) ensures that you can safely add the cocoa to your ingredients — enjoying the antioxidant health benefits and the rich cocoa flavor at the same time. You can even add a little pure cinnamon to the mix for increased flavor and nutrition!

Almonds and Almond Flour

I like to swap almond flour for white all-purpose flour in many of my recipes. It increases the flavor, texture, and nutritional value of many baked goods. It's also been a go-to secret of mine for years to make recipes gluten-free and delicious. In diabetes-friendly desserts, this addition has a special appeal because almonds contain both healthful fats and protein, which serve to balance out the natural sweeteners in the recipes.

Some research suggests that eating almonds can help lower and stabilize blood sugar levels in people with prediabetes and type 2 diabetes. One study found that eating 20 grams (.7 ounces) of almonds 30 minutes before meals for three months led to lower body weight and improved glucose variability. In addition, consuming almonds before a meal helps you to eat less and absorb more nutrients from the food that you eat. Chapter 2 discusses in greater detail the ways that almonds are good for you.

Other Nuts

Nuts contain enough protein, fiber, and fat to help you feel full. Nuts contain healthy mono-and polyunsaturated fats. One ounce of nuts contains 13 to 22 grams of these heart-healthy fats. Walnuts, Brazil nuts, cashews, pecans, hazelnuts, and peanuts (which are actually considered legumes) contain more monounsaturated fats. Although the fat in nuts is predominantly these healthy fats, any fat is calorie dense. A 1-ounce serving of unsalted nuts contains 150 to 200 calories.

A Louisiana State University study involving 13,000 subjects found consumers of tree nuts (the study excluded peanuts) had smaller waist measurements, lower weight, lower blood pressure, lower fasting blood glucose, higher levels of HDL good cholesterol, and lower levels of inflammatory proteins. Regular nut eating was also linked with higher consumption of whole grains and fruits and lower consumption of alcohol and sugar.

In addition, peanut butter has been shown to improve blood glucose control, prevent blood glucose spikes, and lower cholesterol levels in people with type 2 diabetes. Freshly ground peanut butter (without added sugar or salt) can be an excellent snack for people with diabetes and a popular ingredient in American baking. Peanuts, almonds, and walnuts are all associated in studies with improved insulin sensitivity and make a great addition to desserts and baked goods.

Extra-Virgin Olive Oil

Good quality EVOO is indispensable for good nutrition, good flavor, and tradition in my kitchen. Lecturing about olive oil and diabetes was what led me to meet the co-author of many of my books in the *For Dummies* series. Dr. Simon Poole and I even wrote an entire book dedicated to it called *Olive Oil For Dummies*, which dedicates 326 pages to our favorite ingredient.

Because olives and olive oil are a common denominator in the countries surrounding the Mediterranean Sea, they're often the ingredients that are analyzed in Mediterranean diet-based research. Antioxidants such as vitamin E, carotenoids, and phenols such as hydroxytyrosol and oleuropein (known for their anti-inflammatory and antibacterial effects) are found in olive oil.

Best of all, adding EVOO to carbohydrates has the remarkable effect of slowing their absorption as well as increasing insulin sensitivity. It also leaves your appetite more satiated sooner and your gut microbes happier. This combination results in a reduced glycemic load of a meal.

For this reason, I swap out EVOO for all other oils in baking and even use it as a replacement for butter. Chapter 18 discusses why I like to use EVOO in place of butter.

Seeds

I use sesame seeds, sunflower seeds, chia seeds, and flaxseeds quite extensively in the recipes in Part 3. Seeds contain protein, fiber, and fat which, like nuts, are filling and can help prevent the body from absorbing sugar and keep glucose levels in check. Seeds are a desirable element of diabetes management because research has found that their consumption can be a favorable replacement for carbohydrate snacks because they improve A1C numbers and lower LDL cholesterol after 3 months.

TIP

Be sure to purchase salt-free seeds when using. Seeds are easy to find. You can mix them into yogurt and whole grain cereals or baked into bread and baked goods to help reduce their glycemic load.

Citrus: Oranges and Lemons

Citrus is what my maternal great grandmother Michela considered a "secret ingredient" that she used in desserts and one that I can't go without. Oranges are a great source of the cholesterol-reducing soluble fiber called pectin, as well as folate and potassium. Oranges also contain the antioxidant hesperidin, which can help prevent damage to cells. And face it, sometimes it's great to have something really sweet like an orange. A medium-sized orange is one 15-gram carbohydrate choice, making one orange or ½ cup of orange juice an effective treatment for moderate hypoglycemia.

Lemons are a great source of vitamin C, and like vinegars, their acidity decreases the glycemic load when combined with carbohydrates in a meal. Adding a squeeze of lemon juice to water is a wonderful way of staying hydrated while balancing the body's PH levels. It's also a wonderful detoxifier and has antimicrobial properties.

In desserts, oranges can add a sweet-holiday flavor whereas lemon zest adds brightness. Lemon juice helps prevent apples and pears from *oxidizing* (turning brown) during baking. Whenever you want to add more flavor to a dessert without adding sugar, think about incorporating citrus zest and a bit of juice.

Plain, Full-Fat Greek Yogurt

If you can eat dairy, plain, full-fat, Greek yogurt should be a staple in your refrigerator. Yogurt, especially plain Greek yogurt that's produced around the world now, is high in protein and vitamin B12, which is mostly found in animal products, making it a great protein choice for people who don't eat meat. The original Greek variety is made from a combination of goat and sheep milk, and those types of milks offer additional nutrient profiles. Even cow-based milk contains a healthful dose of calcium, vitamin B2 and B12, potassium, and magnesium.

Yogurt with live active cultures (known as *probiotics*) is known to help maintain the natural balance of organisms, known as *microflora*, in the intestines. Gut health, which I discuss in Chapter 2, is essential for well-being in all people, but especially for individuals with diabetes.

When making diabetes desserts, you can swap Greek yogurt out for sour cream and heavy cream in baking and in desserts. Greek yogurt provides body in recipes (see Part 3) while giving them protein and a healthful source of fat that helps to balance the sugars in desserts.

DOCTOR SAYS

According to Dr. Simon Poole, a recent study at the University of Illinois found that adding raw honey to Greek yogurt increases the probiotic content in it, making it even better for gut health than was originally thought. Honey and Greek yogurt is a classic combination for many diabetes-friendly desserts in Part 3.

Fruit

Many people with diabetes and prediabetes think that they can no longer eat fruit. Fortunately, that isn't true. You can still eat fruits; just keep the following in mind as you incorporate fruits into your diabetes-friendly desserts:

>> Spend some time learning which fruits have the highest glycemic load and avoid those. Chapters 2 and 3 discuss which fruits are best.

>> Opt for fruits, such as the ones in the recipes in Part 3, that are better choices for those seeking to balance their blood sugar. Most of the recipes are based on or incorporate fresh fruit or unsweetened dried fruit. The recipes in Chapter 9 use the best fruits for diabetes and discuss why they are good for you.

Index

A

A1C test, 47–48

adenosine triphosphate (ATP), 44, 67

agave nectar, 99

allulose, 98

almonds

benefits of, 33

overview, 32, 305

in recipes

Almond and Apricot Tart, 253

Almond and Banana Smoothie, 267

Almond and Cherry Clafoutis, 208

Almond Orange Biscotti, 173

Baked Spice & Almond Stuffed Apples, 132

Chocolate Almond Pudding, 188

Chocolate Chip Almond Butter Cookies, 165

Date, Almond, and Cocoa Balls, 211

Grape, Goat Cheese, and Almond Skewers, 146

Orange, Almond, and Olive Oil Cake, 280

Orange and Almond Bars, 155

alternative sweeteners, 95

amino acids, 65

Angel Food Cake, 276

apples

Apple, Cinnamon, and Olive Oil Cake, 279

Apple, Raisin, and Nut Strudel, 249–250

Apple Cinnamon Crisp, 199

Baked Spice & Almond Stuffed Apples, 132

Cinnamon-Scented Apple Pie, 254

Spiced Hot Cider, 270–271

apricots

Almond and Apricot Tart, 253

Apricot and Ginger Cooler, 265

Turkish-Stuffed Apricots, 139

Yogurt Custard with Apricots and Pistachios, 193

artificial sweeteners, 95

ATP (adenosine triphosphate), 44, 67

avocados

Avocado, Yogurt, and Mango Salad, 144

Moroccan Avocado Smoothie, 261

B

Baked Spice & Almond Stuffed Apples, 132

baking, 105–106, 112–113, 157

balsamic vinegar

Broiled Figs & Balsamic Reduction, 133

Cantaloupe in White Balsamic Vinegar, 131

Strawberry, Yogurt, and White Balsamic Semifreddo, 228

bananas

as ingredient, 31

in recipes

Almond and Banana Smoothie, 267

Banana and Peanut Butter "Ice Cream," 235

Banana Chocolate Chip Cake, 283

Blackberry Banana Soft Serve, 242

Papaya, Banana, and Orange Smoothie, 266

bark (chocolate), 215–218

bars

overview, 14

recipes

Blackberry Lemon Bars, 154

Blueberry and Lemon Oatmeal Bars, 156

Orange and Almond Bars, 155

Quinoa, Cranberry, and Pecan Bars, 158

Strawberry-Studded Blondies, 153

base recipes

crusts, 117–120

custards, 121–122

ganaches, 123–125

recipes

Basic Tart Crust, 120

Dark Chocolate Ganache, 124

Homemade Pie Crust, 119

Light Fruit "Ganache," 125

Vanilla Cream Custard, 122

basil, 200

berries

Almond and Cherry Clafoutis, 208

Blackberry Banana Soft Serve, 242

Blackberry Lemon Bars, 154

Blackberry Lemon Pie Pots, 257

Blueberry and Lemon Oatmeal Bars, 156

Blueberry Cream Cobbler, 197

Cherries with Goat Cheese and Pistachios, 142

Cherry Chocolate Bread Pudding, 189

Chocolate, Pistachio, and Cranberry Biscotti, 166

Dark Chocolate–Covered Cherries, 222

berries *(continued)*

Kiwi and Raspberry Trees with Honey, 135

Mixed Berry and Mascarpone Parfaits, 205

Mixed Berry Compote, 134

Mixed Berry Crostata, 247

Oatmeal Cranberry Cookies, 183

Quinoa, Cranberry, and Pecan Bars, 158

Raspberry Sorbet, 239

Ricotta and Berry Cheesecake Tart, 206–207

Strawberry, Citrus, and Ricotta Tart, 252

Strawberry, Yogurt, and White Balsamic Semifreddo, 228

Strawberry Basil Crisp, 200

Strawberry Shortcake, 203

Strawberry Swirl Ice Cream, 231

Strawberry-Studded Blondies, 153

Summer Berry and Fresh Fig Salad, 136

Vanilla Pudding with Berries, 191

beverages

cold, 263–267

fruit, 260–262

hot, 267–271

overview, 15

recipes

Almond and Banana Smoothie, 267

Apricot and Ginger Cooler, 265

Creamy Chai, 269

Espresso Granita, 238

Hot Spiced Chocolate, 268

Moroccan Avocado Smoothie, 261

Papaya, Banana, and Orange Smoothie, 266

Pineapple Cardamom Crush, 262

Spiced Hot Cider, 270–271

Zero-Proof Sgroppino, 264

bioactive compounds, 37–39

biscotti

Almond Orange Biscotti, 173

Chocolate, Pistachio, and Cranberry Biscotti, 166

Lemon and Walnut Biscotti, 168–169

bite-sized desserts

chocolate, 215–218

overview, 209–210

recipes

Chocolate Peanut Clusters, 212

Chocolate Swirl Bark, 218

Coconut Chocolate "Fudge," 216

Date, Almond, and Cocoa Balls, 211

Peanut Butter and Coconut Bombs, 213

Quinoa and Macadamia Clusters, 217

Yogurt Kisses, 214

blackberries

Blackberry Banana Soft Serve, 242

Blackberry Lemon Bars, 154

Blackberry Lemon Pie Pots, 257

blondies, 153

blood glucose

affects of in mind and body, 8, 17–18

checking before meals, 74

comparing testing for type 1 and type 2 diabetes, 47–48

exercising and, 28, 75

fasting and, 45

measuring, 46–47

mental health and, 53–54

monitoring, 9, 75, 290

myths regarding, 296–297

overview, 7–10

problematic foods and, 51–55

regulating, 9–10, 43–44

science behind, 44–46

sleep affecting, 75

stress, negative effects on, 75

symptoms of unregulated, 8

blueberries

Blueberry and Lemon Oatmeal Bars, 156

Blueberry Cream Cobbler, 197

body

blood glucose affecting, 8

macronutrients effects on, 64

sugar and, 17–20

bombs (recipe), 213

brain, 8, 17–20

bread pudding, 189

Broiled Figs & Balsamic Reduction, 133

Broiled Pineapple with Yogurt and Honey, 140

brownies

overview, 14, 148

recipes

Dark Chocolate & Extra-Virgin Olive Oil Brownies, 149

Date, Dark Chocolate, and Cashew Bars, 150

Ricotta, Chocolate, and Orange Brownies, 151

Strawberry-Studded Blondies, 153

butter, substituting with extra-virgin olive oil, 292

C

cakes

chocolate, 284–286

fruit and, 278–283

history of, 274

overview, 15

recipes

Angel Food Cake, 276

Apple, Cinnamon, and Olive Oil Cake, 279

Banana Chocolate Chip Cake, 283

Carrot Pecan Spice Cake, 277

Chocolate and Pumpkin Snack Cake, 282

Gluten-Free Chocolate Cupcakes, 286

Italian Sponge Cake, 275

Mini Flourless Olive Oil and Chocolate Cakes, 285

Orange, Almond, and Olive Oil Cake, 280

Strawberry Shortcake, 203

Upside-Down Kiwi Cake, 281

Watermelon "Cake," 137

cantaloupes

Cantaloupe in White Balsamic Vinegar, 131

Watermelon, Cantaloupe, Kiwi, Feta, and Mint Mosaic, 129

cantucci (recipe), 172

carbohydrates

choosing, 69–70

complex, 68

counting, 70–72

glycemic index and load, effect on, 27–28

in nutrition labels, 90–91

overview, 67–72

starches and, 68

sugars and, 7–8

cardamom

Pineapple Cardamom Crush, 262

Poached Pears with Vanilla and Cardamom Cream, 141

Vanilla Cardamom Panna Cotta, 187

carrots

Carrot Cookie Bites, 177

Carrot Pecan Spice Cake, 277

cashews, 150

CDC (Centers for Disease Control and Protection), 294

Chai tea, 269

cheese

Cherries with Goat Cheese and Pistachios, 142

Grape, Goat Cheese, and Almond Skewers, 146

Mixed Berry and Mascarpone Parfaits, 205

Ricotta, Chocolate, and Orange Brownies, 151

Ricotta and Berry Cheesecake Tart, 206–207

Roasted Plums with Mascarpone Cheese, 143

Strawberry, Citrus, and Ricotta Tart, 252

Watermelon, Cantaloupe, Kiwi, Feta, and Mint Mosaic, 129

cheesecake, 206–207

cherries

Almond and Cherry Clafoutis, 208

Cherries with Goat Cheese and Pistachios, 142

Cherry Chocolate Bread Pudding, 189

chia seeds, 36

chocolate

bark, 215–218

benefits of, 164, 304

bite-sized desserts, 215–218

clusters, 215–218

dipping fruits in, 219–222

fudge, 215–218

as ingredient, 34

polyphenols in, 39

in recipes

Banana Chocolate Chip Cake, 283

Cherry Chocolate Bread Pudding, 189

Chocolate, Pistachio, and Cranberry Biscotti, 166

Chocolate Almond Pudding, 188

Chocolate and Pumpkin Snack Cake, 282

Chocolate Chip Almond Butter Cookies, 165

Chocolate "Ice Cream," 233

Chocolate Oatmeal No-Bake Cookies, 182

Chocolate Orange Rice Pudding, 190

Chocolate Peanut Clusters, 212

Chocolate Swirl Bark, 218

Chocolate-Covered Stuffed Dates, 220

Dark Chocolate & Extra-Virgin Olive Oil Brownies, 149

Dark Chocolate Ganache, 124

Dark Chocolate–Covered Cherries, 222

Date, Almond, and Cocoa Balls, 211

Date, Dark Chocolate, and Cashew Bars, 150

Gluten-Free Chocolate Cupcakes, 286

Hot Spiced Chocolate, 268

Mini Flourless Olive Oil and Chocolate Cakes, 285

Ricotta, Chocolate, and Orange Brownies, 151

Stuffed Figs Dipped in Chocolate, 221

cider, 270–271

cinnamon

benefits of, 304

as ingredient, 32–33

in recipes

Apple, Cinnamon, and Olive Oil Cake, 279

Apple Cinnamon Crisp, 199

Cinnamon-Scented Apple Pie, 254

Citrus and Cinnamon Rice Pudding, 194

citrus fruits

benefits of, 307

as ingredient, 31–32

in recipes

Almond Orange Biscotti, 173

Blackberry Lemon Bars, 154

Blackberry Lemon Pie Pots, 257

Blueberry and Lemon Oatmeal Bars, 156

Chocolate Orange Rice Pudding, 190

Citrus and Cinnamon Rice Pudding, 194

Creamy Lemon Crostata, 248

Honey Citrus Cookies, 176

citrus fruits *(continued)*

 Key Lime Pie Jars, 256

 Lemon and Walnut Biscotti, 168–169

 Lemon Granita, 237

 Orange, Almond, and Olive Oil Cake, 280

 Orange and Almond Bars, 155

 Orange and Greek Yogurt Creamsicles, 229

 Papaya, Banana, and Orange Smoothie, 266

 Ricotta, Chocolate, and Orange Brownies, 151

 Strawberry, Citrus, and Ricotta Tart, 252

clafoutis (recipe), 208

closed loop technology and monitors, testing blood glucose with, 46

clusters (chocolate), 215–218

cobblers

 crisps versus, 196

 recipes

  Blueberry Cream Cobbler, 197

  Sweet Peach Cobbler, 198

coconuts

 in recipes

  Coconut Chocolate "Fudge," 216

  Peanut Butter and Coconut Bombs, 213

 as sweetener, 98

coffee, 238

cold beverages, 263–267

compote (recipe), 134

cookies

 baking, 161–163

 bar, 162

 chocolate, 163–166

 confectionery, 162

 drop, 161

 icebox, 162

 molded, 162

 nuts in, 167

 oatmeal, 180–184

overview, 14

piped, 162

pressed, 162

recipes

 Almond Orange Biscotti, 173

 Carrot Cookie Bites, 177

 Chocolate, Pistachio, and Cranberry Biscotti, 166

 Chocolate Chip Almond Butter Cookies, 165

 Chocolate Oatmeal No-Bake Cookies, 182

 Hazelnut Cookies, 170

 Honey Citrus Cookies, 176

 Italian Pine Nut Cookies, 179

 Lemon and Walnut Biscotti, 168–169

 Meringues, 178

 Moroccan Sesame Cookies, 175

 Oatmeal Cookies, 181

 Oatmeal Cranberry Cookies, 183

 Pistachio Macaroons, 171

 Tuscan Cantucci, 172

refrigerator, 162

rolled, 162

sandwich, 162

international, 174

couscous, 192

cranberries

 Chocolate, Pistachio, and Cranberry Biscotti, 166

 Oatmeal Cranberry Cookies, 183

 Quinoa, Cranberry, and Pecan Bars, 158

cream

 creme anglaise, 121

 pastry, 121

 recipes

  Blueberry Cream Cobbler, 197

  Creamy Chai, 269

  Creamy Lemon Crostata, 248

  Orange and Greek Yogurt Creamsicles, 229

  Poached Pears with Vanilla and Cardamom Cream, 141

Red, White, and Blue Creamsicles, 243

 Vanilla Cream Custard, 122

crisps

 cobblers versus, 196

 recipes

  Apple Cinnamon Crisp, 199

  Strawberry Basil Crisp, 200

crostata

 overview, 245–246

 recipes

  Creamy Lemon Crostata, 248

  Mixed Berry Crostata, 247

crusts

 overview, 117–118

 recipes

  Basic Tart Crust, 120

  Homemade Pie Crust, 119

cupcakes, 286

cups (recipe), 241

custards

 creme anglaise, 121

 pastry cream, 121

 recipes

  Almond and Cherry Clafoutis, 208

  Vanilla Cardamom Panna Cotta, 187

  Vanilla Cream Custard, 122

  Yogurt Custard with Apricots and Pistachios, 193

D

dark chocolate

 bark, 215–218

 benefits of, 164, 304

 bite-sized desserts, 215–218

 clusters, 215–218

 dipping fruits in, 219–222

 fudge, 215–218

 as ingredient, 34

 polyphenols in, 39

 recipes

Banana Chocolate
  Chip Cake, 283
Cherry Chocolate Bread
  Pudding, 189
Chocolate, Pistachio, and
  Cranberry Biscotti, 166
Chocolate Almond
  Pudding, 188
Chocolate and Pumpkin
  Snack Cake, 282
Chocolate Chip Almond Butter
  Cookies, 165
Chocolate "Ice Cream," 233
Chocolate Oatmeal No-Bake
  Cookies, 182
Chocolate Orange Rice
  Pudding, 190
Chocolate Peanut Clusters, 212
Chocolate Swirl Bark, 218
Chocolate-Covered Stuffed
  Dates, 220
Dark Chocolate & Extra-Virgin
  Olive Oil Brownies, 149
Dark Chocolate Ganache, 124
Dark Chocolate–Covered
  Cherries, 222
Date, Almond, and Cocoa
  Balls, 211
Date, Dark Chocolate, and
  Cashew Bars, 150
Gluten-Free Chocolate
  Cupcakes, 286
Hot Spiced Chocolate, 268
Mini Flourless Olive Oil and
  Chocolate Cakes, 285
Ricotta, Chocolate, and Orange
  Brownies, 151
Stuffed Figs Dipped in
  Chocolate, 221
dates
  in recipes
    Chocolate-Covered Stuffed
      Dates, 220
    Date, Almond, and Cocoa
      Balls, 211
    Date, Dark Chocolate, and
      Cashew Bars, 150
  as sweetener, 98–99

DAWN (Diabetes Attitudes,
    Wishes, and Needs) study, 48
dentists, 49
desserts
  bars, 14
  beverages as, 15
  bite-sized, 215–218
  brownies, 14
  cakes, 15
  calming shame and guilt, 82–85
  cookies, 14
  eating, 13–15
  enjoying, 289–294
  fitting into diet, 10–11
  frozen, 14
  fruits as, 13–14
  homemade, 87
  identifying for diabetics, 36–39
  ingredients and, 11
  lifestyle choices and, 10–13, 75
  macronutrients and, 10
  meal planning
    example, 78–83
    scheduling, 109–111
    strategizing, 76–77
  myths regarding, 298–302
  non-problematic, 54–55
  pies, 14
  planning, 293, 300
  portion sizes and, 291
  preparing, 77–78, 302
  problematic, 51
  protein in, 65
  puddings, 14
  regulating blood
    glucose and, 9–10
  remaking, 40–41
  restaurants and, 11, 86–87, 291
  snacks and, 14
  spoon, 14
  store-bought, 86–87
  tarts, 14
  timing, 73–75

diabetes
  artificial sweeteners
    and, 298–299
  blood glucose and
    checking before meals, 74
    comparing testing for type 1
      and type 2 diabetes, 47–48
    effects of in mind and
      body, 8, 17–18
    exercising and, 28, 75
    fasting and, 45
    measuring, 46–47
    mental health and, 53–54
    monitoring, 9, 75, 290
    myths regarding, 296–297
    overview, 7–10
    problematic foods and,
      51–55
    regulating, 9–10, 43–44
    science behind, 44–46
    sleep affecting, 75
    stress, negative effects on, 75
    symptoms of unregulated, 8
  chocolate, benefits of, 164
  desserts and
    calming feelings of shame and
      guilt, 82–85
    identifying suitable, 36–39
    planning, 293
  exercising and, 296–297
  glycemic index and load, 27–28
  ingredients impacting, 27–30
  medical care, choosing, 48–51
  medications and, 297–298
  mental health and, 19–20
  overview, 18–19
  planning after diagnosis, 50–51
  prediabetes, 44
  receiving help from others, 292
  type 1 and type 2, 18, 33, 47–48
Diabetes Attitudes, Wishes, and
    Needs (DAWN) study, 48
diabetologists, 49
dietitians, 49

diets
  characteristics of healthy, 64
  fad, 63
  fats in, 30
  fiber in, 29–30
  fitting desserts into, 10–11
  mental health and, 21
  problematic foods and, 52
disaccharides, 44, 69
dopamine, 26
D-psicose, 98

E

eating out, 11, 86–87, 291
Emotional Guidance Scale
    (EGS), 26–27
endocrinologists, 49
endorphins, 25
energy density of fruits, 291
Espresso Granita, 238
exercising
  incorporating into lifestyle, 10
  insulin sensitivity and, 75
  lowering blood glucose with, 28
  meals and, 11
  myth regarding, 296–297
  recommended amount of, 294
extra-virgin olive oil (EVOO)
  benefits of, 210, 306
  butter, substituting with, 292
  as ingredient, 34
  in recipes
    Apple, Cinnamon, and Olive
        Oil Cake, 279
    Dark Chocolate & Extra-Virgin
        Olive Oil Brownies, 149
    Mini Flourless Olive Oil and
        Chocolate Cakes, 285
    Orange, Almond, and Olive
        Oil Cake, 280

F

fad diets, 63
fasting, blood glucose and, 45

fats, 30, 72
feta cheese, 129
fiber, 29–30
figs
  Broiled Figs & Balsamic
      Reduction, 133
  Stuffed Figs Dipped in
      Chocolate, 221
  Summer Berry and Fresh Fig
      Salad, 136
flaxseed, 36
flours, 32, 36
Fresh Fruit Kabobs, 130
frozen desserts
  granitas, 236–238
  Greek yogurt and, 224–229
  ice cream, 230–235
  overview, 14
  recipes
    Banana and Peanut Butter
        "Ice Cream," 235
    Blackberry Banana Soft
        Serve, 242
    Chocolate "Ice Cream," 233
    Coffee Ice Cream, 232
    Espresso Granita, 238
    Frozen Peanut Butter and
        Vanilla Cups, 241
    Lemon Granita, 237
    Mixed Berry and Mascarpone
        Parfaits, 205
    Orange and Greek Yogurt
        Creamsicles, 229
    Pineapple Frozen
        Yogurt Pops, 227
    Pistachio Honey Ice Cream, 234
    Raspberry Sorbet, 239
    Red, White, and Blue
        Creamsicles, 243
    Strawberry, Yogurt, and White
        Balsamic Semifreddo, 228
    Strawberry Swirl Ice
        Cream, 231
    Vanilla Frozen Yogurt, 225
    Vanilla Gelato, 226
  sorbets, 236–239
fruits. See also citrus fruit

bananas, 31
  benefits of, 210, 308
  beverages, 260–262
  choosing, 29
  incorporating into
      lifestyle, 290–291
  dates, 98–99
  desserts and, 13–14
  dipping in chocolate, 219–222
  energy density of, 291
  as ingredient, 30–32
  monk fruit sugar, 99
  overview, 127–128
  in recipes
    Almond and Apricot Tart, 253
    Almond and Banana
        Smoothie, 267
    Almond and Cherry
        Clafoutis, 208
    Almond Orange Biscotti, 173
    Apple, Cinnamon, and Olive
        Oil Cake, 279
    Apple, Raisin, and Nut
        Strudel, 249–250
    Apple Cinnamon Crisp, 199
    Apricot and Ginger Cooler, 265
    Avocado, Yogurt, and Mango
        Salad, 144
    Baked Spice & Almond Stuffed
        Apples, 132
    Banana and Peanut Butter
        "Ice Cream," 235
    Banana Chocolate
        Chip Cake, 283
    Blackberry Banana Soft
        Serve, 242
    Blackberry Lemon Bars, 154
    Blackberry Lemon Pie Pots, 257
    Blueberry and Lemon
        Oatmeal Bars, 156
    Blueberry Cream Cobbler, 197
    Broiled Figs & Balsamic
        Reduction, 133
    Broiled Pineapple with Yogurt
        and Honey, 140
    Cantaloupe in White Balsamic
        Vinegar, 131

Cherries with Goat Cheese and Pistachios, 142

Chocolate Orange Rice Pudding, 190

Chocolate-Covered Stuffed Dates, 220

Cinnamon-Scented Apple Pie, 254

Citrus and Cinnamon Rice Pudding, 194

Creamy Lemon Crostata, 248

Dark Chocolate–Covered Cherries, 222

Date, Almond, and Cocoa Balls, 211

Date, Dark Chocolate, and Cashew Bars, 150

Fresh Fruit Kabobs, 130

Grape, Goat Cheese, and Almond Skewers, 146

Honey Citrus Cookies, 176

Key Lime Pie Jars, 256

Kiwi and Raspberry Trees with Honey, 135

Lemon and Walnut Biscotti, 168–169

Lemon Granita, 237

Light Fruit "Ganache," 125

Mixed Berry and Mascarpone Parfaits, 205

Mixed Berry Compote, 134

Mixed Berry Crostata, 247

Moroccan Avocado Smoothie, 261

Oatmeal Cranberry Cookies, 183

Orange, Almond, and Olive Oil Cake, 280

Orange and Almond Bars, 155

Orange and Greek Yogurt Creamsicles, 229

Papaya, Banana, and Orange Smoothie, 266

Passionfruit Tiramisu, 202

Pineapple Cardamom Crush, 262

Poached Pears with Vanilla and Cardamom Cream, 141

Quinoa, Cranberry, and Pecan Bars, 158

Raspberry Sorbet, 239

Ricotta, Chocolate, and Orange Brownies, 151

Ricotta and Berry Cheesecake Tart, 206–207

Roasted Plums with Mascarpone Cheese, 143

Seasonal Italian Fruit Platter, 145

Spiced Hot Cider, 270–271

Strawberry, Citrus, and Ricotta Tart, 252

Strawberry, Yogurt, and White Balsamic Semifreddo, 228

Strawberry Shortcake, 203

Strawberry Swirl Ice Cream, 231

Strawberry-Studded Blondies, 153

Stuffed Figs Dipped in Chocolate, 221

Summer Berry and Fresh Fig Salad, 136

Sweet Peach Cobbler, 198

Turkish-Stuffed Apricots, 139

Upside-Down Kiwi Cake, 281

Watermelon, Cantaloupe, Kiwi, Feta, and Mint Mosaic, 129

Watermelon "Cake," 137

Wheat Berry Pomegranate Pudding with Pistachios, 195–196

Yogurt Custard with Apricots and Pistachios, 193

spoon desserts and, 201

fudge, 215–216

G

ganaches
Dark Chocolate Ganache, 124

Light Fruit "Ganache," 125

gelato, 226

ginger
Apricot and Ginger Cooler, 265

Gingerbread Spice Squares, 159

Pumpkin Gingerbread Trifle, 204

glucose, 18–19. *See also* blood glucose

Gluten-Free Chocolate Cupcakes, 286

glycemic index and load, 27–28

glycogen, 45, 67

goals, keeping track of, 55–57

goat cheese
Cherries with Goat Cheese and Pistachios, 142

Grape, Goat Cheese, and Almond Skewers, 146

granitas
overview, 236

recipes
Espresso Granita, 238

Lemon Granita, 237

Grape, Goat Cheese, and Almond Skewers, 146

Greek yogurt
benefits of, 210, 307–308

frozen desserts and, 224–229

as ingredient, 35

in recipes
Avocado, Yogurt, and Mango Salad, 144

Broiled Pineapple with Yogurt and Honey, 140

Orange and Greek Yogurt Creamsicles, 229

Pineapple Frozen Yogurt Pops, 227

Strawberry, Yogurt, and White Balsamic Semifreddo, 228

Vanilla Frozen Yogurt, 225

Yogurt Custard with Apricots and Pistachios, 193

Yogurt Kisses, 214

grocery shopping, 90–94

guilt, calming feelings of, 82–85

H

Hazelnut Cookies, 170

hbA1C test, 47–48

hemoglobin A1C test, 47–48

herbs
  Strawberry Basil Crisp, 200
  Watermelon, Cantaloupe, Kiwi, Feta, and Mint Mosaic, 129
homemade desserts, 87
Homemade Pie Crust, 119
homeostasis, 18
honey
  overview, 97
  in recipes
    Broiled Pineapple with Yogurt and Honey, 140
    Honey Citrus Cookies, 176
    Kiwi and Raspberry Trees with Honey, 135
    Pistachio Honey Ice Cream, 234
hormones
  dopamine, 26
  endorphins, 25
  mental health and, 25–26
  oxytocin, 26
  serotonin, 25
  insulin, 8, 19, 28
hot beverages, 267–271
Hot Spiced Chocolate, 268

I

ice cream. *See also* sorbets
  overview, 230–235
  recipes
    Banana and Peanut Butter "Ice Cream," 235
    Blackberry Banana Soft Serve, 242
    Chocolate "Ice Cream," 233
    Frozen Peanut Butter and Vanilla Cups, 241
    Pineapple Frozen Yogurt Pops, 227
    Pistachio Honey Ice Cream, 234
    Red, White, and Blue Creamsicles, 243
    Strawberry, Yogurt, and White Balsamic Semifreddo, 228

Strawberry Swirl Ice Cream, 231
  Vanilla Gelato, 226
impulsive eating, 20–21, 76
ingredients
  dark chocolate, 34, 304
  diabetes and, 303–308
  extra-virgin olive oil, 34, 306
  fats and, 30
  fiber and, 29–30
  freezing, 93–94
  fruits
    citrus, 307
    dates, 98–99
    diabetes and, 308
    overview, 30–32
  Greek yogurt, 35, 307–308
  grocery shopping, 90–94
  impacting diabetes, 27–30
  in nutrition labels, 90–91
  nuts, 32, 35, 305
  overview, 11
  peanut butter, 34–35
  seeds, 35–36, 306
  spices, 32–33, 304
  stocking fridge with, 92–93
  sweeteners
    agave nectar, 99
    allulose, 98
    coconut sugar, 98
    honey, 97
    maple syrup, 97
    molasses, 99–100
    monk fruit sugar, 99
    stevia, 98
    swapping out in recipes, 100–103
    table sugar, 95–96
  vanilla, 98
  whole-grain flours, 36
insoluble fiber, 29
insulin, 8, 19, 28, 75
international desserts

Almond and Cherry Clafoutis, 208
Almond Orange Biscotti, 173
Apple, Raisin, and Nut Strudel, 249–250
Apricot and Ginger Cooler, 265
Carrot Cookie Bites, 177
Chocolate, Pistachio, and Cranberry Biscotti, 166
Chocolate-Covered Stuffed Dates, 220
Creamy Lemon Crostata, 248
Espresso Granita, 238
Honey Citrus Cookies, 176
Italian Pine Nut Cookies, 179
Italian Sponge Cake, 275
Lemon and Walnut Biscotti, 168–169
Lemon Granita, 237
Meringues, 178
Mixed Berry and Mascarpone Parfaits, 205
Mixed Berry Crostata, 247
Moroccan Avocado Smoothie, 261
Moroccan Sesame Cookies, 175
Passionfruit Tiramisu, 202
Pistachio Honey Ice Cream, 234
Pistachio Macaroons, 171
Red, White, and Blue Creamsicles, 243
Seasonal Italian Fruit Platter, 145
Strawberry, Yogurt, and White Balsamic Semifreddo, 228
Stuffed Figs Dipped in Chocolate, 221
Turkish-Stuffed Apricots, 139
Tuscan Cantucci, 172
Vanilla Gelato, 226
Zero-Proof Sgroppino, 264
Italian Pine Nut Cookies, 179
Italian Sponge Cake, 275

J

jars
  overview, 255
  pie recipe, 256
journaling about food and
  exercise, 55–56

K

kabobs
  Fresh Fruit Kabobs, 130
  Grape, Goat Cheese, and
    Almond Skewers, 146
Key Lime Pie Jars, 256
kiwi
  Kiwi and Raspberry Trees with
    Honey, 135
  Upside-Down Kiwi Cake, 281
  Watermelon, Cantaloupe, Kiwi,
    Feta, and Mint Mosaic, 129

L

lemons
  benefits of, 307
  as ingredient, 32
  in recipes
    Blackberry Lemon Bars, 154
    Blackberry Lemon Pie Pots, 257
    Blueberry and Lemon
      Oatmeal Bars, 156
    Creamy Lemon Crostata, 248
    Lemon and Walnut
      Biscotti, 168–169
    Lemon Granita, 237
lifestyle choices
  desserts and, 10–13, 75
  exercising
    incorporating into lifestyle, 10
    insulin sensitivity and, 75
    lowering blood glucose with, 28
    meals and, 11
    myth regarding, 296–297
    recommended amount of, 294
  fruits, incorporating, 290–291

journaling about food and
  exercise, 55–56
  keeping track of goals, 55–57
  macronutrients, consuming
    during meals, 290
  monitoring blood glucose, 75
  noticing patterns, 56–57
  portion sizes, 291
  sleep, 75
Light Fruit "Ganache," 125
limes, 256

M

macadamia nuts, 217
macaroons, 171
macronutrients
  balancing, 10
  carbohydrates
    choosing, 69–70
    complex, 68
    counting, 70–72
    glycemic index and load,
      effect on, 27–28
    in nutrition labels, 90–91
    overview, 67–72
    starches and, 68
    sugars and, 7–8
  consuming during meals, 290
  eating meals with, 76
  effects on body, 64
  fats, 30, 72
  identifying best, 64
  overview, 62–64
  protein, 65–67
mangoes, 144
maple syrup, 97
mascarpone cheese
  Mixed Berry and Mascarpone
    Parfaits, 205
  Roasted Plums with Mascarpone
    Cheese, 143
meal planning
  including baking into, 105–106
  desserts, 109–110

example, 78–83
  strategies for, 76–77, 110–111
medical care for diabetes, 48–51
medications, myth
  regarding, 297–298
mental health
  blood glucose and, 53–54
  calming feelings of shame and
    guilt, 82–85
  diabetes and, 19–20
  Emotional Guidance Scale, 26–27
  hormones, 25–26
  improving, 24–25
  professionals, 49
  sugar cravings and, 21
Meringues, 178
Mini Flourless Olive Oil and
  Chocolate Cakes, 285
mint, 129
Mixed Berry and Mascarpone
  Parfaits, 205
Mixed Berry Compote, 134
Mixed Berry Crostata, 247
molasses, 99–100
monk fruit sugar, 99
monosaccharides, 69
Moroccan Avocado Smoothie, 261
Moroccan Sesame Cookies, 175

N

National Center for Chronic
  Disease Prevention and
  Health Promotion, 291
no-bake cookies, 182
non-problematic desserts, 54–55
nutrition labels, 90–91
nutrition specialists, 49
nuts
  almonds, 32–33
  benefits of, 210, 305
  coconuts, 98
  overview, 35
  in recipes
    Almond and Apricot Tart, 253
    Almond and Banana
      Smoothie, 267

nuts (continued)

Almond Orange Biscotti, 173

Apple, Raisin, and Nut Strudel, 249–250

Carrot Pecan Spice Cake, 277

Cherries with Goat Cheese and Pistachios, 142

Chocolate, Pistachio, and Cranberry Biscotti, 166

Chocolate Almond Pudding, 188

Chocolate Chip Almond Butter Cookies, 165

Chocolate Peanut Clusters, 212

Coconut Chocolate "Fudge," 216

Date, Almond, and Cocoa Balls, 211

Date, Dark Chocolate, and Cashew Bars, 150

Hazelnut Cookies, 170

Italian Pine Nut Cookies, 179

Lemon and Walnut Biscotti, 168–169

Orange, Almond, and Olive Oil Cake, 280

Orange and Almond Bars, 155

Peanut Butter and Coconut Bombs, 213

Pistachio Honey Ice Cream, 234

Pistachio Macaroons, 171

Quinoa, Cranberry, and Pecan Bars, 158

Quinoa and Macadamia Clusters, 217

Wheat Berry Pomegranate Pudding with Pistachios, 195–196

Yogurt Custard with Apricots and Pistachios, 193

O

oatmeal

benefits of, 180

in recipes

Blueberry and Lemon Oatmeal Bars, 156

Chocolate Oatmeal No-Bake Cookies, 182

Oatmeal Cookies, 181

Oatmeal Cranberry Cookies, 183

OGTT (oral glucose tolerance test), 46

oligosaccharides, 69

olive oil

benefits of, 210, 306

butter, substituting with, 292

as ingredient, 34

in recipes

Apple, Cinnamon, and Olive Oil Cake, 279

Dark Chocolate & Extra-Virgin Olive Oil Brownies, 149

Mini Flourless Olive Oil and Chocolate Cakes, 285

Orange, Almond, and Olive Oil Cake, 280

oral glucose tolerance test (OGTT), 46

oranges

benefits of, 307

as ingredient, 31–32

in recipes

Almond Orange Biscotti, 173

Chocolate Orange Rice Pudding, 190

Orange, Almond, and Olive Oil Cake, 280

Orange and Almond Bars, 155

Orange and Greek Yogurt Creamsicles, 229

Papaya, Banana, and Orange Smoothie, 266

Ricotta, Chocolate, and Orange Brownies, 151

oxytocin, 26

P

panna cotta, 186–187

pantry, stocking, 91–94

parfait (recipe), 205

Passionfruit Tiramisu, 202

pastry cream, 121

peaches, 198

peanut butter

as ingredient, 34–35

in recipes

Banana and Peanut Butter "Ice Cream," 235

Chocolate Peanut Clusters, 212

Frozen Peanut Butter and Vanilla Cups, 241

Peanut Butter and Coconut Bombs, 213

pears, 141

pecans

Carrot Pecan Spice Cake, 277

Quinoa, Cranberry, and Pecan Bars, 158

pharmacists, 49

pies

overview, 14, 251

recipes

Blackberry Lemon Pie Pots, 257

Cinnamon-Scented Apple Pie, 254

Key Lime Pie Jars, 256

tarts versus, 251

pine nuts, 179

pineapples

Broiled Pineapple with Yogurt and Honey, 140

Pineapple Cardamom Crush, 262

Pineapple Frozen Yogurt Pops, 227

pistachios

Cherries with Goat Cheese and Pistachios, 142

Chocolate, Pistachio, and Cranberry Biscotti, 166

Pistachio Honey Ice Cream, 234

Pistachio Macaroons, 171

Wheat Berry Pomegranate Pudding with Pistachios, 195–196

Yogurt Custard with Apricots and Pistachios, 193

platter (recipe), 145

plums, 143

Poached Pears with Vanilla and Cardamom Cream, 141

podiatrists, 49

polyphenols, 37–39

polysaccharides, 44

pomegranate, 195–196

Poole, Simon, 110

portion sizes, 291

pots (recipe), 255–257

prediabetes, 44

primary physicians, 48

problematic desserts, 51

protein, 65–67

puddings

  overview, 14, 186

  recipes

    Cherry Chocolate Bread Pudding, 189

    Chocolate Almond Pudding, 188

    Chocolate Orange Rice Pudding, 190

    Citrus and Cinnamon Rice Pudding, 194

    Vanilla Pudding with Berries, 191

    Wheat Berry Pomegranate Pudding with Pistachios, 195–196

pumpkins

  Chocolate and Pumpkin Snack Cake, 282

  Pumpkin Gingerbread Trifle, 204

Q

quinoa

  Quinoa, Cranberry, and Pecan Bars, 158

  Quinoa and Macadamia Clusters, 217

R

raisins, 249–250

raspberries

  Kiwi and Raspberry Trees with Honey, 135

Raspberry Sorbet, 239

  Strawberry, Citrus, and Ricotta Tart, 252

Red, White, and Blue Creamsicles, 243

restaurants, 11, 86–87, 291

rice pudding

  Chocolate Orange Rice Pudding, 190

  Citrus and Cinnamon Rice Pudding, 194

ricotta cheese

  Ricotta, Chocolate, and Orange Brownies, 151

  Ricotta and Berry Cheesecake Tart, 206–207

  Strawberry, Citrus, and Ricotta Tart, 252

Roasted Plums with Mascarpone Cheese, 143

S

salads

  Avocado, Yogurt, and Mango Salad, 144

  Summer Berry and Fresh Fig Salad, 136

saturated fats, 72

Seasonal Italian Fruit Platter, 145

seeds

  benefits of, 306

  chia, 36

  flaxseed, 36

  as ingredient, 35–36

  sesame, 36, 175

  sunflower, 36

semifreddo (recipe), 228

serotonin, 25

sesame seeds, 36

sesame seeds, 175

sgroppino (recipe), 264

shame, calming feelings of, 82–85

shortcakes (recipe), 203

simple sugars, 7

sleep, 75

smoothies

  Almond and Banana Smoothie, 267

  Moroccan Avocado Smoothie, 261

  Papaya, Banana, and Orange Smoothie, 266

snack cake (recipe), 282

snacks, 14

sodium, 90–91

soft serve (recipe), 242

soluble fiber, 29

sorbets, 236, 239

Spiced Hot Cider, 270–271

spices

  as ingredient, 32–33

  in recipes

    Apple, Cinnamon, and Olive Oil Cake, 279

    Apple Cinnamon Crisp, 199

    Apricot and Ginger Cooler, 265

    Baked Spice & Almond Stuffed Apples, 132

    Carrot Pecan Spice Cake, 277

    Cinnamon-Scented Apple Pie, 254

    Citrus and Cinnamon Rice Pudding, 194

    Gingerbread Spice Squares, 159

    Hot Spiced Chocolate, 268

    Pineapple Cardamom Crush, 262

    Poached Pears with Vanilla and Cardamom Cream, 141

    Pumpkin Gingerbread Trifle, 204

    Spiced Hot Cider, 270–271

    Vanilla Cardamom Panna Cotta, 187

sponge cake (recipe), 275

spoon desserts

  cobblers, 196

    Blueberry Cream Cobbler, 197

    Sweet Peach Cobbler, 198

  couscous, 192

spoon desserts *(continued)*
  crisps, 196
    Apple Cinnamon Crisp, 199
    Strawberry Basil Crisp, 200
  custard, 193
  fruits, 201
    Almond and Cherry
      Clafoutis, 208
    Mixed Berry and Mascarpone
      Parfaits, 205
    Passionfruit Tiramisu, 202
    Pumpkin Gingerbread
      Trifle, 204
    Ricotta and Berry Cheesecake
      Tart, 206–207
    Strawberry Shortcake, 203
  overview, 14
  panna cotta, 186–187
  puddings, 186
    Cherry Chocolate Bread
      Pudding, 189
    Chocolate Almond
      Pudding, 188
    Chocolate Orange Rice
      Pudding, 190
    Citrus and Cinnamon Rice
      Pudding, 194
    Vanilla Pudding with
      Berries, 191
    Wheat Berry Pomegranate
      Pudding with
      Pistachios, 195–196
squares
  overview, 157
  recipe, 159
stevia, 98
store-bought desserts, 86–87
strawberries
  Strawberry, Yogurt, and White
    Balsamic Semifreddo, 228
  Strawberry Basil Crisp, 200
  Strawberry Shortcake, 203
  Strawberry Swirl Ice Cream, 231
  Strawberry-Studded
    Blondies, 153

strudels, 246, 249–250
sugars
  artificial, 95
  body and, 17–20
  brain and, 17–20
  cravings, 20–24
  disaccharides, 44, 69
  glucose, 18–19
  glycogen, 45, 67
  history of, 100
  monosaccharides, 69
  oligosaccharides, 69
  polysaccharides, 44
  simple, 7
  substituting unhealthy, 102–103
  insulin and, 8
Summer Berry and Fresh Fig
  Salad, 136
sunflower seeds, 36
Sweet Holiday Couscous, 192
Sweet Peach Cobbler, 198
sweeteners
  agave nectar, 99
  allulose, 98
  alternative and artificial, 95
  coconut sugar, 98
  dates, 98–99
  D-psicose, 98
  good versus bad, 94–96
  healthy, 96–100
  honey, 97
  maple syrup, 97
  molasses, 99–100
  monk fruit sugar, 99
  myths regarding, 298–299
  overview, 94–95
  stevia, 98
  substituting sugars
    with, 102–103
  swapping out in recipes, 100–103
  table sugar, 95–96
  vanilla, 98

T
tarts
  overview, 14
  pies versus, 251
  recipes
    Almond and Apricot Tart, 253
    Basic Tart Crust, 120
    Ricotta and Berry Cheesecake
      Tart, 206–207
    Strawberry, Citrus, and
      Ricotta Tart, 252
tea, 269
test strip method (blood
  glucose test), 46
tiramisu, 202
tree nuts, 35
trifles, 204
truffle recipes
  Chocolate Peanut Clusters, 212
  Chocolate Swirl Bark, 218
  Chocolate-Covered Stuffed
    Dates, 220
  Coconut Chocolate "Fudge,"
    216
  Dark Chocolate–Covered
    Cherries, 222
  Date, Almond, and Cocoa
    Balls, 211
  Peanut Butter and Coconut
    Bombs, 213
  Quinoa and Macadamia
    Clusters, 217
  Stuffed Figs Dipped in
    Chocolate, 221
  Yogurt Kisses, 214
Turkish-Stuffed Apricots, 139
Tuscan Cantucci, 172
type 1 and type 2 diabetes
  benefits of almonds, 33
  calming feelings of shame and
    guilt, 82–85
  comparing testing for, 47–48
  overview, 18

U

unsaturated fats, 72
Upside-Down Kiwi Cake, 281

V

vanilla
coconut sugar and, 98
in recipes
Frozen Peanut Butter and
Vanilla Cups, 241
Poached Pears with Vanilla and
Cardamom Cream, 141
Vanilla Cardamom Panna
Cotta, 187
Vanilla Cream Custard, 122
Vanilla Frozen Yogurt, 225
Vanilla Gelato, 226
Vanilla Pudding with
Berries, 191
vegetables
choosing, 29
nonstarchy, 68
in recipes
Carrot Cookie Bites, 177
Carrot Pecan Spice Cake, 277
Chocolate and Pumpkin
Snack Cake, 282
Pumpkin Gingerbread
Trifle, 204
vegetarian desserts
Almond and Apricot Tart, 253
Almond and Banana
Smoothie, 267
Almond and Cherry
Clafoutis, 208
Almond Orange Biscotti, 173
Angel Food Cake, 276
Apple, Cinnamon, and Olive
Oil Cake, 279
Apple, Raisin, and Nut
Strudel, 249–250
Apple Cinnamon Crisp, 199
Apricot and Ginger Cooler, 265
Avocado, Yogurt, and Mango
Salad, 144

Baked Spice & Almond Stuffed
Apples, 132
Banana and Peanut Butter
"Ice Cream," 235
Banana Chocolate
Chip Cake, 283
Basic Tart Crust, 120
Blackberry Banana Soft
Serve, 242
Blackberry Lemon Bars, 154
Blackberry Lemon Pie Pots, 257
Blueberry and Lemon
Oatmeal Bars, 156
Blueberry Cream Cobbler, 197
Broiled Figs & Balsamic
Reduction, 133
Broiled Pineapple with Yogurt
and Honey, 140
Cantaloupe in White Balsamic
Vinegar, 131
Carrot Cookie Bites, 177
Carrot Pecan Spice Cake, 277
Cherries with Goat Cheese and
Pistachios, 142
Cherry Chocolate Bread
Pudding, 189
Chocolate, Pistachio, and
Cranberry Biscotti, 166
Chocolate Almond Pudding, 188
Chocolate and Pumpkin
Snack Cake, 282
Chocolate Chip Almond Butter
Cookies, 165
Chocolate "Ice Cream," 233
Chocolate Oatmeal No-Bake
Cookies, 182
Chocolate Orange Rice
Pudding, 190
Chocolate Peanut Clusters, 212
Chocolate Swirl Bark, 218
Chocolate-Covered Stuffed
Dates, 220
Cinnamon-Scented
Apple Pie, 254
Citrus and Cinnamon Rice
Pudding, 194
Coconut Chocolate "Fudge," 216
Coffee Ice Cream, 232

Creamy Chai, 269
Creamy Lemon Crostata, 248
Dark Chocolate & Extra-Virgin
Olive Oil Brownies, 149
Dark Chocolate Ganache, 124
Dark Chocolate–Covered
Cherries, 222
Date, Almond, and Cocoa
Balls, 211
Date, Dark Chocolate, and
Cashew Bars, 150
Espresso Granita, 238
Fresh Fruit Kabobs, 130
Frozen Peanut Butter and
Vanilla Cups, 241
Gingerbread Spice Squares, 159
Gluten-Free Chocolate
Cupcakes, 286
Grape, Goat Cheese, and
Almond Skewers, 146
Hazelnut Cookies, 170
Homemade Pie Crust, 119
Honey Citrus Cookies, 176
Hot Spiced Chocolate, 268
Italian Pine Nut Cookies, 179
Italian Sponge Cake, 275
Key Lime Pie Jars, 256
Kiwi and Raspberry Trees with
Honey, 135
Lemon and Walnut
Biscotti, 168–169
Lemon Granita, 237
Light Fruit "Ganache," 125
Meringues, 178
Mini Flourless Olive Oil and
Chocolate Cakes, 285
Mixed Berry and Mascarpone
Parfaits, 205
Mixed Berry Compote, 134
Mixed Berry Crostata, 247
Moroccan Avocado
Smoothie, 261
Moroccan Sesame Cookies, 175
Oatmeal Cookies, 181
Oatmeal Cranberry Cookies, 183
Orange, Almond, and Olive
Oil Cake, 280

vegetarian desserts *(continued)*

Orange and Almond Bars, 155

Orange and Greek Yogurt Creamsicles, 229

Papaya, Banana, and Orange Smoothie, 266

Passionfruit Tiramisu, 202

Peanut Butter and Coconut Bombs, 213

Pineapple Cardamom Crush, 262

Pineapple Frozen Yogurt Pops, 227

Pistachio Honey Ice Cream, 234

Pistachio Macaroons, 171

Poached Pears with Vanilla and Cardamom Cream, 141

Pumpkin Gingerbread Trifle, 204

Quinoa, Cranberry, and Pecan Bars, 158

Quinoa and Macadamia Clusters, 217

Raspberry Sorbet, 239

Red, White, and Blue Creamsicles, 243

Ricotta, Chocolate, and Orange Brownies, 151

Ricotta and Berry Cheesecake Tart, 206–207

Roasted Plums with Mascarpone Cheese, 143

Seasonal Italian Fruit Platter, 145

Spiced Hot Cider, 270–271

Strawberry, Citrus, and Ricotta Tart, 252

Strawberry, Yogurt, and White Balsamic Semifreddo, 228

Strawberry Basil Crisp, 200

Strawberry Shortcake, 203

Strawberry Swirl Ice Cream, 231

Strawberry-Studded Blondies, 153

Stuffed Figs Dipped in Chocolate, 221

Summer Berry and Fresh Fig Salad, 136

Sweet Holiday Couscous, 192

Sweet Peach Cobbler, 198

Turkish-Stuffed Apricots, 139

Tuscan Cantucci, 172

Upside-Down Kiwi Cake, 281

Vanilla Cardamom Panna Cotta, 187

Vanilla Cream Custard, 122

Vanilla Frozen Yogurt, 225

Vanilla Gelato, 226

Vanilla Pudding with Berries, 191

Watermelon, Cantaloupe, Kiwi, Feta, and Mint Mosaic, 129

Watermelon "Cake," 137

Wheat Berry Pomegranate Pudding with Pistachios, 195–196

Yogurt Custard with Apricots and Pistachios, 193

Yogurt Kisses, 214

Zero-Proof Sgroppino, 264

vegetarians and vegans, 66–67

vinegar. *See* balsamic vinegar; white balsamic vinegar

W

walnuts, 168–169

watermelon

Watermelon, Cantaloupe, Kiwi, Feta, and Mint Mosaic, 129

Watermelon "Cake," 137

Wheat Berry Pomegranate Pudding with Pistachios, 195–196

white balsamic vinegar

Cantaloupe in White Balsamic Vinegar, 131

Strawberry, Yogurt, and White Balsamic Semifreddo, 228

whole grains

baking with, 157

flour, 36

overview, 29

Y

yogurt

benefits of, 210, 307–308

frozen desserts and, 224–229

as ingredient, 35

in recipes

Avocado, Yogurt, and Mango Salad, 144

Broiled Pineapple with Yogurt and Honey, 140

Orange and Greek Yogurt Creamsicles, 229

Pineapple Frozen Yogurt Pops, 227

Strawberry, Yogurt, and White Balsamic Semifreddo, 228

Vanilla Frozen Yogurt, 225

Yogurt Custard with Apricots and Pistachios, 193

Yogurt Kisses, 214

Z

Zero-Proof Sgroppino, 264

About the Author

Best-selling author **Amy Riolo** is also an award-winning chef, television host, and Mediterranean diet ambassador. The author of 20 books, she has been named Knight of the Order of the Star of Italy by the Italian government, "The Ambassador of Italian Cuisine in the US" by The Italian International Agency for Foreign Press, "Ambassador of the Italian Mediterranean Diet 2022-2024" by the International Academy of the Italian Mediterranean Diet in her ancestral homeland of Calabria, Italy, and "Ambassador of Mediterranean Cuisine in the World" by the Rome-based media agency *We The Italians*.

In 2019, she launched her own private label collection of premium Italian imported culinary ingredients called **Amy Riolo Selections** and include extra-virgin olive oil, balsamic vinegar, and pesto sauce from award-winning artisan companies. Amy also co-authored *Diabetes For Dummies, Diabetes Meal Planning and Nutrition For Dummies,* and the *Diabetes Cookbook For Dummies* (John Wiley & Sons, Inc.) with Dr. Simon Poole.

Dedication

This book is dedicated to the memory of my Nonna Angela who taught me the power of desserts to transform everyday into a special occasion, and for her unconditional love and support.

Author's Acknowledgments

My earliest memories of cooking were with my mother, Faith Riolo, who taught me that food wasn't just something we eat to nourish ourselves, but an edible gift that could be given to express love. When she was later diagnosed with diabetes, it was my love for her and desire to create delicious and nutritious meals for my parents that eventually led me to write books on the topic. I owe much of my professional culinary success to my father, Rick Riolo, for always believing in my talent and supporting my career goals. To my beloved little brother, Jeremy, I love baking with you, and I'm grateful to be able to pass our family's knowledge down to you.

My nonna, Angela Magnone Foti, taught me to cook and bake, as well as valuable lessons that served me outside of the kitchen. My Yia Yia, Mary Michos Riolo, shared her beloved Greek traditions with me as well. I would probably never have published a cookbook if it weren't for my mentor, Sheilah Kaufman, who patiently taught me much more than I ever planned on learning. I'm proud to pass her knowledge to others. Without the assistance and guidance of my late friend, spirit sister, and healer Kathleen Ammalee Rogers, I'd never have been able to realize my professional writing goals. I'm very thankful to Chef Luigi Diotaiuti for his support and for always believing in me and for encouraging me to foster my dreams and goals.

There are dozens of people whom I'm proud to call friends and colleagues that I interact with daily and whom each indirectly enable me to achieve my goals. I'm grateful to each of you. I want to thank Italian President Matarella, Minister Gonzalez of the Embassy of Italy in the United States, and Counselor Michela Carboniero of the Italian Cultural Institute for giving me the honor of being titled Knight of the Order of the Star of Italy. I also thank my dear friends and importers of my Amy Riolo Selections products Stefano and Davide Ferrari of Cibo Divino and Vince Di Piazza of DITALIA for distributing them. Many thanks to all of my wonderful producers: Tenute Cristiano, Olio Anfosso, Pasta Marella, and Acetaia Castelli for their partnerships.

In Calabria, Italy, I want to thank my cousins Angela Riolo, Pina Macrì and Franco Riolo, Tonia Riolo, and Mario Riolo for their support. I thank Chefs Salvatore Murano and Enzo Murano of Max Trattoria Enoteca for including me in their culinary-cultural pursuits in Italy and for naming me an honorary member of ARCP (the Regional Association of Pythagorean Cooks). I thank Alessandro Cuomo for naming me the Director of A.N.I.T.A. (The Italian Academy of Traditional Italian Foods). Mille grazie to Dr. Battista Liserre for his inspirational work on nourishing both the mind and soul and to Silvestro Parise for including me in projects that promote Calabria.

To my dear friends Jonathan Bardzik, Gail Broeckel, Ann Hotung, Sharon Wolpoff, Pina Dubbio, Francesco Marra, Chef Jeff Fritz, Paul Kolze, Edward Donnelly, Sedrick Crawley, Stu Hershey, Maria Fusco, and Kim Foley, you are my spirit family, and I'm blessed to have you in my life. Many thanks to Melissa's Produce for their generous donation of produce for recipe development. And finally, I want to thank my co-author, and in the case of this book, technical editor Dr. Simon Poole, for his tremendous knowledge and commitment to the cause of promoting health and happiness, for always inspiring me, and for valuing my voice. It's a pleasure and an honor to collaborate with you.

I'm especially grateful to Tracy Boggier for being so enthusiastic, efficient, and great to work with. I truly appreciate the expert and efficient editorial support and guidance of Chad Sievers, Wendy Jo Peterson, and Grace Geri Goodale for their fantastic photography and support as well.

Publisher's Acknowledgments

Executive Editor: Tracy Boggier

Project Editor and Copy Editor: Chad R. Sievers

Technical Editor: Simon Poole, MD

Recipe Tester and Nutritional Analyst: Rachel Nix

Production Editor: Tamilmani Varadharaj

Photographers & Stylists: Wendy Jo Peterson and Grace Geri Goodale

Cover Images: Courtesy of Wendy Jo Peterson and Grace Geri Goodale